Dear Betty and Ne...

It's been a pleasure getting to know you and your wonderful family. Hold onto that faith — I know things will continue to get better.

All the best.

Bob Woehrle

INTERNAL BLEEDING

THE TRUTH BEHIND AMERICA'S TERRIFYING
EPIDEMIC OF MEDICAL MISTAKES

ROBERT M. WACHTER, M.D.
KAVEH G. SHOJANIA, M.D.

MORE ADVANCE PRAISE FOR *INTERNAL BLEEDING*

"The authors have achieved something quite special. *Internal Bleeding* is full of insights, learning and guidance that will help health care professionals create and keep a 'culture of safety'... Read this book."
—Dick Davidson, President, American Hospital Association

"The first rule is 'physician, do no harm,' but American medicine now feels like a terrifying crapshoot. Wachter and Shojania give us the first honest appraisal of just how dangerous a visit to your hospital can be — and offer solutions to our medical crisis. Internal Bleeding has arrived — not a moment too soon!"
—Laurie Garrett, Author of *Betrayal of Trust: The Collapse of Global Public Health*, and the only writer ever to have won journalism's three major prizes: The Peabody, The Polk, and The Pulitzer

"*Internal Bleeding* is a gripping and incisive account of why errors are so likely in America's hospitals and clinics and what can be done to reduce them. This book may make you a bit more nervous about your next visit to the doctor, but it will also tell you what can and must be done to insure your visit is far safer than it is today."
—Arthur Caplan, Ph.D., Director of the Center for Bioethics, University of Pennsylvania, and author of *Due Consideration: Controversy in the Age of Medical Miracles* and *Am I My Brother's Keeper? The Ethical Frontiers of Biomedicine*

"*Internal Bleeding* is a beautifully written book that is chock-full of dramatic and engaging stories about medical errors... This is a book of seminal importance that is likely to become a classic. In the same way that *Unsafe at Any Speed* transformed the automobile industry and *Silent Spring* launched the environmental movement, *Internal Bleeding* could become the catalyst for creating a better and safer system of health care."
—Kenneth M. Ludmerer, M.D., author of *Time to Heal* and *Learning to Heal*, and Professor of Medicine and History, Washington University in St. Louis

"Approximately once a week, a menace sweeps through America and exacts a toll in human life and suffering equal to our 9/11 tragedy. With elegance and simplicity, *Internal Bleeding* explains how this happens and why we allow it to continue. More importantly, it will help trigger the informed public pressure needed to stop the carnage."
—Arnold Milstein, M.D., M.P.H., Co-Founder, The Leapfrog Group, and Medical Director, Pacific Business Group on Health

"Wachter and Shojania have performed a remarkable feat. They have clearly set forth the complicated medical, sociological and policy issues surrounding the epidemic of medical injuries. *Internal Bleeding* is a book that will be of incredible importance for every patient, while also informing the academic debate about medical errors for years to come."
—Troyen Brennan, M.D., J.D., M.P.H., Professor, Harvard Schools of Medicine, Law, and Public Health, and co-author of *A Measure of Malpractice: Medical Injury, Malpractice Litigation, and Patient Compensation*

"*Internal Bleeding* documents the perils that await unsuspecting patients, why it is so difficult to design a fail-safe system for hospital care, and how the culture of medicine resists becoming a culture of safety. This fascinating book manages to be provocative and entertaining while simultaneously being insightful and even-handed. It is must reading for everyone who walks into a hospital, either as a worker or a patient."
—Steven Schroeder, M.D., Immediate Past-President, The Robert Wood Johnson Foundation

"Critical care nurses will want to read this riveting book as it tells the truth—in brutally honest language—about the current reality of medical errors... Wachter and Shojania don't just analyze and criticize—they offer thoughtful and viable solutions to fix the systems errors and change the culture of hospitals to prevent catastrophic mistakes. It is past time for us all to work together to ensure this happens."
—Dorrie Fontaine, R.N., D.N.Sc., President, American Association of Critical Care Nurses

"*Internal Bleeding* should be mandatory reading for medical professionals… and everybody else who plans to set foot in a hospital. Wachter and Shojania have pried open our eyes, and have managed to do so with compassion, clarity, and insight. Let's hope that this engaging and important book leads to a tipping point, in which we all demand that our health care system finally puts quality and safety first."
—Larry Wellikson, M.D., Executive Director, Society of Hospital Medicine

"This is a timely and exceptionally readable book that sorts out the many threads that lead to the tangled issues of patient safety. With wit as well as depth and compassion, the authors explore the elements of modern health care delivery that present risks along with their dazzling benefits; and they develop constructive suggestions that can reduce those risks, both through systems change and improved teamwork, along with intelligent patient participation in individual care."
—June Osborn, M.D., President, The Josiah Macy Jr. Foundation, and the first chairperson of the U.S. National Commission on AIDS

"*Caveat aeger.* Let the patient beware. Unexpected tragedy awaits. *Internal Bleeding* should further energize a rightfully fearful population of activist patients to demand safe medical care."
—George Lundberg, M.D., Editor-in-Chief, *Medscape General Medicine*, and former Editor, *Journal of the American Medical Association*

"It's been four years and arguably almost 400,000 lives lost since the 1999 Institute of Medicine study galvanized the nation's focus on medical errors and patient safety. *Internal Bleeding* gives the reader the compelling stories about how this happens, coupled with the facts needed to understand this serious problem and find a rational solution. Drs. Wachter and Shojania are to be complimented for their contribution to patient safety."
—The Honorable James M. Jeffords, United States Senator (I-VT)

"In this beautifully written book, Robert Wachter and Kaveh Shojania combine personal experience, scholarly insight, and gut-wrenching clinical examples to take us into the dark side of a health care system gone seriously awry. With a compelling blend of sensitivity and irreverence, they demystify the complex world of medical error. Most importantly, they show how cognitive psychology and human factors engineering provide the way out by shifting attention from blaming individuals to fixing faulty systems. *Internal Bleeding* is a morality tale for our time. You will never forget its leading actors: suffering patients and struggling doctors. As the authors remind us, we are all in this together."

—Lucian L. Leape, M.D., Adjunct Professor of Health Policy, Harvard School of Public Health

"Internal Bleeding is long overdue. Finally, a book that doctors and patients can read together, with equal amounts of fear about the current state of affairs, and optimism about how much safer medical care could be. Wachter and Shojania are the kind of smart, sensible doctors we all want treating us and running our hospitals. Their prescription for the future of American health care is well crafted, provocative and, unlike many things written by physicians, completely legible."

—Stephen Fried, Author of *Bitter Pills: Inside the Hazardous World of Legal Drugs*, and Adjunct Professor, Columbia University Graduate School of Journalism

RUGGED LAND | 401 WEST STREET · SECOND FLOOR · NEW YORK CITY · NY 10014 · USA

Published by Rugged Land, LLC

401 WEST STREET · SECOND FLOOR · NEW YORK CITY · NY 10014 · USA

RUGGED LAND and colophon are trademarks of Rugged Land, LLC.

Cataloging-in-Publication Data

Wachter, Robert M.

Internal bleeding : the truth behind America's

terrifying epidemic of medical mistakes /

Robert M. Wachter, Kaveh G. Shojania. -- 1st ed.

p. cm.

LCCN 2003097138

ISBN 1-59071-0738

1. Medical errors--Case studies.

I. Shojania, Kaveh G. II. Title.

R729.8.W33 2004   610

QBI03-200769

Book Design by

HSU+ASSOCIATES

RUGGED LAND WEBSITE ADDRESS:WWW.RUGGEDLAND.COM

MAY 2005

3   5   7   9   10   8   6   4

Second Edition

For the patients and caregivers let down

by the system they trusted

It may seem a strange principle to enunciate

as the very first requirement in a Hospital

that it should do the sick no harm.

—Florence Nightingale
Notes on Hospitals, 1859

CONTENTS

PART IV: CURES

A NEW EPIDEMIC

F or years we've tracked the growth of a terrible disease. It has killed millions of people, in locations all over the world. Its symptoms appear only after the major damage has been done. It can affect anyone, anywhere, at any time, but it often strikes the weak and the helpless, usually without warning. The authors of this book first became aware of the disease through two terrifying cases that happened a decade apart.

In the first case, the reporting physician was a former resident in internal medicine at the University of California, San Francisco (UCSF). After residency, he spent a quiet year working the ER in a comfortable, homey community hospital nestled in the hills of Northern California. The caregivers at the little hospital were pleasant and competent. Physicians shared gossip with the nurses during breaks over microwave popcorn. After endless years of formal training in an academic mecca and a rough-and-tumble, big-city hospital, the "Mayberry" quality of the doctor's new assignment was as refreshing as a dip in the local swimming hole.

But charm, the young physician discovered, came with a price.

Local community hospitals deliver babies, treat infections, and set broken arms, but they lack the specialists and high-tech devices critically ill people often need and expect. As a result, patients are routinely transferred from these mom-and-pop facilities to bigger, regional teaching hospitals: those high-tech temples of modern medicine found in and around our major cities and (sometimes) affectionately referred to by rural caregivers as the "Big House."

This poses a practical problem for ER physicians: How do

you get a really sick patient safely from the smaller hospital to the Big House? On TV, a jet helicopter lands on a windblown rooftop and heroic doctors rush around spouting lifesaving lines over the whoop-whoop of whirling rotor blades. In real life, such dramatic transfers are rare. Usually, the staff simply slides the needy patient into the back of an ordinary ambulance—and off they go.

On this particular balmy evening, back in the mid-1980s, the young physician was confronted by Carlos, a fourteen-year-old Latino boy big enough to be an NFL linebacker. He was dragged in—rubber-legged and semiconscious—by a smaller friend about the same age. With the help of two nurses, the doctor heaved the huge boy onto a gurney and began a preliminary assessment, which included an attempt to establish—as quickly as possible—the nature of the emergency and a bit of the patient's medical history.

Eyelids fluttering, Carlos mumbled answers to the doctor's questions in a mixture of Spanish and English—not much help to the ER staff, but at least it showed the patient's brain wasn't completely fried. His friend, speaking mostly in Spanish, tried to fill in the gaps. What he said fit with the clinical symptoms: rapid heartbeat, widely dilated pupils, skin dry and flushed, with a strangely quiet bowel (even an empty gut gurgles into a stethoscope), and an EKG whose big lazy loops looked like a preschooler's crayon drawing. Carlos, it seemed, had taken a major league overdose of an antidepressant drug.

In those days, even modest overdoses of tricyclic antidepressants such as Elavil could cause life-threatening, runaway heart rhythms (whereas overdoses of modern antidepressants, like Prozac or Paxil, seldom do). So the young doctor's job now was to stabilize the patient, verify his preliminary diagnosis with a couple of blood tests, and begin administering oxygen, IV fluids, and sodium bicarbonate to keep the poisoned heart beating. The doctor stood ready to insert a breathing tube deep into the lungs but, thankfully, that proved unnecessary. Carlos continued to breathe on his own—but barely.

The next order of business was to get the boy out of Mayberry and into the pediatric ICU of the nearest regional hospital, a "mere" ten miles away. The young physician knew that even a short ambulance trip could be deadly for a patient in Carlos's condition, so he decided to ride along. That way, he would at least be on hand to administer some powerful cardiac meds if they were needed, or even use those famous high-voltage paddles if Carlos's heart began to flutter. He ordered the ambulance and alerted his backup to cover him in the ER.

The ambulance, provided by a local service, arrived promptly and the young doctor and his patient boarded quickly. Lights flashing, siren blaring, the vehicle pulled onto the freeway and immediately got bogged down in the evening commute. Drivers, some cursing, tried desperately to be good citizens and scrambled into nonexistent spaces. The ambulance took turns trying the shoulder and the median divide, but both dead-ended. What was supposed to be a ten-minute trip threatened to drag out to twenty, thirty, forty minutes, or more.

The young doctor, faced with a youngster whose heart could stop without notice, began ticking through various contingencies in his mind. He would hook Carlos up to the on-board heart monitor and watch for early signs of cardiac instability. If the machine showed the slightest arrhythmia, he would inject the appropriate drug and restore an acceptable heart rate. If Carlos didn't respond to medications and his heart went completely haywire, there were always the emergency paddles.

Or were there?

The doctor glanced quickly around the ambulance's interior— tubes and wires swaying, cabinet doors rattling as the vehicle accelerated and braked. His own heart began to beat faster.

"Hey guys," he shouted to the paramedics, "where's the cardiac monitor?"

One EMT turned and answered, "Oh, we don't carry them."

"Then what about the defibrillator?" The doctor's voice was an octave higher.

"Don't have those either."

The physician looked back at his patient, whose young life now seemed to hang by an even narrower thread. Slowly, deliberately, a bit impatiently—like a prosecuting attorney at trial—he asked, "Well, what exactly *do* you have back here?"

The paramedic shrugged. "We have bandages."

The following silence was deafening. The young doctor exploded, "Are you telling me I'm riding in the back of a *fucking taxicab?!*"

The paramedic turned and stared out the window.

The doctor slid closer to Carlos, as if mere proximity might help. He started taking the boy's pulse manually—a position he'd hold for the rest of the ride. Sweat popped out on the doctor's forehead, but there was no nurse to blot it away; no cardiologist to swoop in with some special, lifesaving technique; no pediatrician to assure him just how much arrhythmia a fourteen-year-old heart can take; no high-tech gadget on board to keep the poor kid's sputtering body on track if it decided to derail. All the young doctor had was basic CPR—the technique of last resort taught by the Red Cross to Boy Scouts and housewives. Unmentioned in those classes was the fact that 90 percent of the time, CPR (unless rapidly followed by defibrillation) makes no difference—it merely gives good Samaritans something to do while nature takes its deadly course.

Fifty minutes later—a lifetime in that rolling metal coffin—the "taxi" arrived at its destination. Carlos was still alive and the young doctor silently thanked that special God who looks out for kids and drunks. His phone call to the "Mayberry" ER was not so quiet, or polite. "What the hell happened to my Priority One ambulance?" he shouted. After a few moments of buck-passing around the ER's clerical staff, a surprisingly calm voice came back, "Got your order right here. It didn't say Priority One, so we ordered a Priority Three. Why—was there a problem?"

Truthfully, the young doctor answered, "No," and hung up. *But there sure as hell might have been!* Knees shaking, he took a seat in the very expensive "taxi" for the much shorter ride home. He decided en route that he would not make an issue of the foul-up. Yeah, he hadn't specified the ambulance type, he thought, but didn't the nurse or the clerk realize that an antidepressant OD had to have a full-service ambulance? Well, he sighed, this was a team blunder. In any case, the catastrophe was avoided, the bullet dodged, so the young doctor kept his mouth shut. He swore he would be more careful next time.

The second case occurred ten years later and half a continent away. A different doctor, also young and relatively new to his art, was in his third month of residency, on his first shift as an "on-call" physician in the ER of a major urban hospital.

Among the stream of walk-in patients, a twenty-nine-year-old man appeared with his wife, complaining of chest pains. The triage nurse tagged his problem as "low acuity"—not life threatening— but thought it warranted examination by a physician. So after a brief wait, the new doctor met the patient and began taking a case history, eyeballing the young man as he spoke—consciously trying to either match or note discrepancies between the words and the clinical signs of injury or disease. The man's wife—a short woman with suspicious eyes and a brusque manner—did most of the talking.

It seems the patient, a computer programmer, had slipped in the shower two days before and hit the tub with his chest. He'd been sore ever since, but this morning the ache had blossomed into full-blown pain—seven or eight on a subjective scale of one to ten—so he asked his wife to call an ambulance.

The young doctor later recalled that the patient "didn't look quite right," but he couldn't put his finger on the problem. The man described his medical history reluctantly, almost evasively, even though there seemed to be nothing to hide. The physical examination was equally perplexing. The doctor applied pressure to the right side of the patient's chest—the place where he reported striking the tub—but got no flinching or cries of pain in response.

Pressing the abdomen, he noticed mild tenderness just under the ribs. Since this was at some distance from the site of the trauma, the doctor was a bit surprised, but these inconsistencies didn't set off any alarms. A more experienced physician might have been sufficiently bothered by these discrepancies to wonder whether this was an unusual presentation of a serious illness. The junior doctor did not... with one notable exception. Having spent his first few months as a resident in the hospital's cardiac care unit, the CCU, the possibility of heart pain fleetingly—almost subconsciously— entered his mind, but exited just as promptly. This young man just didn't fit a heart patient's profile.

Following hospital procedure, the resident reviewed his findings and preliminary diagnosis—posttraumatic chest pain, complicated by "gastritis" (an upset stomach) brought on by several days' use of over-the-counter pain relievers—with the ER's attending physician, a very experienced practitioner. The "attending" gave the patient a quick once-over—asking a couple of questions and listening through the stethoscope to the heart and lungs—and concurred with the diagnosis. The resident prescribed a low dose of codeine and bed rest, plus advice to avoid drugstore pain relievers that might irritate the stomach.

Prescription in hand, the man and his wife left the building and the young doctor returned to the growing crowd of patients.

A few days later, the resident was walking through the CCU and, to his astonishment, saw the same young man being prepped for emergency heart catheterization. He looked at the patient's "chart" (mostly handwritten notes by doctors and nurses, plus computer printouts of various tests) with mounting horror. As he read, the events of the last few days unfolded before his eyes.

A day after leaving the ER, he learned, the patient saw his primary care physician, who suspected a gastric ulcer and ordered an upper-gastrointestinal (GI) X-ray. The test was negative. Two days later, the young man consulted a cardiologist who, lacking any other explanation for the patient's persistent pain, ran an EKG. To the amazement of everyone, it showed that the young programmer had suffered a massive heart attack! He was admitted immediately to the CCU for an angiogram, a prelude to either angioplasty (reopening a clogged coronary artery with a tiny balloon) or even coronary bypass surgery.

The young physician closed the chart, shut his eyes briefly to steel his nerves, then approached the patient, who was pale and perspiring like a rag doll in the thin hospital gown. The resident felt a flood of conflicting emotions. His initial reaction had been anger at himself—even shame for blowing a serious diagnosis. On the other hand, he had followed all the rules, asked all the right questions—even consulted a senior physician—and used his very best judgment. Was this a royal screwup or "just one of those things" that, unfortunately, can happen in any profession?

He identified himself as the ER physician who had sent the young man away with a codeine prescription for "rib trauma and gastritis," and offered a lame smile and effusive apology. The patient acknowledged the apology but was already groggy with the tranquilizers used before catheterization. Outside the CCU, the resident encountered the man's wife, whose accusing stare flashed, *"incompetent, uncaring bumbler."*

After enduring this quiet, but unmistakable, penitential abuse, the resident went to the ER to tell the attending physician—the doctor who had concurred with his original diagnosis—that they had both been as wrong as wrong could be. The older doctor shrugged and started to speak. The resident waited to hear some words of wisdom about the fallibility of God's children and the mysteries of the human body—even another chewing out might have been good for his soul—but what came out was totally unexpected.

"Well," the veteran said phlegmatically, "I guess we better call our lawyers."

Sadly, cases like these—in which mistakes cause, or nearly cause, grave harm to patients—are not unique. In fact, they are distressingly common and spin out, in one way or another, thousands of times each day in hospitals all over the country. These two cases, though, have special significance for us.

The young doctor in the glorified taxicab was Bob Wachter. The young resident who missed the heart attack was Kaveh Shojania. We have seen the enemy and it is us.

Or is it?

*　*　*

A 1999 report by the prestigious Institute of Medicine made clear what doctors have long known: Hospitals can be dangerous. The report highlighted the now-famous statistic that 44,000–98,000 Americans die each year of medical errors, numbers that led reporters to reach for their word processors, politicians for their microphones, and patients for their Valium. But after five years and lots of activity, even the most optimistic observer would say that health care is not much safer than it was in 1999.

Media reports of medical errors would lead one to believe that the problem is relatively straightforward and could be solved if all errors were reported to newspapers and to regulators, bad-apple physicians and nurses were purged, and sleep-deprived residents and interns were allowed to get a little shut-eye. Moreover, patients have been reassuringly told that they themselves can prevent errors by simple steps that essentially amount to an exaggerated state of vigilance. These solutions seem so straightforward that many see incompetence, malfeasance, and conspiracy in the fact that this all wasn't solved decades ago.

The problem is that these simple-minded analyses and solutions are largely wrong.

This book presents an alternative approach. Decades of research, mostly from outside health care, has confirmed our own medical experience: Most errors are made by good but fallible people working in dysfunctional systems, which means that making care safer depends on buttressing the system to prevent or catch the inevitable lapses of mortals. This logical approach is common in other complex, high-tech industries, but it has been woefully ignored in medicine. Instead, we have steadfastly clung to the view that an error is a moral failure by an individual, a posture that has left patients feeling angry and ready to blame, and providers feeling guilty and demoralized. Most importantly, it hasn't done a damn thing to make health care safer.

There is a better way. We and others have called this new approach "systems thinking," by which we mean a carefully developed and applied set of rules, standards, checklists, technologies, and training programs that helps good caregivers give good care and prevents them from inadvertently harming their patients. We also mean a culture that prizes safety, focuses on it as a core professional value, and is open to discussing errors and learning from them. It is both proactive—built into the way care is delivered so as to avoid errors in the first place—and reactive—guiding the way we respond to our errors when they do occur. Both elements are vital, but neither has been our strong suit. As organizational psychologist Karl Weick observes, "postmortems of medical errors tend to focus too much on the last few minutes and the last error just before the adverse event, and too little on the contributions to error that were laid down in the preceding days and decisions and that made these last few minutes so harrowing and inevitable."

"SURGEON REMOVES WRONG PART OF BRAIN!" shouts the newspaper headline. The knee-jerk response to simply fire the surgeon might feel like closure but leaves unfixed the various underlying factors that could place the next one hundred patients at risk for a sequel. On the other hand, the systems approach would begin by investigating the hospital's procedures for verifying surgical sites (not just the brain but right versus left eyes, legs, and arms as well), for identifying X-rays, and for training doctors and nurses. Firing the surgeon simply won't do the trick. Think of your doctors and nurses as actors in a grand play. Sure, the play is different when King Lear is played by Sir Laurence Olivier or Robin Williams. But Lear dies in both stagings. *If we want the patient to live, we must change the script!*

The principal message of this book is that most medical mistakes can be prevented by *thoughtfully* applying principles of systems thinking. The word "thoughtfully" is key here. Although there is much we can learn from industries that have long embraced the systems approach (like commercial aviation—and we will point out parallels and differences with this and other industries throughout the book), medical care is much more complex and customized than flying an Airbus: At 3 A.M., the critically ill patient needs superb and compassionate doctors and nurses more than she needs a better checklist. We take seriously the awesome privileges and responsibilities that society grants us as physicians, and don't believe for a second that individual excellence and professional passion will become expendable even after our trapeze swings over netting called a "safer system." In the end, medical errors are a hard enough nut to crack that we need excellent doctors *and* safer systems.

Our enthusiasm for systems thinking must also be tempered by the inevitability of unintended consequences and trade-offs. One of the key lessons from other, "safer" industries is this: Virtually every fix has a dark side, and some staggering errors spin out from what appeared to have been straightforward remedies. This does not mean that these fixes are bad ideas (they're often not), but rather that we can't fall asleep at the wheel once we've implemented them. We'll crash.

For example, we'll show you how increased technology and specialization—generally good things—can create errors by fragmenting care. Even ensuring that residents in teaching hospitals get some sleep may lead to more mistakes by generating more handoffs to fumble. And you'll learn why hospitals are often forced to make Solomonic safety trade-offs, such as whether to invest the next $30 million in a spiffy new computer system to prevent medication errors or in shoring up the ICU with more nurses.

You'll also see how the interpersonal and cultural milieu of the hospital—proud but stubborn—provides rich soil for millions of errors every year. Without appreciating this culture, it is difficult to fathom why we don't fire incompetent doctors, how a nurse can remain silent rather than question a physician's order she suspects is fatally wrong, or why hospitals sometimes seem powerless to force their providers to follow even simple rules that might prevent deadly errors.

As we pull back the curtain on medical errors, you'll read some cases that are profoundly disturbing—we expect you'll feel natural sympathy for the patient and, surprisingly, empathy for (or at least a better understanding of) some of the caregivers who let them down. Other cases are just plain ludicrous—as if the Marx Brothers or Keystone Kops had wandered onto the hospital floor, though the suffering they cause is no laughing matter. Although every case is based on fact (a few, which we clearly identify, are drawn from published accounts), we've disguised the details of some to respect the privacy of those involved. The anonymity serves two purposes. First, without it, few doctors, nurses, and institutions, operating under the Sword of Damocles that is the American malpractice system, would have shared their errors with us. Second, we strongly believe that virtually all of the errors we describe *could have happened* at virtually any hospital, and to virtually any caregiver. Particularizing them unnecessarily focuses attention onto these individuals and institutions and away from their general lessons, a distraction we wish to avoid.

We first presented some of these cases in two academic series on medical errors that we are privileged to edit: "Quality Grand Rounds" in the *Annals of Internal Medicine*, and *AHRQ Web M&M*. Others came from colleagues around the country. As you've already seen, a few were drawn from our own experiences. Be assured (not reassured, unfortunately) that all hospitals—from the marquee academic medical center to the rural hospital that doubles as a community center for Friday night Bingo—commit errors every day and are trying to figure out, at this very moment, how to commit fewer.

We divide the book into four major parts. The first, called "The System," begins with the dramatic case of a patient who received another patient's invasive heart procedure. It goes on to describe the systems approach to errors, and introduces you to the 1999 report by the Institute of Medicine, the blockbuster that catapulted medical mistakes onto the public's radar screen. In Part II, "The Errors of Our Way," you'll read dramatic cases of all types of medical mistakes, from medication errors to misdiagnoses, from botched resuscitations to wrong-site surgery. Through these cases, you'll gain a deep understanding of why errors happen, a prelude to the third section, "Consequences," in which you'll learn about various ways of responding to errors (public reporting, media coverage, the malpractice system). We end with "Cures," our prescription for curing the epidemic of medical errors—of stanching the bleeding—although by that time we expect you'll have some new ideas of your own.

Through it all, our aim is to take you into the secret world of the hospital to show you an insider's view of medical mistakes. The truth is that neither the public nor the media—nor, truth be told, most health care professionals and administrators—fully appreciates why errors happen. This lack of understanding is attributable partly to the media's tendency to tackle complex issues with one-dimensional intensity—to depict errors as rousing tales of human suffering, of good versus evil, of heroes versus villains—but also to the difficulty that outsiders have in breaking through our culture, language, and, yes, our code of silence.

One caveat before we begin. As we sat down to write this book, we struggled with how we could share troubling, often fatal cases of medical errors with you without being overly sensational or scaring you away from getting the medical care you need. This is a book about medical errors, and it would not be surprising for you to emerge a little gun-shy as you approach your next hospitalization or surgery. We hope and trust you will not overlook several important points:

Most American hospitals are safe for the vast majority of patients, the vast majority of the time. Even when mistakes are factored in, you are safer in an American hospital than in virtually any care-giving facility on the planet.

The vast majority of our caregivers are well trained and conscientious. Even if all the bad apples—the incompetents, the addicts, and the pathologically sloppy—were removed from practice overnight, we'd still have errors in our ICUs, laboratories, operating rooms, and pharmacies. This is one of the things that makes *our* epidemic so vexing, and the need to tackle it with a fresh approach so great.

Western medicine's ability to save and extend life, and to improve the quality of life for the chronically ill, is nothing short of miraculous. This applies not just to extraordinary procedures like heart transplants, but also to our ability to prevent, diagnose, treat, and often cure diseases that only a generation ago were routinely fatal.

Taken together, this means that a strategy of staying away from the hospital when you need to be there, for fear of a mistake, will put you at far greater risk than that caused by errors. Like peace officers, firefighters, and members of other lifesaving professions, most medical caregivers will be there when you need them, will know what they are doing, and will try to do the right thing—and usually succeed.

In fact, our cases are less horror stories of malfeasance or incompetence than cautionary tales about misguided priorities, mixed signals, and mass denial. From congressional decisions about what kinds of research to fund, to choices by hospitals about where to focus their attention and dollars, to judgments by medical and nursing schools about how to train the healers of tomorrow—safety has always been an afterthought. It is the problem you tackled after all the high-tech, profitable, and sexy stuff was taken care of (which, of course, it never was). We all know that our arsenal of clot-busters, MRI scanners, gene therapies, and columns of specialists maim and kill the patients we aim to heal with shocking regularity, but our profession has reacted to this knowledge mostly with a collective shrug of its shoulders. We have become inured to and paralyzed by it, coming to think of medical errors as the unavoidable collateral damage of a heroic, high-tech war we otherwise seem to be winning. It's as if we spent the last thirty years building a really souped-up sports car, but barely a dime or a moment making sure it has bumpers, seat belts, and air bags.

You may be wondering what patients themselves can do about medical mistakes. While there *are* some simple strategies you can use to prevent certain kinds of errors (and we'll describe them in the book), and on-the-ball patients or their caffeinated loved ones *will* occasionally intercept a mistake, we need to be realistic: In general, patients are no more able to protect themselves from hospital errors than passengers can protect themselves on commercial airplanes. In this particular Oz, there is simply too much going on behind our curtain for you, the patient, to save yourself from most of our mistakes.

And yet—because this book is designed to be a call for action— it really *is* about what patients can do. Patients—individually and collectively—must insist that caregivers, administrators, and politicians get deadly serious about making health care safer. It will take tremendous determination and leadership to transform the way doctors and nurses think about, organize, and carry out their work. This may sound daunting, but consider the alternative. If we continue to focus on errors as individual screwups—as human failings to be managed with shaming and suing—the only way we can prevent mistakes is by redesigning the human condition. Compared to divine intervention, creating new systems to prevent medical errors seems downright simple.

PART I: THE SYSTEM

CHAPTER 1: THE WRONG PATIENT

The mistakes are all there, waiting to be made.

—Chessmaster Savielly Tartakower (1887–1956)

Joan Morris was asleep. A no-frills, high school educated woman of sixty-seven years, she was exhausted from yesterday's procedure and ready to go home.

She had been well until a few months earlier, when she passed out without warning. A brain CAT scan revealed not one, but two brain aneurysms, each a small outpouching in a cerebral blood vessel. Left untreated, these marble-sized aneurysms are time bombs that can burst without warning. Although they are often clipped off surgically, her daughter, a physician as it happens, had recommended that she have a newer procedure, called *embolization*, in which tiny platinum coils are injected into the aneurysm through a thin catheter to starve it of blood.

Two days earlier she had checked into the academic medical center, said to be one of the best places in the country to undergo the delicate procedure. Located in the heart of a major city, the teaching hospital was surrounded by a park-like setting of mature eucalyptus trees, tony shops and microbreweries, and the independent bookstores that sprout like mushrooms around any big academic facility. If any health care complex displayed—or, more accurately, radiated—an aura of orderly professionalism, it was this one. It was a shrine to high-tech competence.

The procedure had gone without a hitch. Although the neurosurgeon told Joan she'd need a second procedure on her other aneurysm, the success of the embolization left her feeling very reassured. Still, she felt drained by the experience and told the doctor she preferred to recuperate for a month before Round Two, and he agreed.

Her daughter had told her what to expect on the morning of checkout. She would wake up, have a breakfast of cool hospital eggs and limp toast, be read some discharge instructions by a doctor "with one foot out the door—these guys are really busy!" and be on her way home by noon. Before going to sleep, Joan mentally reviewed the list of things she'd do the next day: get her cat back from the neighbor, water the plants, and make a dozen phone calls to worried friends to tell them all was well and that her prognosis was excellent.

One floor below, Jane Morrison was also asleep. Morrison, a seventy-seven-year-old grandmother of eight, had been transferred to the Big House from a rural community hospital after passing out from an erratic heartbeat. Medications hadn't controlled the runaway rhythm, and she had been referred for a cardiac electrophysiology study (or EPS). She had been waiting for two days, as her semielective procedure had been bumped from the schedule a few times by emergency cases. But she was set to be the first case this morning. All night, she tossed and turned in her creaky hospital bed, anxious to get it over with.

The EPS procedure is a remarkable example of the advances in medical technology over the past thirty years. A generation ago, someone with Jane Morrison's arrhythmia would have been placed on toxic medications for the rest of his or her life. In addition to typical side effects like stomach upset, these medications sometimes *caused* the very type of rhythm disturbances they were meant to prevent. With the advent of EPS, many of these patients could enjoy the rest of their lives free of both runaway heartbeats and noxious pills.

In the EPS procedure, a team of cardiac super-specialists threads a slender catheter from an incision in the groin, through a major blood vessel, and ultimately into the cavity of the heart. Once the catheter has arrived there, the beating muscle is stopped and restarted, its electrical secrets mapped by ultrasensitive probes. If a single area of overly twitchy heart cells is found, the offending tissue is literally fried with a "hot" wire using high-frequency radio waves. The procedure is generally safe, though rare complications include unintended puncture of the heart's wall and inability to kick-start the quivering organ. Both can be fatal.

EPS encapsulates the story of modern medicine: dazzling in its complexity, breathtaking in its hubris, extraordinarily expensive, generally effective and periodically risky. It can literally be a lifesaver... for the right patient.

At 6:15 A.M., the first nurse arrived in the EPS lab to check the morning schedule. She saw a "Jane Morrison" listed on the informal schedule kept by the EPS laboratory. The EPS doctors and nurses liked the flexibility of their e-mail-generated, homegrown scheduling system, since a doctor could easily add a new patient by sending an e-mail to the lab ("Hold the 3 P.M. slot for McGuire on Thursday"). Of course, this "system," which frequently omitted patients' first names and never included hospital numbers or birthdays, was riddled with typos. The hospital periodically asked the EPS lab to "play ball" and use the main hospital computers, but that system was old, often down for maintenance, and perennially awaiting upgrades "next year, when the budget is better." So they stuck with the tried and true.

The EPS nurse telephoned the floor where Ms. Morrison, the patient scheduled for the EPS procedure, was sleeping, but was told—incorrectly—that she had been moved from the cardiac ward to the cancer ward. Such errors are common—it is tricky to keep track of who is where at any given time, especially given the rapid turnover of patients in contemporary American hospitals, and their ever-increasing propensity to be filled to the brim.

Few hospitals have given a moment's thought to the safety trade-offs involved in running fast and full, so desperate are they to meet the bottom line. This tension is not unique to the medical business. At San Francisco International Airport, planes take off and land on two parallel runways only 750 feet apart. Airlines would love it if the FAA allowed them to send the next plane off just as the previous plane was clearing the runway, or let them land side-by-side even in terrible weather—the technology exists to permit it. But the FAA's charge is not only to make air travel fast and convenient, it is to make it safe as well. The time between arriving and departing aircraft, as well as the distance between those en route, is closely regulated—not just by pilots, but by controllers on the ground. Violation of these regulations—even once, if it is serious enough—can cost pilots their wings. In the battle between safety and efficiency, safety wins. The stakes are too high to allow it to be otherwise.

Less than a mile from SFO is an International House of Pancakes. Show up any weekend morning and you'll see a crowd out front, spilling onto the sidewalk, parents herding their kids away from the parking lot. An interminable wait? Well, no: Once you sit down a waiter appears within seconds, and your food is on the table eight minutes later. Drop your fork and exhale, and your waiter asks if you'd like the check. As you walk to the cash register—your kids' faces slathered with raspberry syrup—look over your shoulder and you'll see the busboy cleaning the table and resetting it for the next group. Sure, he'll forget the crayons or napkins every now and then, but the priority is clear—throughput is king.

In most hospitals, the effort to manage a full census is no more systematized than a panicky 7 A.M. e-mail from the chief of nursing to the entire medical staff: "We're packed this morning. Fifteen admitted patients spent the night in the ER, and we may have to cancel nine elective surgeries today. Please discharge your patients as early as possible." The pressure of production (we sometimes call it "The Tyranny of the Slot") trumps all other considerations, even safety. In the modern hospital, the EPS suite is a precious resource that can't be wasted. Unfortunately, we approach it more often like the IHOP table than the SFO runway.

This was one of those crazy, overflow days. When the hospital is full, it is common practice to admit new patients to the first available bed, even if it is not on the floor that specializes in the patient's condition. Once the dust settles, things get sorted out: Heart patients are "repatriated" from urology to the cardiac ward, and cancer patients move from ob-gyn to oncology. Conversely, stable patients—like Jane Morrison—may leave their "correct" floor to make room for sicker or more specialized patients. All of this bouncing around makes the hospital's system of tracking patients' whereabouts a critical element in avoiding errors.

You might think that hospitals would have accurate, up-to-the-minute information about where every patient is, perhaps using high-tech gizmos like GPS wristbands, but you'd be wrong. Like most hospitals, this one used an Eisenhower-era system in which nurses or clerks write patients' names, room numbers, and sometimes the names of their physician and nurse on a big whiteboard behind the main desk of each nursing unit. Errors on these boards are common, and it is easy to see how patients could be subject to mix-ups.

Things sometimes get even more complicated when the cultural or language background of a clerk or nurse differs from that of the patient, or that of other caregivers. In America's increasingly diverse big cities, it's not unusual to see non-native English speakers from one country struggle to decipher the unfamiliar name of a non-native English speaker from another—Ellis Island in reverse.

Finally, added to this dangerous melding of "Musical Chairs" with "Telephone" is the fact that patients may have similar sounding and/or appearing names. On a recent (random) day on two floors at UCSF Medical Center, for example, we found two patients with the same last name, Chan, and three other pairs of similar sounding last names (like Pena and Pineda).

So—given the semiorganized chaos of patient flow—it didn't surprise the EPS nurse to hear that her patient had been moved from the cardiac floor to another. At 6:20 A.M. she called the cancer floor, and quickly explained that she needed "Morrison" for her electrophysiology procedure, without giving a first name or hospital number.

Dutifully, the ward clerk—typically a high school graduate with one or two years of health care training, in a tough job that is usually underpaid and overworked—pivoted in her chair, glanced at the whiteboard, saw "Morris," and told Joan Morris's nurse that the EPS lab was ready for her patient.

Joan Morris's nurse picked up the chart and started toward her room, then paused. Her notes said that Morris was recovering from a cerebral aneurysm procedure and would be discharged later in the day. No one had mentioned an EPS procedure, and there was no written order for one in the chart. *Another snafu*, she thought. But she was used to this—patients were always being carted off the floor for procedures she or her fellow nurses hadn't been told about. She knew that if she took the time to verify the order, the EPS folks would be incensed, not just for wasting precious minutes of their heavily scheduled time, but for questioning their instructions. They were incredibly busy and when slots were available, you hustled.

So Joan Morris's nurse woke her patient from a deep sleep and, instead of the cold eggs and toast she'd been promised, told her in a gentle but authoritative voice that it was time to go for her procedure.

Morris later described the scene this way:

> I was half-awake—I was sound asleep actually—
> and this lady comes in and she says, "Oh you have
> an appointment in room so-and-so." And I said,
> "No I don't." I told her, "I would like to go home,
> and give me a chance to breathe a little, catch up
> with myself and then we'll come back and get the
> other done. I told my family, my children, and the
> doctors that I just could not take anything else. I
> need to go home. Then I will come back."

The nurse later recalled that Morris said that she didn't know anything about an EPS procedure, and that she was feeling sick to her stomach. This too was common—pre-procedure anxiety—so the nurse reassured her that she could refuse the procedure after she got down to the EPS laboratory. The patient later remembered little of this conversation.

"I don't remember what she even looked like, to tell you the truth," Morris said. Then, recalling the ride on the hospital gurney to the EPS suite and the preparation for the catheter, she added, "I got up on that thing and the next thing I know, I am going here and there, and all of a sudden there's something in between my legs and I thought, "What are they doing? It's my head!""

Once in the EPS lab, four floors above her hospital room, Morris told the EPS nurse that she felt nauseated and again said she didn't want the procedure. The nurse phoned the EPS attending physician, Dr. Andy Robbins (who had met Jane Morrison, the correct patient, the previous night), and let him speak to the patient, who, unbeknownst to him, was Joan Morris. Her anxiety was odd, Robbins thought, since she'd expressed no concerns in their prior meeting. Still, a chilly cath lab can be a pretty scary place, and Dr. Robbins prided himself on his ability to talk down jittery patients.

"You'll be OK," he reassured her. "It'll be over quickly and we'll fix the problem. You'll be glad you had it done."

After a little more cajoling, Morris agreed to the procedure, returned the phone to the nurse, and received some anti-nausea medication.

Shortly thereafter, the EPS fellow arrived to prepare for the morning's first case. A "fellow" is a physician who has completed training as a generalist (usually in pediatrics or internal medicine) and is now training to specialize in a body part (such as nephrology, to become a kidney specialist) or a disease (like oncology, to become a cancer specialist). Some large subspecialties like cardiology have their *own* specialties (in essence, sub-sub-specialties) like electrophysiology.

This EPS fellow had already qualified as a regular cardiologist and was in her final year of EP training. This meant she was building experience by doing more and more EPS procedures—direct hands-on manipulation of the catheter and wire—with less and less direction from a supervising physician, the "attending." So, unlike in surgical procedures, where the fellow and attending generally stand across the table (and the patient) from each other, the EPS fellow would usually manipulate the catheter around the inside of the heart while the attending stood behind a computer console in the next room and watched the catheter's progress on a monitor, barking instructions, when necessary, into a microphone.

This morning, the fellow was surprised to find no information about the planned procedure in Joan Morris's chart. However, like the ward nurse, she had seen plenty of charts with little or no documentation and shrugged it off. It must be right, she thought. After all, the folks downstairs sent the patient up here for the procedure.

So, assuming the patient had already given permission to the nurse or the attending, the fellow went through the motions of filling out the "informed consent" paperwork. She explained the procedure in a breezy monologue, her arcane medical jargon punctuated by soothing reassurance and gentle petting of the patient's shoulder. Joan Morris, still reeling from the morning's events and now slightly tipsy from the nausea medicine, placed her ragged signature on the form, legally indicating that she had agreed to an "EP Study with possible ICD and possible PM placement." Of course, she had no way of knowing the translation: an electrophysiology study with possible implantation of a cardiac defibrillator (a device, now inside Vice President Dick Cheney, that shocks the heart out of potentially fatal, rapid rhythms) or a cardiac pacemaker. Not surprisingly, Morris said later that she recalled none of this conversation either.

At 7:10 A.M., the EPS lab's charge nurse arrived for work. A "charge nurse" is an experienced nurse who performs extra administrative chores during her shift. He or she is something like a corporal to the "head nurse," who is the ward's top sergeant—a very senior nurse who often has extra academic credentials, such as a master's degree. While head nurse is a title attached to the person, the charge nurse can be any qualified nurse working the shift. The job—and the role—gets passed around.

In the EPS lab, the charge nurse checked to see that the lab's daily paperwork was in order. She settled down in her seat, and was told that the morning's first patient was "teed up" and ready to go. No names were used in this conversation.

At 7:15 A.M., another EPS nurse transferred Joan Morris from the gurney to the cold steel table on which the procedure would be performed. Partly to keep the patient calm, she made small talk, asking why the patient needed the procedure. Morris answered that she had fainted, which was true—ironically fainting can be both a symptom of a cerebral aneurysm *and* a serious heart arrhythmia. Consequently, the EPS nurse just smiled and nodded understandingly.

Downstairs, neurosurgery resident Dr. Ajay Singh, an athletic young man in his early thirties, hustled to compete his morning rounds before his first surgical case. In his left hand he held his usual double espresso—the eye-opener that allowed him to function at 6 A.M. after completing a difficult surgery at 10 P.M. the previous night. In his right was the steel clipboard containing his list of patients: each name followed by several tasks related to their care, including a box for checking them off. One of them said, "Discharge Mrs. Morris."

Dr. Singh was running a bit late, so he was happy to see the discharge checkbox. All it involved was the standard doctor's benediction—take it easy, don't overdo it, take your meds, keep an eye out for unusual bleeding, and so on. Then, after completing a few forms, the patient was in a wheelchair heading out the door, and he could cross her name off his dance card.

Joan Morris was his ninth patient of the morning. Singh entered her room at about 7:30 and was surprised to find an empty bed.

"Where is she?" he asked the nearest nurse.

"Oh, she's up in the cardiac cath lab, getting her EPS," came the blithe reply.

Concerned, Singh parked his espresso and hustled to the stairs. He was a bit out of shape—his high school tennis days seemed like a lifetime ago—and the lab was four floors up. He ran to the main EPS desk, and breathlessly asked the first nurse he saw, "Why is my patient here?"

Matter-of-factly, the nurse told him that his patient had already been bumped twice from the schedule, so they made sure she'd get the first slot that morning.

"Oh—" Singh paused, still not sure that she had answered his question. But the reply was reassuring. After all, Singh was just a resident—a full-fledged MD, but working under the supervision of an attending. Perhaps his attending had ordered the test without telling him. He made a note on his clipboard: "Check Morris EPS results," and left the EPS lab to complete his rounds.

At 8 A.M., Dr. Robbins, the electrophysiology attending physician, arrived, and was told the morning's first procedure was ready to start. Although Robbins liked to enter the procedure room to greet his patients, "Jane Morrison" had already been draped and mildly sedated. Besides, the fellow and her assisting nurse were poised to insert the catheter through the groin incision, so he went directly to his seat at the computer console and waited for the telltale blips of an ailing heart to begin their march across the oscilloscope. The case began.

Back on the cardiology floor, the nurses were puzzled. After their patient had been bumped from the EPS schedule two days running, they had been assured that Jane Morrison would be this morning's first case. Now it was after 8:30 A.M. and nobody from the lab had called for her.

Morrison's floor nurse called the EPS lab and asked, a bit tersely, when they would be ready for *her* patient. The EPS nurse who took the call shouted to the nurse in the procedure room, where by now

Joan Morris's heart had been stopped and restarted several times by puzzled doctors looking for an electrical short-circuit that didn't exist. They yelled back that the morning's first case was turning out to be a tough one and would take at least another ninety minutes.

"Send your patient down about ten," the EPS nurse told the floor. "We'll be ready for her by then."

While this exchange was going on, the EPS charge nurse was rhythmically stamping patient stickers from the laminated plastic cards that accompany each patient as they move through the hospital labyrinth—the way administrators keep track of patient services for billing purposes. Whenever a sticker with a patient's name appears on a lab report or specimen, the hospital cash register goes *ka-ching*.

This time, the charge nurse paused. The name on the sticker said "Joan Morris"—yet there was no "Morris" on the lab's informal e-mail schedule for the day.

She left her desk and went into the procedure room. This act alone was a minor breach of protocol—no doctor wants to be interrupted during a delicate procedure, but the nurse's sixth sense told her that something awful was about to happen—or perhaps already had. She asked the EPS fellow about the person on the table.

"This is my patient!" the fellow snapped, never taking her eyes from the monitor that showed the catheter snaking through the patient's heart.

Like a sailor reamed out by the captain, the charge nurse slunk back to her desk. "Joan Morris," whoever she was, must've been added after that day's advance schedule was distributed. It happened all the time.

At 9 A.M., the attending who had performed the embolization on Joan Morris's brain aneurysm the previous day, Dr. Singh's boss, went to Morris's room to say good-bye—and make sure his resident had completed the necessary discharge briefing and paperwork. Like Singh, he was surprised to find the room empty. Even more surprising, he went to the floor's main nursing station and found the

Morris chart was missing.

"Well, has anyone seen the patient?" he asked.

Nobody knew where she was. He asked the ward secretary.

"Oh, she's gone for her procedure."

That's when the attending felt the short hairs rise on his neck. He was Joan Morris's attending physician. Nothing was supposed to happen to her without his knowledge and approval. The odor of panic began to waft through the ward.

"I think I heard that she's up in the EPS lab," another nurse offered.

The attending picked up the phone, punched in the lab's extension, and asked to speak to the EPS attending. Dr. Robbins was still at his console watching the "Jane Morrison" case come to its maddening conclusion. They'd not found any twitchy patch of myocardium to explain her blackout, and so there was nothing they could fix.

After listening for a minute, Robbins covered the phone's mouthpiece and spoke through the mike to the team in the procedure room. "Neurosurgery's on the horn asking about a patient named Morris. Does anybody know that patient?"

"We're *doing* Joan Morris," the charge nurse corrected him. That's her on the table. I just stamped her sticker."

Robbins grabbed the patient's chart, opened it, and slumped into his chair.

Joan Morris later recalled, "Yeah, it was about halfway through, I think, the doctor said... 'How do you spell your name?' And so then I told him what my name was and I told him how to spell it, you know. And that was about it. But then I was glad to go back to my room."

* * *

If you were CEO of the hospital and were hell-bent to fire somebody for the Morris fiasco, who would it be? The EPS nurse who failed to identify the patient fully when she called the ward for Jane Morrison? The ward nurse who released Joan Morris for somebody else's procedure? The EPS attending, who is "captain" of the crew and therefore responsible for what happens on his watch? How about the neurosurgery resident who ran up to the EPS lab to find out why this patient was undergoing an unscheduled, unrelated procedure, then satisfied himself—without asking—that somebody higher in the hospital pecking order must have ordered it?

The fact is, there was enough blame to go around for everyone. Analyzing this case in our *Annals of Internal Medicine* series, Drs. Mark Chassin and Elise Becher of New York's Mount Sinai Hospital found no fewer than seventeen separate errors in the Morris case (they're listed in Appendix I). Taken alone, none of them was irredeemable—most were even understandable, given the circumstances. But in combination, they became the ingredients for a life-threatening blunder.

Thankfully, Joan Morris emerged from her ordeal undamaged, except for a little scar on her groin where the catheter was inserted. In fact, a few months later she charitably allowed, "I'm glad that my heart checked out OK." But her case illustrates many of the key principles of medical errors, and why fighting mistakes will depend on a new and deeper understanding of why they happen.

CHAPTER 2: IT'S THE SYSTEM, STUPID

I hate the goddamn system, but until someone comes along with some changes that make sense, I'll stick with it.

—Clint Eastwood as "Dirty Harry," *Magnum Force,* 1973

The British psychologist and professor James Reason didn't set out to study health care. His background was in aviation safety, especially looking at the human factors that caused many plane crashes. Trim and good-humored, Reason had become the guru of industrial safety on both sides of the Atlantic by the late 1990s. His brilliantly argued "theory of error" was used by airlines, navies, railroads, truckers, maritime shippers, nuclear power plants, and financial services companies—just about everywhere but medicine.

Most human endeavors, he believed, could be compared to a chisel, with a sharp end that splits the wood and a blunt end that receives the hammer blows to drive it. After major accidents, people generally blame those operating at the "sharp end" of the activity: the surgeon slicing his scalpel through a patient's skin, the pilot adjusting a plane's rudder, the pharmacist dispensing a medication, and the oil rig worker operating a massive drill. The "blunt end" of the process—managers setting priorities, supervisors preparing schedules, administrators processing forms, regulators enforcing rules—is seldom examined; usually only after a failure pattern has become so obvious that it can no longer be ignored.

Workers in the meatpacking industry who carve the meat are, quite literally, operating at the sharp end, as they wield glistening knives while standing shoulder to blood-spattered shoulder with other meat carvers and machines. To any victim of a Sunday morning bagel slice-a-thon, it should come as no surprise that these workers are injured frequently. Of course, some of these injuries are indeed due to failures at the sharp end—a careless worker, perhaps, or a defective knife. But Eric Schlosser, writing in *Fast Food Nation*, suggests that the reasons behind the disturbing rate of injuries go deeper, and can only be fully understood by watching the frenetic pace of the meatworkers' assembly lines. This furious pace reflects a blunt end comprised of administrators putting profit over safety and incentives that pay for speed above everything else. The sharp end of the chisel may be where the chips fly, but in most dangerous industries the blunt end is where the power to make mistakes—or avoid them—begins.

"Human fallibility," Reason notes, "is like gravity, weather and terrain, just another foreseeable hazard." Thus, while sharp-end workers at all levels must have adequate training, motivation, and self-discipline to do their jobs safely, it's up to the blunt-end managers to see that the sharp-end workers have all the tools they need, whether it's up-to-date navigational charts for pilots or a reliable patient ID system for hospitals—and to make sure that they use them.

Making these changes—all of which take time, money, and attention—before an error happens is the fundamental conundrum of safety, in every industry, and coming to terms with this is at the core of our message. All businesses, whether they produce widgets or Happy Meals, fly airplanes or treat the sick and wounded, face an inevitable tension between production pressures and safety. Production usually wins hands down. How many CEOs are hired to improve safety (versus enhance the bottom line, levitate the stock price, or get beyond the scandal of the week)? Whose job has more sizzle: the plant's VP for sales or its safety czar? Even after some buffing up of the safety system after an accident or a near-miss, what business can resist stealing dollars or people from the safety cookie jar after a long period of no foul-ups? The subordinate who blows the whistle on an unsafe situation or supervisor is branded "fussy," a "malcontent," or (either ironically or aptly, depending on your point of view) "insubordinate." All of this makes sustaining a robust safety system a tremendous organizational challenge, one that depends on creating a culture that prizes safety and frets about it incessantly.

With this as background, let's take a new, "systems-oriented" look at the Joan Morris debacle described in the previous chapter.

The case chillingly illustrates James Reason's "Swiss cheese" model, in which multiple small errors in a complex system reach patients only when many holes in the protective barriers align to let them through. Each of the "safety checks"—the nurse releasing her patient off the floor, the fellow obtaining informed consent, the EPS attending speaking to the patient—has a small, but non-zero, rate of error. On most days, the holes would not have aligned: Somebody would have caught the mistake and protected Joan Morris from having the wrong procedure. But notice that the redundancy of the "system" is mostly a mirage: Once Morris got closer and closer to the moment of truth, caregivers became increasingly inclined to blow off inconsistencies, assuming that "someone must have checked this" at an earlier step.

This means that counting on individual competence and good intentions to prevent errors is destined to fail—not always, but often enough. To make a meaningful difference—not just in the cardiac lab but in the operating room, the colonoscopy suite, and other areas where patient identification is the name of the game—the hospital will need to fix its operational blunt end: its highly flawed process for checking patient IDs, the pressure to send patients to procedures the moment a slot opens up, its ever-growing hyperspecialization (which makes it likely that patients will be seen by seven different doctors, none of whom could ID them in a police lineup), and—most importantly—the poverty of communication across departments.

Communication is critical, both because poor communication makes organizations far worse than the sum of their specialized parts, and because communication is the main bridge between sharp-end and blunt-end workers. Here, we refer not just to verbal communications—face-to-face or phone conversations—or written communications—e-mails, forms, memos, even Post-its stuck to patient charts—but even the body language used to convey these messages. Is safety valued? Are questions and cross-checks encouraged or merely tolerated, and in some cases not even that? The expectations and preoccupations of the giving and receiving parties are encoded in every message, whether we realize it or not, and have tremendous power over how that message is interpreted.

In the Morris case, hospital communications—both verbal and nonverbal—were geared to just about everything *other* than patient safety. Everyone knew that it was not impossible for the wrong patient to be subjected to an invasive procedure, but everyone quickly set aside their concerns. Why? Chassin and Becher conclude:

> We suspect that these physicians and nurses had become accustomed to poor communication and teamwork. A "culture of low expectations" developed in which participants came to expect a norm of faulty and incomplete exchange of information, [which] led each of them to conclude that these red flags signified not unusual, worrisome harbingers but rather mundane repetitions of the poor communication to which they had become inured.

One way to penetrate this culture of noncommunication after an error is with a technique borrowed from other industries but superbly suited to medical systems: *root cause analysis*, or RCA. In health care, RCA attempts to write a "second story" about the actions that led to error—to look past the obvious, sharp-end scapegoats and find the other culprits, however deeply they may be embedded in the system or lost in the labyrinth of procedures and traditions. RCA converts obvious, "first story" questions like "who did it" and "who is responsible" to subtler inquiries, such as "how did this happen?" or "why did they do what they did?"

This is critical, since catastrophic failures almost always reflect deep, widespread problems—with the morale and cohesiveness of workers, how information is shared across departments, whether employees feel safe to question the actions of their bosses, and the "safety culture" of the organization. In the case of Joan Morris, the hospital's RCA involved a dozen meetings of nurses, doctors, technicians, administrators, and key leadership. Blackboards were filled with weblike diagrams, sketching out each step—no matter how small—in the process of moving a patient through the hospital ("OK, the EPS nurse calls the floor. Who answers the phone? What does she say? Does the EPS nurse identify the patient by last name, first name, or hospital number?"). The ultimate result was a new, and far more robust, system of error-proofing the process.

To further illustrate the value of RCA and some other key principles of error theory, let's look briefly at a couple of very well-known nonmedical mistakes.

September 11, 2001

In the initial, terrible days after September 11, there was an effort to pin the tail on FBI director Robert Mueller, who had been at his job, overseeing the bureau's 27,000 employees and fifty-six field offices, for all of one week. The passage of time and careful analyses of the events leading to 9/11 now confirm their similarity to the events leading up to most major organizational failures, whether in the realm of intelligence, politics, business, or foreign affairs. This "intelligence failure" had its roots in decades-old problems with communication between various intelligence and law-enforcement agencies. Not surprisingly, the FBI, CIA, NSA, and other national security agencies discovered many "second stories" of morale problems and lack of cohesiveness among workers. They found administrative firewalls that prevented cross talk between departments and a culture that made it unacceptable to question the decisions of supervisors—even though everyone shared the same goal of national safety.

NASA: The Challenger and Columbia Disasters

The 1986 space shuttle Challenger disaster illustrates a similar culture and communications divide. The well-known first story involved the now infamous "O-rings"—rubber seals on the solid fuel booster whose failure on lift-off precipitated the catastrophic explosion. The O-ring problem had been known for some time, and was, in fact, the subject of a dramatic teleconference between NASA managers and engineers from Morton Thiokol, the manufacturer of the solid rocket booster, hours before the launch. In a nutshell, NASA took a calculated risk that the O-rings—which were known to crack under certain, low-temperature conditions—wouldn't fail that day. In the interest of keeping on schedule, they rolled the dice but came up "snake eyes," tragically ending the lives of the crew and NASA's myth of infallibility. The launch-site managers were blamed—villains in the disaster's "first story"—and the Thiokol engineers became heroes for their plucky insistence on safety over "the tyranny of the slot." End of story. Or is it?

Boston College sociologist Diane Vaughan, writing a decade later in *The Challenger Launch Decision*, discovered a much deeper and darker "second story" than the one accepted at the time by the popular press. According to Vaughan's RCA, two factors beyond NASA's highly touted preoccupation with schedule contributed to the accident.

First, knowledge tended to be compartmentalized at NASA, and its departmental keepers were quite possessive and secretive about what they knew. Second, the "go-oriented" NASA culture not only insisted on keeping to schedules, it actively attacked anything that threatened delays—including bad news and the people bearing it. Thus unfavorable or inconclusive test results were either minimized or explained away, and engineers, scientists, or managers who asked for repeated tests, or who questioned positive results, were criticized and sometimes shunted into organizational dead ends. Among these were workers who voiced concerns about the wisdom of launching under certain conditions, including those involving the fatally flawed O-rings.

"No fundamental decision was made at NASA to do evil,"

Vaughan writes. "Rather, a series of seemingly harmless decisions were made that incrementally moved the space agency towards a catastrophic outcome."

The disaster led to a thorough investigation by a blue ribbon commission chaired by former Secretary of State William Rogers, and a set of no-holds-barred recommendations that were designed to not just fix the O-rings, but to remake NASA's safety culture. The agency blessed the report and chanted "never again" in unison, but Vaughan was skeptical. Writing in 1997, she noted that the "supportive political environment has changed. NASA is again experiencing the economic strain that prevailed at the time of the disaster. Few of the people in top NASA administrative positions exposed to the lessons of the Challenger tragedy are still there. The new leaders stress safety, but they are fighting for dollars and making budget cuts."

Perhaps most eerily, one space center engineer told her, "We'll blow another one, but it won't be the solid rocket booster that does it."

Tragically, in February 2003, he was proved right.

The sharp-end cause of the Columbia crash is now clear: a piece of foam insulation, breaking off from the booster and striking and damaging the thermal tiles on the leading edge of the shuttle's wing. The breach in the tiles allowed the heat of reentry to penetrate the wing and melt its structure, leading to the vehicle's breakup. Again, NASA's "go-oriented" mission controllers and launch managers were initially singled out as probable villains in this "first story": There might have been ways to repair the damaged tile or rescue the stranded crew in space, but managers brushed aside those options, quashing repeated requests by engineers to look for foam damage by having spy satellites photograph the wing while the shuttle was aloft.

The deeper RCA—carried out by a thirteen-member independent panel at a cost of $400 million—revealed that blunt-end problems were, as usual, at the root of the catastrophe. The analysis, detailed in a devastating 248-page report released in August 2003, showed that NASA engineers and managers ignored evidence, from at least six prior flights, that flying foam could damage the fragile tiles. More insidiously, the culture of safety—whose absence was so clearly documented by Vaughan after Challenger—had eroded over time, the victim of competing priorities, massive budget cuts, and human nature. By the time of the Columbia crash, wrote the board, the bad habits "that were in effect at the time of the Challenger accident—like inadequate concern over deviations from expected performance, a silent safety program and schedule pressure—had returned to NASA… [and] history became cause."

In essence, in the seventeen years that separated the Challenger and Columbia crashes, NASA had forgotten to be afraid. Admiral Harold Gehman, Jr., the Columbia investigation chair, said that the space agency's prevailing posture had changed from "one in which you had to prove that it was safe to fly to one in which you had to prove it was unsafe to fly."

This letting down the guard, unfortunately, is as predictable as it is human. "If eternal vigilance is the price of liberty, then chronic unease is the price of safety," writes James Reason. The University of Michigan's Karl Wieck, who calls safety a "dynamic nonevent," adds, "When things are going right, nothing adverse is happening. The huge trap here is the inference that because nothing adverse is happening, nothing is being done to create this nonoccurrence. That inference is wrong… Hubris is the enemy."

* * *

The second stories of the shuttle crashes, and of their medical siblings like Joan Morris's cardiac procedure, show us humans who have become accustomed to small errors and routine malfunctions, and, as a result, ignore what *in retrospect* are obvious red flags. This kind of adaptation is not exceptional; it is in fact just the opposite. Accommodating frequent glitches is part of what allows workers to continue functioning—if we investigated every signal or alarm, we would never get any work done. It's not just Homer Simpson who cares more about his next doughnut than the warning light flashing on the nuclear power plant monitor.

This "hindsight bias" problem, which also bedevils medical RCAs, should give us pause before we shout *voilà* after unearthing "smoking-gun" precrash e-mails warning of flawed O-rings or damage from flying foam. Admiral Gehman was particularly sensitive to ensuring that any so-called warning signs implicated by his Columbia investigation could in fact have been detected in advance. "So if these flaws are out there laying around and everybody should have seen them," he challenged, "well, tell me what the next one is if you're so smart."

Psychologist Baruch Fischhoff coined the term "creeping determinism" to describe this tendency to see events that were unexpected as having been completely obvious in hindsight. This tendency also reared its head after September 11. Writing in the *New Yorker*, Malcolm Gladwell pointed out the numerous "red flags" known to the FBI prior to the 9/11 attacks, such as the flight school reports from the FBI's Phoenix and Minneapolis field agents. But, he warns, "what we don't hear about is all the other people whom American intelligence had under surveillance, how many other warnings they received, and how many other tips came in that seemed promising at the time but led nowhere." In fact, the FBI's counterterrorism division had sixty-eight *thousand* outstanding leads at the time of the terrorist attacks. With this much noise, it is inconceivable that any type of attack, no matter how outlandish, would *not* have been followed by the exposure of a smoking gun that made the attack inevitable, had "they" just "connected the dots."

In many ways, creeping determinism represents our attempt to make sense of a terrible paradox. Most safe procedures are defined in terms of the actions they prohibit. But over time, the procedures we use and the precautions we take—as physicians or nurses, astronauts or airline pilots—accumulate like barnacles on a ship. After a while, they begin to slow us down and, because we've been safe and successful so often, we feel it's OK to scrape them off.

For example, it takes a fine touch to thread an intravenous catheter into a patient's vein, particularly if the patient is elderly or has had many prior catheters. In these tough cases, the caregiver must palpate the skin (tap or push it lightly) with the touch of a safecracker to discover the vein, which is often hidden below the surface. With heightened concerns over blood-borne diseases like AIDS and hepatitis, doctors and nurses now wear latex gloves when they draw blood or place IVs—some so thick that the tactile clarity needed to feel the vein is lost. So, this "safer practice" can both slow down the provider and cause patients to feel like pincushions after several botched IV attempts. Ultimately, some caregivers say, "To hell with it!" and strip off the gloves, subjecting themselves to the dangers of an inadvertent needle stick or spatter of blood. They have committed a "routine rule violation"—breaking the "safety rule" either to get their work done or, ironically, because they find the rule fundamentally *un*safe.

As you can see, the challenges of trying to put safety first are daunting. Whether our aim is to prevent shuttle crashes, terrorist plots, or invasive procedures on wrong patients, human beings start with more than two strikes against them. We tend to ignore alarms because of "noise," to let our guards down over time, to jettison safety practices when they are costly or inefficient, to oversimplify the causes of errors by mindlessly invoking sharp-end explanations, and to misinterpret blunt-end problems that we view through the distorted lens of hindsight. Notice that none of this has anything to do with bad apples: Most organizational errors are made by well-intentioned human beings—most highly educated, well trained, and experienced—who have become accustomed to small glitches, routine foul-ups, and a culture that suppresses doing much about them in the name of an overriding goal. The saga of human error is not a story about people who aren't good enough, but merely one about people.

Admittedly, shifting the perspective from bad apples to bad systems is not entirely intuitive, so teaching workers and managers to approach errors this way takes some heavy lifting. Armies, airlines, and power plants learned this lesson long ago, and have made many of the required curricular changes. But until very recently, in thousands of hours of lectures, seminars, and hands-on training, the average medical or nursing student would have been taught precisely nothing about how errors happen, how they should be investigated, and how they can be prevented.

Yet the lessons learned from other industries can take us only so far in health care. First, although our medical system kills tens of thousands of people each year, we register these deaths one at a time, not by the hundreds, as in airline disasters; and behind closed doors in hospital rooms, not on national television, as when a shuttle orbiter explodes. Because of this, it's easy to sweep them under the rug and, like NASA, maintain our "go orientation."

Second, if we ever felt that flying manned space shuttles or generating nuclear power were simply too dangerous (as some clearly do), we could simply choose to forsake these activities. Or, at very least, we could suspend our practice for a year while we reflected on our errors and fixed what we could. But we can't take a hiatus from health care. The pressure to perform without reflection is relentless and gets worse with each passing year.

Finally, medicine's history over the last fifty years is that of ever-increasing complexity—and with it, a parallel growth in the opportunity for errors. Over the past decade, news stories have made patients increasingly worried about receiving the wrong medicine, or the right medicine in the wrong dose, or having the wrong leg or breast removed in surgery, or developing a hospital-acquired infection with some brand-new superbug. All that remained was for a spark to strike the kindling of their anxiety. From this perspective, the electrifying 1999 report on medical mistakes by the Institute of Medicine—which we'll examine in the next chapter—was like a bolt of lightning. The conflagration it started was at once terrifying and illuminating.

CHAPTER 3: JUMBO JETS CRASHING

Facts are stubborn, but statistics are more pliable.

—Mark Twain (Samuel Clemens, 1835–1910)

The Institute of Medicine (IOM), founded in 1970 as the National Academy of Sciences' think tank for health care issues, has a venerable history. Its mission statement could hardly be more sober and bureaucratic: to provide "objective, timely, authoritative information and advice concerning health and science policy to government, the corporate sector, the professions and the public." It has tackled issues ranging from the mundane ("Dietary Reference Intakes: Calcium, Phosphorus, Magnesium, Vitamin D, and Fluoride") to the futuristic ("Stem Cells and the Future of Regenerative Medicine"). Its members are the royals of American academia, and the tone of its fifty or so reports per year is measured, erudite, and miles above the fray. It is an alabaster-pillared, sherry-sipping, Washington institution.

So one could not help but be taken aback by the screaming headlines that leapt off the book jacket of the IOM's 1999 report, *To Err Is Human: Building a Safer Health System*. One part Constitution Avenue to three parts Madison Avenue, its tone instantly caught the attention of the general populace and the media. Just consider the breathless prose of the book jacket, more like the trailer for a Hollywood blockbuster than the synopsis of an academic report:

> Experts estimate that as many as 98,000 people die in any given year from medical errors that occur in hospitals. That's more than die from motor vehicle accidents, breast cancer, or AIDS—three causes that receive far more public attention.... Faced with

these stunning statistics, the IOM has initiated a
project.... This volume reveals the often startling
truth of medical error and the disparity between the
incidence of error and public perception of it...

Even the timing of the report's release seemed to be managed
more by Saatchi and Saatchi than MacNeil and Lehrer. Originally,
it was to be published on December 1, 1999, concurrent with a press
conference in which its authors would attempt to put the report's
sexy marketing handle ("the equivalent of a jumbo jet crashing
every day!") in a less emotional perspective. The real message, like
ours, was that despite an unacceptably high rate of medical errors,
most mistakes were the result of bad systems, not bad people.

On November 29, however—two days before the conference—
Robert Bazell, Tom Brokaw's telegenic medical correspondent, broke
the story on national TV, scooping his rival networks. Immediately,
other broadcasters followed suit and the press conference turned into
a media feeding frenzy.

It was later revealed that IOM officials, knowing they had a
potential hot potato on their hands, consulted several veteran health
care reporters as to how best to handle the release. Whether Bazell's
"exclusive" was planned, was payback for advice, or was simply
good old-fashioned journalistic one-upmanship has never been
explained. But the premature scoop was enough to catapult the story
from routine B-section medical news to front-page headlines that
nobody could ignore.

After saturation coverage for two days, 51 percent of the American public said they now knew about the epidemic of medical
mistakes. Headlines like, MEDICAL ERRORS KILL THOUSANDS, PANEL
SAYS and DOCTORS' DEADLY MISTAKES, all generated by the IOM
report, were seen by more than 100 million Americans. For a while,
medical errors became a cottage industry, with TV specials, feature
stories in slick-cover magazines—even a spate of congressional

hearings. Medical mistakes now joined airline and food safety (and, two years later, terrorism) as omnipresent sources of angst in the American zeitgeist.

Before the shouting died down, $50 million was added to the federal budget for medical error abatement, and that amount has increased—modestly—each year since. Accrediting agencies now require hospitals to meet certain basic safety standards, and a consortium of Fortune 500 companies, the "Leapfrog Group," is promoting other practices designed to reduce mistakes. Each year, new bills are introduced in Congress and in state legislatures to advance hospital safety, including a "patients' bill of rights," though most fail to pass and none have had a substantial impact on injury or mortality rates.

Oddly enough, for all the hoopla, the IOM report actually introduced no new data or statistics—it simply consolidated a number of old reports and repackaged them in a dramatic way. Its most startling "finding"—that 44,000 to 98,000 Americans die annually from medical errors in U.S. hospitals—was derived from two previous studies, one more than fifteen years old. In fact, five years earlier, Dr. Lucian Leape, a Harvard pediatric surgeon and long time patient safety advocate, had published an article in one of the world's most prominent medical journals, the *Journal of the American Medical Association (JAMA)*, which contained all of the IOM's statistics and anticipated its key findings—yet it received no media attention at all and drew yawns from health care professionals. Years later, *JAMA* editor Dr. George Lundberg admitted he wanted to make more of the issue, "but feared that I would lose my job if the public media hit hard on it."

These facts raise certain troubling questions. Why did the IOM choose to publish its report in the form of a quasi-political manifesto under the guise of a white-paper study? Why did all this information, which had been circulating for years, suddenly catch the media's attention? For that matter, how accurate is the "one jumbo jet per day" statistic and—in a larger sense—do such numbers really matter? Wouldn't "one commuter airliner" crashing each day be enough, or "one Greyhound bus" going over a guardrail?

At the bottom of it all, we think, is the mystery and mythology of medical mistakes. Just what *are* medical errors, anyway, and are handsome TV anchormen and flashbulbs the most effective way to combat them?

Like every serious reform, the seeds of the patient safety movement were planted years before they took root in the public imagination. The original crusaders' creed was twofold: (1) that patient safety deserved a place on the public policy agenda—that it wasn't just a problem for experts and individual practitioners; and (2) that medical errors themselves were only part of the problem. The bigger, overarching issue was the *quality* of patient care.

The distinction between quality and errors can be tricky. Overdosing a diabetic patient on insulin is a medical error, whereas failing to control a patient's diabetes tightly enough over years of office visits, raising the patient's risk for a stroke or heart attack, is a quality problem. A brisk postoperative hemorrhage following a hysterectomy because of botched surgical technique is clearly an error, while performing a hysterectomy unnecessarily because the doctor hasn't kept up with the latest guidelines on who should and shouldn't have the procedure is a quality issue. Finally, and perhaps most distressingly, overlooking a subtle fetal abnormality on a prenatal ultrasound is an error, but the complete absence of prenatal care for millions of women is a shameful quality problem. When compared with optimal care—care that is timely, skillfully delivered, and scientifically based—there is little question that these broader quality problems kill hundreds of thousands of people each year in the United States.

These quality crusaders—including Harvard's Leape, pediatrician Don Berwick of Boston's Institute for Healthcare Improvement, and former New York State Health Commissioner

Mark Chassin—sought to engage both academics and the public in the quest for quality. The ammunition in their armory was compelling:

- Research by Dartmouth's Jack Wennberg showed that a patient's chance of receiving a cardiac bypass operation or back surgery, or a woman's chance of having a C-section (Caesarian delivery) during childbirth, varied by up to a *factor of ten* depending on where they lived.

- Tens of thousands of lives were lost annually because high-risk surgeries were performed in hospitals that had inadequate experience with the specific procedure.

- First and second heart attacks could be dramatically reduced simply by administering cheap, lifesaving drugs like aspirin and beta-blockers.

- Thousands of people could be saved from the ravages of colorectal cancer with regular screening for polyps and early cancers.

To make these and other quality findings public, Chassin began publishing a yearly report card on New York hospitals showing their track records for a variety of common procedures. If people took the time to read *Consumer Reports* before buying a refrigerator or car, he reasoned, wouldn't they want to know the postoperative complication and mortality rates of competing doctors and hospitals?

Well, no.

As it turned out, the Chassin reports (and the handful of others that followed) were met with indifference from a public that, apparently, preferred to look the other way. A 2002 Harris poll found that while 26 percent of consumers had seen hospital report cards, only 3 percent considered a change in their care based on those ratings, and only 1 percent had made a change. Quality ratings of HMOs and doctors had even less impact, if that were possible.

It appeared that real people either didn't understand how the health care system really worked, or didn't care much about it when they did. Of course, in an industry that consumes nearly 1.5

trillion dollars per year, the absence of competition on quality just caused hospitals to compete in other areas. So while few providers marketed themselves on credible quality statistics, hospitals, doctors, and health plans avidly showcased their amenities and whiz-bang technology. Brochures showing polished hardwood floors and Jacuzzis in "birthing suites" (Vivaldi playing softly in the background, of course) proliferated. While unmet medical needs and major quality defects remained bountiful, people flocked for Botox injections, laser keratotomies, and total body scans.

Naturally, the quality experts were stunned by their failure to capture the public's imagination with the facts—especially since the market for cosmetic do-overs and even risky "cures" for pseudo-illnesses was booming. To them, it appeared to be a vicious cycle. Without increased quality awareness among caregivers, old habits would never change. Without encouragement and resources from blunt-end administrators, sharp-end quality awareness would never catch on. Without public outrage aimed at lawmakers and regulators, administrators would have no incentive to change their priorities and there would be no research dollars to catalyze quality improvement programs. It was a deadly spiral that left the quality crusaders utterly demoralized—several talked despairingly of leaving the field or of changing the direction of their research. Their dog just didn't hunt.

Before throwing in the towel, they decided to give it one last try. Perhaps the issue of medical mistakes—a subset of the larger issue of health care quality but one that packed more visceral wallop—would resonate with the public and the press when these broader questions of quality had not. After all, everyone likes a good drama, particularly when it's accompanied by a pungent morality play featuring heroes and villains.

The result of all this was the IOM report: their Hail Mary pass, thrown more out of desperation than indignation. But it certainly caught the public's fancy, and in doing so fundamentally altered the terms of the whole debate.

Why did the issue of medical errors catch such a wave when broader quality concerns had not? (As Chassin, one of the IOM report's authors, later lamented to *The New York Times*, "Talk about overuse and underuse of health care, issues that are as important as errors, and everybody goes to sleep.") Perhaps psychologist Abraham Maslow had it right: Humans are unable to focus on complex needs until their basic needs—particularly safety and security—are reasonably satisfied. Although Maslow was mainly concerned with psychological and social wants like self-esteem, the health care analogy seems apt: It is tough to concentrate on postoperative infection rates when you're worried that they'll operate on the wrong leg.

Moreover, whereas errors feel like dramatic, singular events (a feeling reinforced by over-the-top media coverage), most people think of quality more probabilistically. Cutting off the wrong leg is a ghastly outcome that cannot be undone. As a patient, it's a risk I didn't sign up for, and knowing that it might happen makes me profoundly insecure and untrusting of the entire medical enterprise. On the other hand, the fact that my surgeon may have a slightly higher mortality or infection rate feels like a matter of the "odds." I know going in that I might die (after all, they said so when I signed the informed consent), but to keep myself sane I've already talked myself out of that possibility. For most operations, the mortality rate is 1-in-100 or even 1-in-1,000, so even if I learn that my surgeon had a threefold higher complication rate, I can still go into the OR with my faith intact. I'm likely to do fine.

The fact that errors resonate more than quality may not be entirely rational, but it is consistent with our approach to many other risks. Mile for mile, airplanes are safer than cars, yet most people would rather drive than fly, provided the distance isn't too far. What goes unspoken is our intuitive sense that auto accidents tend to be more survivable than air crashes, and that we somehow feel more "in control" strapped in a car than in an airliner five miles up.

For all of these reasons, medical mistakes captivated the public's imagination in a way that quality never did, and perhaps never will.

This lesson was relearned when the IOM published its broader indictment of overall health care quality in 2001, *Crossing the Quality Chasm*. The media *did* pick up on this report... but mostly to ask why it wasn't as exciting as the 1999 medical errors report. We shouldn't have been surprised: Errors are the cute younger sibling who gets all the attention.

If the IOM Report was the tipping point for the issue of medical errors, the "44,000 to 98,000 yearly deaths" statistic was what tipped the report itself. (The accuracy of these numbers has been hotly debated in health care circles, but the debate is a bit arcane—we have placed its highlights in an endnote for those who are interested). Like the infamous *Newsweek* article that mistakenly claimed that a forty-year-old single woman had better odds of being killed by a terrorist than getting married, or the misleading statistic that 1 in 8 women will ultimately get breast cancer, the mortality statistics changed how everyone viewed medical errors. It was not much of a stretch to move from the inevitable comparisons with AIDS and motor vehicle accidents to the far more vivid (even pre–September 11) jumbo-jet-a-day comparison. Virtually every story on the IOM report was spiced with this or an equally dramatic analogy.

Why did these statistics, largely drawn from the fifteen-year-old Harvard Medical Practice Study, cause such an uproar? It was partly timing. In late 1999, the U.S. economy was flying high, the country was at peace, and no one had yet heard of hanging chads or Osama bin Laden. "Nine-eleven" was the number you dialed to call the police. *Time* magazine covers around the time of the IOM Report featured "Jesus at 2000," "The Simple New Year's Eve," and "Can the Pokémon Onslaught Be Bad for Your Kids."

Context also matters. *To Err Is Human* struck fertile soil in a public that had lost patience with managed care, and by extension the entire health care system. A 1999 Harris poll found that less than 40 percent of Americans had confidence in "the people in charge of running medicine," and a study the previous year ranked hospitals just below the post office—and, whew, just above the IRS—in customer satisfaction. The notion that patients might be hurt by their doctors and nurses now seemed distressingly plausible.

Finally, although relatively few Americans had heard of the Institute of Medicine prior to the report, it seemed a credible institution, and the media certainly accepted it as such (by the way, this perception is accurate). So we had a formula for a tipping point: a trustworthy messenger, a compelling statistic, and a receptive populace. Moreover, physicians, congenitally poised to reject any discussion of medical errors as a thinly veiled overture to a symphony of malpractice suits, found the IOM's emphasis on systems thinking rather than "the blame and shame game" liberating. In the hope (mostly wishful thinking, as it later turned out) that the report would herald a new public attitude toward errors, doctors became an important part of the IOM's cheering section.

But they were sorely disappointed. In part *because* the mortality statistics were so alarming, the public was not inclined to sit still for the IOM's no-blame, "It's the System, Stupid" approach. In a 2002 survey, 1,200 citizens and 800 physicians were asked about the most effective ways to prevent medical mistakes. Half the general public wanted to suspend the licenses of professionals who made errors, while slightly less (40 percent) favored government fines. One in four liked the idea of more lawsuits.

In contrast to lay opinion, fewer than 3 percent of doctors favored any of these solutions. Only 14 percent of physicians thought information about medical mistakes should be released, while 62 percent of the public thought that was a good idea. Clearly, the gulf between practice and preferences—for both groups—has never been wider.

So—now that the frightening reality of medical errors has caught the attention of patients, providers, and politicians—our task is to reorient the whole debate; to level the playing field between sensationalism and fact, and to move us all from the startling realization of the scope and complexity of the problem to a new understanding that will actually help us fix it.

That is the job of Part II of this book. Even those well versed in patient safety will find that these dramatic stories of people and systems will turn many of their cherished beliefs upside down.

PART II: THE ERRORS OF OUR WAY

CHAPTER 4: DOCTORS' HANDWRITING AND OTHER PRESCRIBING ERRORS

I firmly believe that if the whole *materia medica* [the list of available drugs] could be sunk to the bottom of the sea, it would be all the better for mankind—and all the worse for the fishes.
—Oliver Wendell Holmes (1809–1894),
addressing the Massachusetts Medical Society, 1860

Even before he fell victim to a medical mistake, Ramon Vasquez knew he was unlucky. In June 1995, at age forty-two, chest pains took him from his hot, dusty home in rural Odessa, Texas, to the local medical center. After a battery of tests, a cardiologist informed him that the chest pains he'd been experiencing were actually angina, the heart's painful plea for more oxygen. He had coronary artery disease. Although men tend to get coronary disease earlier than women, Vasquez was definitely at the younger end of the spectrum. He left the doctor's office and went home to tell his wife, Teresa, and their three teenage children the bad news.

He also left with something else: a prescription for a new heart medicine. But what was this prescription for? Why don't *you* try your hand at "prescription roulette": Look closely at Vasquez's actual prescription, reproduced below, and decide for yourself if the doctor is prescribing Plendil (a powerful calcium-channel blocking drug sometimes used to treat angina) or Isordil (a longer lasting version of the tiny nitroglycerin tablets heart patients slip under their tongues for temporary relief from angina).

If you had trouble deciding, welcome to the club. We asked 158 physician colleagues to interpret this prescription. Half thought it was for Plendil; about a third voted for Isordil. And the rest thought it was for a third drug, Zestril, a medication for high blood pressure. Even knowing Vasquez's diagnosis wouldn't be much help, since all three are used to treat heart patients.

Ramon Vasquez's doctor actually intended to prescribe 120 tablets of Isordil, at its typical dose of 20 milligrams (*mg*) by mouth (*po*) every (*Q*) six hours. Tragically, like the majority of our colleagues, Vasquez's local pharmacist also "flunked" this test, sending him home with a bottle of Plendil. The instructions told him to take 20 mg at breakfast, lunch, dinner, and bedtime—a total of 80 mg a day.

Even more tragically, the usual and safe dose of Plendil is 10 mg a day.

Just as the doctor ordered, Ramon began taking the pills immediately—and immediately began to feel terrible. His wife, Teresa, later testified that "after he took it, he would complain that his heart was pounding real fast, but after a while it would go away." Still, he stuck with his doctor's instructions, and continued to overdose himself with the wrong drug.

Twenty-four hours later, his blood pressure had plunged so low that his already ailing heart could no longer deliver enough oxygen to keep itself going. He suffered a massive heart attack and was taken to a local hospital, where he died a few days later.

Teresa Vasquez filed a malpractice suit against both the cardiologist who scrawled the prescription and the pharmacist who filled it (and who should have realized that the "Plendil" dose was absurdly high). The jury awarded her $450,000—the full amount her attorney asked for—with payment to be split between the defendants. One juror later said that if Mrs. Vasquez had asked for a bigger award, they would have gladly granted it. After the trial, Mrs. Vasquez explained that she had taken legal action less for the money than "because if the doctors don't change their writing, then it could happen again with my kids, or even me."

Poor physician handwriting and illegible prescriptions leap to many people's minds when they think about medication errors, and understandably so. But are doctors uniquely sloppy in their penmanship? A study published in the *British Medical Journal* tried to answer this question. During a break at a conference attended by doctors, managers, and health care executives, the 209 participants were each given ten seconds to write the same sentence. Judges, who did not know the scribbler's profession, graded each note on legibility. It turned out that the physicians' handwriting *was* terrible, scoring 7.1 out of a possible 13 points, leaving lots of room for improvement. But the nonphysicians' notes were nearly as indecipherable.

Of course, these results give small comfort to patients. Legible writing on a prescription is vastly more important than on a hastily scribbled business memo. And there's another land mine in the prescribing world: Many popular medications have remarkably similar names. The antidepressant Zyprexa and the antihistamine Zyrtec; the anticonvulsant Cerebyx and the anti-inflammatory Celebrex; and the mood stabilizer Lamictal and the antifungal Lamisil are but three of many examples where even good penmanship is no substitute for an alert and functioning brain in those who write and those who fill prescriptions. Only recently has the FDA pushed manufacturers to avoid sound-alike names. The pharmaceutical giant Eli Lilly, for one, was compelled to change the name of a new drug for attention-deficit disorder from tomoxetine to atomoxetine because the former resembled the anticancer drug, tamoxifen, to a dangerous degree. Simple labeling changes can also help pharmacists and patients distinguish between these deceptive duos, such as using "tall man" lettering for the suffixes of drugs that begin with the same prefix, like "ClomiPHENE" and "ClomiPRAMINE."

Although doctors' bad handwriting will undoubtedly remain a staple for stand-up comics, more insidious prescription problems—

wrong doses, overlooked drug interactions, misleading instructions, and so on—represent an even graver threat to patients.

In 1994, Betsy Lehman, the popular health columnist for the *Boston Globe*, received experimental treatment for recurrent breast cancer at the Harvard-affiliated Dana-Farber Cancer Institute, where her husband was a scientist. With short, dark curly hair and a ready smile despite her condition, the thirty-nine-year-old mother was understandably anxious to conquer her disease and get back to her career and two children. Of course, as a medical journalist, she had more than the average cancer patient's interest in and knowledge about her treatment, and in the way care was delivered at Dana-Farber, one of the world's top cancer hospitals.

The experimental protocol required patients to receive unusually high doses of a powerful but toxic drug called cyclophosphamide—a cousin of nitrogen mustard, which in turn is closely related to the deadly mustard gas used in World War I—followed by a bone-marrow transplant. The ordering physician wrote—legibly but imprecisely—"cyclophosphamide 4 g/sq m over four days," intending that Lehman receive a total of four grams ("g") per square meter ("sq m")—a commonly used measure of body size in oncology—spread out over four days. Instead, the nurses administered the intended *total* dose, 4 grams, on *each* of the four days, a terrible error—quite literally—of execution.

Soon after treatment, Lehman's stomach began to churn. Nausea consumed her, and her muscles felt like Jell-O. These were familiar chemotherapy side effects, so her doctors ignored them and Betsy simply gritted her teeth and determined to ride them out—she had written about such patient fortitude often enough in her medical column. However, the toxic symptoms continued. Her condition grew worse and she entered an inexorable downward spiral that ended in her death three weeks later, likely of heart failure brought on by the unintentional overdose. Her autopsy revealed no visible signs of residual cancer. The treatment was successful, but the patient died.

If any of us paid much attention to the small print on most drugs, we'd never take another pill. No matter how benign-sounding the medication, the potential side effects always seem impossibly broad. Some of these reactions are merely annoying: dry mouth, diarrhea, upset stomach, and fatigue. Others are terrifying: "In rare cases, this laxative may cause coma or death."

Although side effects are nearly always undesirable, there are some interesting exceptions. For instance, minoxidil is a potent blood pressure medication that fell out of favor in the 1980s when many patients noticed an unusual "side effect": The drug caused them to grow more hair. Now, one man's poison is another man's meat, and Pharmacia & Upjohn knew a good thing when they saw it. They reformulated minoxidil into a medication called Rogaine and made a bundle selling it to the balding.

An even more profitable topsy-turvy success story came in 1991, when Pfizer researchers in England ran clinical trials of a new drug called sildenafil for the treatment of angina—the same type of chest pain that afflicted Ramon Vasquez. A year into the trials, it was clear that the drug was not terribly effective, so the investigators were surprised when many test patients told them they were reluctant to quit. Questioning the participants about their unexpected passion for this apparently ineffectual drug, male patients whispered that they had experienced the "side effect" of increased erectile function. Nobody talks about sildenafil these days, but everyone knows it by its trade name, *Viagra*.

One of the challenges of studying and understanding medication errors is just this: All drugs—even when used properly—can have side effects, and some side effects (like minoxidil's and sildenafil's) may even prove to be advantageous.

But the task of creating safer and better drugs is a story for another day, and another book. Our main concern here is with medication misadventures: when a drug is used improperly, or when a doctor miscalculates and prescribes an excessive dose, or when the pharmacist misreads a scrawled prescription and prescribes the wrong medicine. To avoid a lot of hairsplitting about side effects versus medication errors, patient safety researchers increasingly use the term *adverse drug event*, or ADE. This broad term includes any problem resulting from a drug, whether it's a side effect, the result of improper usage, or the consequence of an out-and-out error.

In large studies of health care complications, ADEs consistently rank as the leading type of harm experienced by patients. At least 5 percent of hospital patients experience an ADE at some point during their stay, and an additional 5–10 percent experience a potential ADE—where they *almost* take the wrong medication, or the wrong dose, or experience some other type of prescription error, but escape unharmed, often by dumb luck. For instance, a relatively healthy patient who incorrectly receives a minoxidil tablet instead of the antiarrhythmic Mexitil might experience no symptoms, and the error would go unrecognized (alas, the hair growth takes weeks). By contrast, a frail elderly patient receiving the same medication in error might see his blood pressure fall suddenly and lose consciousness, a life-threatening problem.

The high frequency of ADEs, both actual and potential, is itself a side effect of the ubiquitous use of drugs in modern medicine. Whereas a patient admitted to the hospital typically undergoes one—or even no—surgical procedure, virtually everyone gets bombarded with an array of medications the whole time they're there. Thus we believe the medical error spotlight should shine even more brightly on ADEs because—whether the unwanted results are either recognized side effects or are the result of true errors—they pose a significant threat to patients. The easy answer to the problem is simply to recount the tragic stories of Ramon Vasquez and Betsy Lehman as iconic cautionary tales. Their stories shout: "Doctor, write legibly!" "Pharmacist, make sure the dose makes sense!" "Nurse, are you sure you understand what this prescription means?!" These admonishments are crucial, and they'll save lives. But the real answer is a better system for prescribing, and there *is* such a system now, ready for prime time, if we only had the will and the money.

The use of Computerized Physician Order Entry, or CPOE, could potentially eliminate most of the medication errors that occur at the prescribing and order-filling stage—whether due to poor handwriting, sloppy instructions, or bad therapeutic choices (the wrong medicine or the wrong dose). At minimum, CPOE's word-processed orders can prevent the handwriting problems that killed Ramon Vasquez. But its breathtaking potential lies in more sophisticated "expert" systems, aptly named "decision support," that include menu-driven dose selection, warnings about possible drug interactions, tracking of patient allergies—systems that would have, for instance, disallowed Betsy Lehman's caregivers from giving her a lethal overdose.

A few examples: The CPOE system at Brigham and Women's Hospital in Boston keeps track of a patient's kidney function by monitoring a lab test called creatinine, alerting the doctor to adjust the dose of any of the many medicines that are excreted by the kidney when it detects evidence that the organ is failing. The Department of Veterans Affairs now has a national system—on-line at every VA hospital—that can tell a doctor in San Francisco what medications a patient received during his last visit to the VA's outpatient clinic in San Antonio. Salt Lake City's LDS Hospital keeps track of which antibiotics work best against certain organisms, taking into account the local bugs' unique and ever-changing antibiotic resistance patterns, giving physicians better tools for fighting infections.

Prescribing doctors can override CPOE suggestions—and sometimes they should. But before they can veto a computerized suggestion, doctors must answer an "are-you-sure?" type of prompt; the way your own desktop computer asks whether you *really* intend to delete an unwanted file. The system may even require the prescriber to obtain approval from a relevant specialist. That may not make health care faster or cheaper than it is now, but it will certainly make it safer.

Unfortunately, the vast majority of U.S. hospitals still lack any form of CPOE system—let alone those that offer doctors sophisticated clinical guidance. Efforts to propagate the handful of successful CPOE systems nationally are too often foiled by user affection for home-grown systems and the problems inherent in adapting new systems to old ones (the supermarket doesn't need to know what you bought three years ago, but, to avoid mistakes, we need to access your entire medical history even after we switch to a computerized system). Moreover, antique laboratory reporting systems (often jury-rigged themselves) may cause intractable hiccups when hooked up to new CPOE systems.

Even the lessons learned from CPOE pioneers like Brigham and LDS may not be transferable to other hospitals. These institutions have built their own systems with blood, sweat, and the passion of committed clinical leaders and researchers. But the average hospital will not share these conditions, any more than your local Gilbert and Sullivan troupe resembles the Met. Many commercial vendors produce and market "off-the-shelf" clinical information systems, claiming they will solve every conceivable problem, but more than one chief information officer has tried to "airlift" a commercial system into her hospital, then stood scratching her head at how slick the system *seemed* to be during the vendor's demo, and how poorly it performed in real life. In medical computing, the purchase is just the starter's gun for the real work.

Cost is an even bigger barrier. The acquisition and implementation cost of a CPOE system for a typical midsized hospital can run from $20 to $30 million. This same amount of money would allow the hospital to hire one hundred nurses and pay their salaries for five years. Small wonder that in the late 1990s, the organization that accredits most American hospitals found that fully one-third of the commercial CPOE systems they endorsed had not yet found a single user. In 2003, fewer than 5 percent of American hospitals had functioning CPOE.

If you're in a charitable mood, you might say, "OK, CPOE is pretty complicated. But what about the rest of medicine?" It's a good question, one that sometimes leaves us scratching our heads as well. Why has the computerization of health care—one of our most information-intensive and risky businesses—been so exasperatingly slow?

Other industries and services, from airlines and department stores to movie theaters and public libraries, have not only computerized, but made the leap onto the Internet; why not your local hospital? Many patients (and, truth be told, many doctors) have asked in frustration how it is that they can go online and book a trip to Maui, choose an aisle seat, and select the vegetarian plate in far less time than it takes to book a doctor's appointment in the clinic across town.

Clearly, the sheer economics of doing a lot of little things more reliably but more expensively is a big part of the problem. As the cost of health care exploded in the 1970s and '80s, payers responded with so-called managed care: a system designed to procure medical services at the lowest possible cost. This put tremendous financial pressure on most hospitals and clinics. In 2000, the average American hospital had an operating margin—the profit pool from which new equipment is purchased—of less than 5 percent, and fully one-third of all hospitals were in the red. The chance of such cash-strapped hospitals squirreling away the tens of millions needed for a basic CPOE system was practically nil, especially since this purchase yielded no compensatory bump in reimbursements, and lacked the marketing cache of a new MRI scanner or laser surgery device. Have you ever seen a hospital ad touting, "Come see our new computerized physician ordering system"?

Local politics enter the equation, too. If a hospital has extra cash at the end of the year, there is usually a donor or advocacy group pushing for a new cancer wing, a surgeon pleading to remodel an outdated operating room, or a head nurse begging for more staff. Amid this sea of supplicants, the physician, nurse, or administrator arguing for a CPOE system has a tough time making the case, coming off as at worst nerdy and at best uninspired.

Organizational passivity and resistance to change are the final, and often the most daunting, obstacles. Initially most new hospital computer systems *create* work rather than simplify things, because the computer forces users to enter far more data than they'd write on their own. So, in addition to the (always underestimated) time it takes to train all the workers, and the awkward transition period when the hospital is partly on the old paper system and partly computerized, the once-enthusiastic CIO must invariably confront active resistance or passive aggression by workers scattered like snipers in disparate units around the institution. The end result is frequently inertia, sometimes interrupted by a few halfhearted mini-programs (a handful of Palm Pilots here, a computerized system for generating patient discharge instructions in the ER there) to answer the critics and give the hospital a patina of space-age modernity. But the illusion is too often only skin deep.

Even when the economic, logistical, and behavioral barriers to CPOE systems are factored in, we're still amazed at modern medicine's failure to fully embrace integrated computerized scheduling, bar-coding, and other information handling and data manipulation technologies used so successfully in other industries. It's tempting to diagnose this unfortunate situation as some fundamental flaw in the medical mind, a deficiency in doctors that somehow rubs off on everyone who works with and around them. But before we leap to that damning conclusion, let's reflect a moment on the expectations customers have about service in other industries, and the nature of these businesses' transactions.

Parcel delivery services use bar codes to track hundreds of thousands, if not millions, of packages from warehouse to doorstep each day; but customers don't expect to reschedule or change the destination of these deliveries en route. If you miss your FedEx or UPS delivery, you know you'll receive it the next day—or you can arrange to pick it up at the local depot—but you *can't* bump another parcel and take its place simply by saying your shipment is more important than the others in the queue. We *expect* certain processes to take a certain amount of time. Similarly, many financial transactions require several business days—or more—before they become effective, even when conducted online. That's just part of the business; and high-volume, high-transaction industries have "trained" their customers to expect nothing less—but nothing more.

In the hospital business, however, we routinely change or add medications not once, but many times each day for each patient; and procedures—often involving expensive machines and highly trained teams—need to react quickly to changing conditions, such as emergency admissions or "crashing" patients. In the airline business, all passengers enter and exit the plane at the same time. At a hospital, the "passengers" board, fly, and deplane one at a time, throughout the day and night—and each one orders from an "in-flight menu" of literally thousands of items—then each disembarks at a unique destination! This is a fundamentally different process, with vastly different record keeping and liability constraints, than airline operations—even though safety is crucial to both. Capturing all of this in a computerized medical system that is both sufficiently flexible and unerringly reliable is harder than getting your package to Tulsa, or you to O'Hare.

Even for health care administrators—those much maligned "paper pushers" we blame for so many costs and inconveniences—the convoluted U.S. medical system creates dyspepsia. Stick your bank card into an ATM and enter your PIN. If the amount you've requested is less than the balance in your account, the machine gives you the cash. By contrast, even the shortest hospital stay requires multiple cross-checks, validations, and rule-based authorizations for services performed and charged. Why? Because controlled substances, such as toxic or potentially addictive drugs, are administered and must be accounted for; procedures must be documented for billing and liability purposes—the requirements are practically endless. After tracking down your insurance carrier (are they still in business?) the system must verify your coverage, or fraction of coverage; whether the treatment you received was proper and allowable for the official diagnosis; whether the payer considers your doctor, or doctors, approved providers; whether time limits apply to your claim (only one general checkup per year, for example, or a cap of twelve visits to a physical therapist); and so on. Compared to this, an ATM is little more than a glorified abacus.

Ultimately, computers will help treat our epidemic of medical mistakes, but they are not a panacea. Although our experience with sophisticated systems, such as CPOE, gives us hope, we mustn't raise those hopes too high, or pin them on technology alone. A few examples will show why. In 1988, an Iranian airliner was destroyed by an American-guided missile cruiser, the U.S.S. *Vincennes*, when the warship's sophisticated Aegis computer system mistook the wide-bodied Airbus A300 for a much smaller F-14 fighter. In 1992, all ambulance service in London was shut down on two occasions—contributing to as many as twenty deaths—because its centralized computer dispatching system had crashed. Well-funded and technically savvy institutions like NASA, the FAA's Air Traffic Control system, phone companies, the Social Security Administration, and the IRS—not to mention the infamous Florida election system and the electrical grid of the northeastern United States—have all experienced computer-related disasters, and the horror stories keep coming.

The prospect of similar snafus in health care only adds to hospitals' trepidation when it comes to laying out big bucks for electronic brains. Even in the hermetically sealed clinical environment, such concerns are real. On November 13, 2002, a state-of-the-art computer system at Harvard's Beth Israel Deaconess Hospital stopped dead in its tracks when the entire network choked on a single researcher's data. For four days, every bit of the medical center's computerized information—from prescriptions and patient histories to hospital bills and routine e-mails (over 100,000 of them each day!)—remained frozen in the log-jammed circuits. In the resulting scramble to keep its doors open and patients alive, Beth Israel's campus was literally papered with, well, paper. Handwritten "DO NOT USE" signs sprouted on every computer monitor and reams of dusty parchment were exhumed from data warehouses. The laboratory began dumping three thousand results slips into plastic bins so that they could be hand-sorted each day, by workers ranging from orderlies to the CEO. Computer SWAT teams from all along the Eastern seaboard were activated and descended on the facility to help cool the digital meltdown. "It's like the Y2K that never happened," said a Beth Israel VP. The headline in the *Boston Globe* asked administrators—and the public—rhetorically: "GOT PAPER?"

A few months later, L.A.'s Cedars-Sinai Hospital pulled the plug on a brand new, house-developed CPOE system when doctors using it—or, rather, refusing to use it—all but threatened to strike. You didn't have to know the price tag—$34 million—to guess that the system spared no expense. Cedars is one of the world's toniest hospitals; partly because it's where Hollywood's glitterati go when they are sick (its address is on Gracie Allen Drive; the pediatric research center is in the Spielberg Building), and partly because it is enormously well endowed. But money can't buy everything; and in this case, it couldn't buy a usable system. One doctor told the *Los Angeles Times* that while it previously took him five seconds to prescribe Vancomycin, a commonly used IV antibiotic, it now took him over two minutes. "If I have to add five to ten minutes to each patient," he complained, "that adds hours to my day. That's time that I either can't read, I can't be with my family, or I can't be with my patients."

Cedars executives insisted that they'd kept their rank-and-file doctors in the loop as the system was developed, but the physicians disagreed. "They poorly designed the system, poorly sold it, and then jammed it down our throats and had the audacity to say everybody loves it and that it's a great system," said one surgeon. Although no fatalities occurred during the fiasco, patient safety problems were plentiful, including that of a baby who received a short-acting anesthetic for his circumcision a day before the procedure.

As you can see, there's nothing wrong with America's medical prescribing and information handling system that an infinite amount of time and money couldn't cure. Of course, we don't have an infinite amount of time and money; and the evolution of truly reliable, standardized, and widespread computer systems, such as sophisticated CPOE, will undoubtedly come too late for many patients.

But it will come.

Just as it has in other industries, the peculiar demands of the health care environment will not only be understood, but harnessed and integrated into information systems that are truly informative— *safe* as well as effective. In fact, computerization of dangerous processes, such as medication and procedure ordering, will probably be mandated for hospitals in the near future—a process that has already begun in California. Even without legislative action, institutional health care customers—premium payers such as the Fortune 500 companies represented by the Leapfrog Group—have put implementation of CPOE at the top of their list of innovations that define high-quality organizations.

If additional studies demonstrate that CPOE and computerized decision support really do make a difference in health care, then pressure will undoubtedly build for an ambitious federal program to computerize, and perhaps link via high-speed Internet connections (in the manner of the VA system), every hospital. This would be the health care equivalent of the Apollo moon shot or the creation of the Internet itself, but the cost would almost certainly be worth it— particularly when a whole category of potent medical errors would be reduced to an occasional, rather than everyday, occurrence.

But without some sort of governmental support or subsidy to get things started and keep them moving, many hospitals already strapped for cash will simply cut caregiver salaries, services, and other necessities to pay for new computers, and our epidemic of medical mistakes will only get worse—in ways we never expected. When it comes to our woefully underfunded efforts to prevent medical errors, we can't afford to rob Peter to pay Paul: Both need the money.

CHAPTER 5: THE FORGOTTEN HALF OF MEDICATION ERRORS

[Only] the right dose differentiates a poison from a remedy.

—Paracelsus (1493–1541), the father of modern pharmacology

Sandra Geller looked far younger than her sixty-eight years. Always careful about her appearance, she loved wearing antique brooches and never left home without a bit of makeup. She visited her hairdresser each Wednesday, and slept in a hairnet to keep her curls in place. After two weeks in a hospital's intensive care unit, though, her hair lay matted against her scalp. A series of life-sustaining tubes and wires was now all that accessorized her faded hospital gown.

For several years, Sandra's angina—the chest pain associated with coronary artery disease—had gotten progressively worse. She finally entered her local hospital for elective cardiac bypass surgery. The procedure went well, but postoperative complications set in almost immediately. The first was a lung infection acquired while she was on a mechanical ventilator. She then suffered a small stroke, some gastrointestinal bleeding, and acute kidney failure that required short-term dialysis. We physicians sometimes indelicately call such patients "train wrecks," and they usually don't survive.

But after two weeks in the ICU, her doctors finally believed she had turned the corner and was starting on the long road to recovery. She "actually told us that she was comfortable and felt good for the first time," her primary physician recalled. "She looked wonderful during rounds."

It was true. Sandra had brushed the tangles out of her hair and pinned it neatly behind her head. She even asked one nurse about lipstick. Doctors have an old adage: You know that a female patient is getting better when she applies makeup (for men, it's when they shave).

So plans were already afoot to move Sandra out of the ICU and back to the regular cardiac ward when, at 8:15 one morning, the ICU nurse heard a loud noise coming from her room. She ran in to see the patient jerking violently on the bed: her head snapping back and forth, back arching, arms and legs thrashing. She was having a seizure.

Few episodes in medicine are as disturbing to watch as a full-blown seizure. The onset of a seizure may be subtle—a twitching finger or fluttering eyelid, or a fleeting grimace—as if the patient is lost in a daydream. Some seizures stop there.

But usually, seizures "generalize." The convulsions move from a single limb to the torso, and then throughout the body. These *grand mal* (basically, French for "big bad") seizures are the stuff of epic drama—the "falling sickness" of Julius Caesar. Eyes roll back in their sockets and the whole body wracks with violent spasms. The patient froths at the mouth; bladders empty; bowels cut loose. It's an ugly, terrifying sight.

Yet even *grand mal* seizures play out after a minute or so, the brain's short-circuit resolving itself before medications can be administered. In fact, the immediate treatment for most seizures consists of little more than removing breakables and gently placing the patient on the floor to prevent injury. However, some seizures don't stop on their own, at least not so quickly. Mercifully, patients subjected to these longer seizures usually lose consciousness; but after about ten minutes of a *grand mal* seizure, the electrical storm surging through the patient's central nervous system can, quite literally, "fry the brain"—causing irreversible damage.

Because these protracted seizures can be life-threatening, doctors give them a special name: *status epilepticus*. Early in our training, we memorize the protocols for treating them, much as we learn the rules for treating cardiac arrest with CPR. These protocols begin with injections of Valium-like drugs, progressing to intravenous administration of antiepileptics like Dilantin and—in the most serious cases—general anesthesia to effectively shut down the brain before the seizure can wreak its ultimate havoc.

But whether the seizure subsides on its own or requires medical intervention, the doctor's next priority is to find out why the seizure happened. In contrast to childhood epilepsy, which traces its pathology mainly to bad luck (genetic heritage or random brain anomaly), seizures beginning in adulthood usually signal some serious, underlying disorder, such as intracranial bleeding, strokes, or brain tumors.

In addition to these traditional sources of seizures, which occur when the orderly flow of electrical impulses constantly traversing our brains hits a physical roadblock, some seizures occur simply because the brain is malnourished—starved of essential nutrients for long periods. For example, both mountain climbers at high altitudes and drowning victims can seize due to lack of oxygen, as can patients who don't have enough of the special blood sugar known as glucose to fuel their brains. This latter condition, sometimes called "insulin shock," occurs when diabetic patients overdose on insulin. As every diabetic knows, the treatment is simple: Eat something sweet. They also know that every minute counts. Brain cells deprived of sugar or oxygen begin to die in minutes.

So even as the doctors and nurses ran to Sandra Geller's bedside to begin their ministrations, they began to wonder: Why had she seized?

Within moments, the ICU "crash" team surrounded Geller. One of the physicians administered an intravenous sedative. Another placed a breathing tube down the patient's already battered throat (a similar tube, needed during her complications, had recently been removed). This would protect her lungs in case she vomited during the seizure. They drew a vial of blood and sent it off to the lab, to check whether the levels of certain important chemicals, such as sodium and glucose, were out of kilter. Oxygen was not the problem, as a quick check of the oximeter—a gadget used in every ICU to monitor O_2

saturation—looked good. They also knew Geller had no history of diabetes, so they didn't think to give her the same 60-second, finger-stick blood sugar test used by millions of diabetics in their homes each day, or to inject her with a concentrated sugar solution.

But they did know she'd had a minor postoperative stroke, and both strokes and intracranial bleeding can cause seizures, so it was logical to whisk her down to radiology for a CAT scan of her brain. It came back negative, and they scratched their heads again: Why *had* she seized?

Thirty minutes after leaving the ICU, as Geller was exiting the CT scanner, the hospital's lab paged Geller's lead physician. Geller's blood sugar (glucose) level was not only low, it was completely undetectable.

Flabbergasted by this news, the doctors immediately injected Geller with a syringe-full of concentrated dextrose, a sugar solution. Thinking the first result may have been in error—she had absolutely no reason to be hypoglycemic—they took another blood sample and rushed it to the lab. She had tested normal for blood sugar upon admission and had not received insulin or other drugs that depress those levels. But the second sample, even after the large injection of "D50," showed only a marginal increase: 18 mg per deciliter. Since the normal reading is about 80 mg per deciliter, this was still brain-threateningly low.

So they slammed in another big dose of concentrated sugar, took more blood, and ran it to the lab. They were amazed: They had only nudged the meter up to 24—still not nearly high enough—and brain cells were dying every minute. They began a continuous intravenous infusion of dextrose and crossed their fingers. Slowly, the patient's blood glucose level rose to normal levels, but the damage had been done. Geller lapsed into a coma from which she would never awaken. After two weeks, in accordance with the patient's "living will"—the important document that states a patient's desires in just such catastrophic circumstances—life support was withdrawn. She died shortly thereafter. For weeks, several of the ICU doctors and nurses had flashbacks of the scene on morning rounds an hour before she seized: the smiling caregivers standing around her bed, congratulating her on her near-miraculous recovery, with Sandra beaming right back at them.

About an hour after the seizure, another nurse tidying up Geller's disheveled ICU room noticed two different medication vials amidst the syringes, tubing, and other flotsam and jetsam that typically clutter a patient's bedside table. One was heparin, a blood thinner routinely injected in small doses through intravenous lines to make sure they don't clot off. The other was insulin. The bottles were about the same size and shape, and their labels were also similar in appearance. Given the nature of Geller's emergency, it did not take a rocket scientist to realize what had happened: The patient's ICU nurse, intending to flush Geller's IV line with heparin two hours earlier, had inadvertently injected a fatal dose of insulin.

In the last chapter, we saw how illegible handwriting, sound-alike drugs, and miscalculated doses can devastate sick, and even not-so-sick, bodies. But not all medication errors start on the prescription pad or at the computer terminal. After all, the prescription process is just beginning when physicians try to pluck from their memory the right drug, in the right dose, from the thousands available—taking care to prevent adverse drug interactions or complications that might arise because of the age or condition of a particular patient. More chances for error occur when that decision, even if it's correct, gets written down or punched into a computer keyboard, conveyed to a pharmacy (sometimes by fax, where new legibility problems can arise), then deciphered by a pharmacist, dispensed, packaged, labeled, and transported back to the ward, or to a patient's home, to be administered by a nurse or by the patients themselves.

One analyst found that *fifty* steps stood between a doctor's decision to order a medication for a hospitalized patient and the actual delivery of that medication to the patient. That's a lot of places where things can go wrong, and even if they each go right 99 percent of the time, the chance that one error will occur in a fifty-step process works out to a stunning 39 percent of the time.

In fact, although errors at the ordering end can certainly harm and kill patients (witness Ramon Vasquez and Betsy Lehman), these mistakes are often *less* treacherous because there are still opportunities to catch and correct them further down the line. But as the drug nears the dispensing and administration stages—that is, the closer it gets to the patient—the chances of trapping a particular error fall precipitously.

The Sandra Geller case illustrates this slow march to the gallows in inexorable, painful detail. The case virtually writes its own headline: NURSE KILLS PATIENT BY ADMINISTERING OVERDOSE OF INSULIN—the first story of the tragedy is complete.

The second story, however, begins and ends quite differently. Like hundreds of thousands of medical errors each year, this story simply cannot be written without understanding the difference between "slips" and "mistakes."

Psychologists have long recognized the difference between *conscious* behavior and *automatic* behavior. Conscious behavior is what we do when we "pay attention" to a task, and it's especially important when we're doing something new, like learning to play the piano or program our DVD. Kids are especially good at many conscious behaviors because virtually everything they do is new; for them, "paying attention" may be tough, but it's a familiar mode of thought. (That's why they seem to catch on to computers and DVD players so quickly while it takes their parents hours of frustration.) The point is, conscious behavior—paying close attention to what we are doing—is a lot of work for anyone, which is one reason we instinctively try to quickly switch over to the alternative: automatic behavior.

Automatic behaviors are the things we do almost uncon- sciously—they may have required a lot of thought originally, but after a while we do them virtually "in our sleep." We humans prefer automatic behaviors because they take less energy, have a predictable outcome, and allow us to "multi-task"—do other things at the same time. Some of these other tasks are automatic behaviors themselves—like driving a car while drinking coffee—but some require conscious thought as well, and that's where we run into trouble, where the distinction between "slips" and "mistakes" rears its ugly head.

Slips are inadvertent, unconscious lapses in the performance of some automatic task. You set out on Saturday to buy groceries from a market you pass every day on your way to work, but drive past it because your automatic behavior—driving to work five days out of seven—kicks in and dictates your actions. Slips like this sound innocent enough—and they usually are—because we usually "snap out of it" to expose the error. Slips happen most often when we put an activity on "autopilot" so we can deal with new sensory inputs, think through a problem, or deal with emotional upset, fatigue, or stress. If this last problem sounds familiar, it should. It's the environment of most high-pressure jobs, including those performed by doctors and nurses in hospitals.

Mistakes, on the other hand, result from incorrect choices. Rather than blundering into them while our mind is someplace else, they usually result from insufficient knowledge, lack of experience or training, insufficient information (or inability to interpret available information properly), or applying the wrong criteria to a decision. If this also sounds like the medical environment, you're right—and mistakes like these can befall beginners and veterans alike.

If we measure safety on an "errors per action" yardstick, conscious behaviors are more prone to mistakes than automatic behaviors are prone to slips. Think about that for a minute. You are far more likely to make a mistake (an incorrect choice) when driving to a new supermarket than you are to inadvertently drive past a familiar market—although both types of errors can happen. But in health care, oddly enough, real mistakes—errors in conscious choices—present a far lesser threat than slips, or inadvertent lapses in familiar behaviors. How can this be?

The answer lies in the relative frequency of conscious versus automatic behaviors. Like most people, you probably drive to work and other familiar places (the supermarket, the dry cleaner, etc.) dozens, if not hundreds, of times for each time you drive to a new location—such as visiting a new acquaintance in an unfamiliar suburb. Consequently, you apply plenty of cognitive reasoning—conscious behavior—to finding that new friend's house; partly because you know you might get lost, and partly because you know you can't trust your usual driving instincts. Automatic behaviors, on the other hand, are so common that we can count on committing many slips during the course of a week, a month, or a year. Over time, those slips can be more than an annoyance: They can put you—and our patients—in real danger.

Thus while most people associate medical errors with untrained, inexperienced, or incompetent caregivers, most of our errors are made by well-trained, experienced, and competent caregivers who perform their tasks *so* well that they have become almost second nature. Doctors and nurses are most likely to slip doing something they have done correctly a thousand times—asking patients if they are allergic to any medications before writing a prescription, for example, or remembering to verify a patient's identity before sending them off to a procedure, or loading a syringe with heparin, and not insulin, before flushing an IV line, or (as we'll discuss later) verifying their blood type before performing a hugely complex transplant procedure.

The big implication of this is that some of the most routine health care tasks paradoxically carry the biggest risk to patients—more, even, than certain exotic procedures. Like pilots, soldiers, and others trained to work in high-risk occupations, doctors and nurses are programmed to do specific tasks, under pressure, with a high degree of accuracy. But unlike many other professions, medical jobs typically combine three very different types of "tasks": lots of conscious behaviors (complex decisions, judgment calls), lots of "customer" interactions, and innumerable automatic behaviors. Our training has traditionally emphasized the decision making, highly cognitive aspects (essentially all of medical school), focused a bit on the human interactions (getting a bit better but still not our strong suit), and completely ignored automatic behaviors. Sadly, neither of the authors of this book can remember a *single* discussion during our own long and arduous medical training that dealt with medical slips and how to prevent them.

How, then, should we respond to the inevitability of slips? Our typical response would be to reprimand (if not fire) a nurse for confusing two otherwise identical-looking vials—one of heparin, the other of insulin—and command her to "look more carefully next time!" Even if she did, she is just as likely to commit a different error while automatically carrying out a different task in a different setting. As James Reason reminds us, "Errors are largely unintentional. It is very difficult for management to control what people did not intend to do in the first place."

Part of the problem is in how practitioners themselves respond to slips after they happen. When we make a slip—a stupid error in something that we usually do perfectly "in our sleep"—we feel embarrassed. We chastise ourselves harder than any supervisor could, and swear we'll never slip like that again. Realistically, though, such promises are almost impossible to keep. Before you know it, one day you forget to check if the top of the salad dressing is screwed on tightly enough, and end up with vinaigrette all over the table... again!

So, if just paying more attention to things is not the answer to preventing slips, what is?

Part of the solution may lie in technology, not all of it computerized or high-tech. Like the "childproof" caps on prescriptions, a few simple mechanical precautions can give an otherwise competent and well-trained practitioner that instantaneous second chance to interrupt an automatic behavior and avoid a deadly error.

For example, in trying to prevent cases like the heparin-insulin mix-up, it seems obvious that a medication administration protocol that includes a mandatory label check could make an enormous difference. You'd think caregivers would do this anyway, but recall the bedside environment: The same vials have been side-by-side for days with no mix-up and, most likely, the administering caregivers were quite conscious of the process when it began, taking care to identify the 'right vial. But gradually, human nature—and its built-in autopilot function—kicks in and we end up relying on past success and rote behavior patterns, such as, "I always leave the heparin on the right, nearest the window, so that's the vial I use to flush the line." In such automatic behaviors, it never occurs to us that someone—even the patient looking for a magazine or hairbrush—might reposition the vials.

In any case, the most effective and foolproof system would be one that physically prevents the administration of one drug when another drug is intended—the way square pegs can't fit into round holes. This strategy, called a *forcing function*, has its roots in human factors engineering and has been used for decades to design cockpit controls. The technique is also used in automobiles. After scores of children were run over by cars lurching backward when sleepy or distracted drivers threw the gears into reverse, designers simply reworked the controls so that the car won't go into reverse without one foot on the brake. In medicine, surgical deaths due to "wrong gas" anesthetics were virtually eliminated by simply redesigning the nozzles that connected different gas canisters to the mask—the same way you can't fill a car designed for unleaded fuel with old-fashioned leaded gasoline: the nozzles for one are simply incompatible with the receptacles of the other.

One notch down on the complexity scale—but equally important to any campaign to prevent harm from slips—are passive protection systems. These don't require action from anyone, and their very presence keeps people from doing harm. In cars, these systems include roll bars and air bags. Detroit toyed with passive seat belts for several years, but the resulting models—complete with electric ceiling tracks for chest straps—were so unappealing they were dropped. Even worse, some drivers (who still had to snap the lap belt in a conventional way to be safe) relied on the chest strap alone and sustained serious injuries when they "submarined" under the strap in collisions, demonstrating once again how real people will undermine safety systems if they are too unwieldy or inefficient. (Another vexing example, which one researcher dubbed the "revenge effect," is that some safer systems seem to actually promote unsafe behaviors, as when we drive faster because we're confident that our air bags and roll bars will protect us.)

So passive systems have their limits, and active safety devices must sometimes come to the rescue. In driving, seat belts were eventually mandated by law and given economic encouragement—such as discounted insurance premiums for safe drivers. Today, in some regions, allowing kids to ride unbelted, aside from being illegal, carries the same social stigma as driving drunk, so peer pressure and culture play a role as well.

One lesson from all of this goof-proofing is that boring, repetitive tasks can be dangerous and are often performed better by machines. In medicine, these tasks include monitoring a patient's oxygen level during a tedious operation, suturing large wounds, holding surgical retractors steady for a long time, and scanning mountains of data for significant patterns. Anesthesiologist Alan Merry and legal scholar Alexander McCall Smith note that

> ... people have no need to apologize for their failure to achieve machine-like standards in those activities for which machines are better suited. They are good at other things—original thought, for one, empathy and compassion for another.... It is true that people

are distractible—but in fact this provides a major survival advantage for them. A machine (unless expressly designed to detect such an event) will continue with its repetitive task while the house burns down around it, whereas most humans will notice that something unexpected is going on and will change their activity...

A trip to your local supermarket demonstrates how modern industries—especially retail chains—have harnessed technology to ensure that boring, repetitive tasks get accomplished with minimum errors. Since your local Safeway or Wal-Mart uses bar-coding to charge you the correct price for milk or toaster ovens, it would seem to be a no-brainer for hospitals to use this technology to reduce the chance of medication mistakes. And if they can bar-code medications, why not patients' bracelets—requiring a match before administering a drug or wheeling you off for that cardiac electrophysiology study?

As of this writing, less than 2 percent of U.S. hospitals have bar-coding systems. This is partly a chicken-and-egg problem. Few hospitals want to be first on the dance floor. They may be willing to make the investment, but only after pharmacies, drug makers, and blood banks make the switch. Conversely, manufacturers and dispensers want to see hospitals install scanners before they retool their labeling systems. This situation, like many others in health care, shows why we can't always rely on the market to solve our safety problems; and where marketers and administrators fear to tread, regulators must eventually lead the way. In March 2003, FDA commissioner Dr. Mark McClellan announced that his agency will soon require pharmaceutical companies to bar-code all medications. Hopefully, this will encourage their institutional customers to follow suit. Will such federally mandated systems work?

One of the few studies examining the impact of bar-coding on medication errors (as opposed to improving inventory management,

Wal-Mart style) found that routine patient ID scanning was circumvented easily and often by busy nurses who could manually override the system. A more recent study of bar-coding in VA hospitals showed that the system itself, while generally helpful, created new errors, including one instance in which the system did not detect a discrepancy between the intended and actual patient. In our view, though, it's probably just a matter of time until bar-coding (along with CPOE) becomes an accepted part of the medical landscape and, as with cell phones and e-mail, we'll all wonder how we ever got along without it.

While we wait for that glorious day, however, there are other things we can do to reduce less visible medication mix-ups.

For one, we can prohibit storing look-alike vials in the same physical space—particularly those close to the site of administration, such as a patient's bedside. It's also a simple, sensible precaution to require potentially lethal medications to be returned to a secure storage area after each administration—although busy caregivers will squawk about that and, in too many cases, "forget" to do it.

That's what happened in the ICU where the Geller heparin-insulin swap occurred. Protocols like these are developed in the bracing, authoritative air of the hospital administration's conference room, only to be routinely violated by the staff. This is not a minor problem—or even one that can be corrected by disciplinary measures, fines, threats, and "brown bag" seminars at lunchtime. Sharp-end workers in most industries become very adept at working around rules they perceive to be superfluous or counterproductive. These "routine rule violations" seem irritating and dangerous to safety-conscious managers—and they are—but they are also a bit of real-world data no manager or administrator can afford to ignore: a gift of valuable feedback about how caregivers *really* think and operate. As such, they are the raw material for making apparent safety fixes more real and reliable.

A classic example of a routine rule violation is what happened after hospitals began forbidding the storage of concentrated potassium on medical wards. Potassium is a vital body mineral that is depleted by such illnesses as prolonged diarrhea, or by powerful diuretics like Lasix. Because of this, many intravenous solutions contain (in addition to a salt, or saline, mixture) a few vials of potassium chloride (KCL). In the old days, nurses kept these vials in cabinets on their wards, which gave them the ability to add potassium to IV solutions at will if morning lab studies showed that a particular patient had developed hypokalemia, or low potassium. But a few high-profile accidental potassium overdoses convinced administrators and regulators that concentrated KCL should not be stored on the hospital floors. (Concentrated potassium, after all, is the agent of death in capital punishment—a big injection short-circuits the heart—so keeping it lying around does seem like asking for trouble.) Instead, the new plan was that nurses would order their IV solutions from the pharmacy, where trained specialists, working with fewer distractions and more fail-safe systems for mixing meds, would add the potassium before the bag itself went to the ward. The only exception would be the ICU, which needs to keep concentrated potassium handy for emergencies.

Sounds sensible enough, right? Problem fixed? Well, not exactly.

In some hospitals, ward nurses soon discovered that they could not get their potassium solutions from the pharmacy quickly enough to meet their patients' needs. Some began surreptitiously hoarding concentrated KCL in cubbyholes, coat closets, or in the ward's refrigerator behind yesterday's half-eaten yogurt. In response, house pharmacists began "raiding" the wards like DEA agents; and ICUs, exempt from the prohibition, became de facto satellite pharmacies, informally dispensing KCL to nurses on other floors. All these hospitals needed was Al Capone, and the miniature drama of bootleggers and speakeasies would be complete.

The take-home lesson for rule-makers here was not to give up and allow everyone but candy-stripers to dispense potentially deadly medications, but that even well-intended, commonsense rules can backfire—and in ways nobody expected. As Dr. Richard Cook (who, with Professor David Woods, conceived the "first story"/ "second story" model we've used throughout the book) observed, the concentrated KCL story is a cautionary tale to all those who think "advancing safety is a straightforward matter of removing hazards and forestalling human error." It's not, and it never will be.

Whatever we do about exposing and controlling the hidden side of medication errors, it had better be soon. Dr. Don Berwick, the Boston pediatrician who has emerged as the nation's most passionate spokesmen for health care quality, speaks eloquently of his wife Ann's harrowing string of hospitalizations for an obscure, progressive neurological illness. Berwick took her to some of America's greatest teaching hospitals, where, as the wife of a famous physician and patient safety advocate, she was greeted as a super VIP. You can be sure that everybody treating Ann felt they were under a microscope. There could be no more fitting close to this chapter than Berwick's account of his wife's harrowing hospitalizations:

> The errors were not rare; they were the norm. During one admission, the neurologist told us in the morning, "By no means should you be getting anticholinergic agents [a medication that can cause neurological and muscle changes]," and a medication with profound anticholinergic side effects was given that afternoon. The attending neurologist in another admission told us by phone that a crucial and potentially toxic drug should be started immediately. He said, "Time is of the essence." That was on Thursday morning at 10:00 A.M. The first dose was given 60 hours later—Saturday night at 10:00 P.M. Nothing I could do, nothing I did, nothing I could think of made any difference. It nearly drove me mad. Colace [a stool softener] was

discontinued by a physician's order on Day 1, and was nonetheless brought by the nurse every single evening throughout a 14-day admission. Ann was supposed to receive five intravenous doses of a very toxic chemotherapy agent, but dose #3 was labeled as "dose #2." For half a day, no record could be found that dose #2 had ever been given, even though I had watched it drip in myself. I tell you from my personal observation, no day passed—not one—without a medication error.

CHAPTER 6: SOLVING THE RIDDLE

Half this game is 90 percent mental.

— Yogi Berra

Annie Jackson, a grandmotherly African-American woman whose throaty alto was the envy of her church choir, coped comfortably, despite her multiple ills. Pills controlled her mild diabetes, high blood pressure, and elevated cholesterol. She quit smoking, saw her doctor regularly, and went for brisk walks in her leafy neighborhood a few days each week.

But just after dinner one evening, she sat in her favorite, overstuffed chair in front of the TV with a decidedly unpleasant feeling. She wasn't in pain, exactly—she just felt uncomfortable somewhere deep inside her chest. After a while, the discomfort settled under her left breast. The thought of a heart attack flitted briefly across her mind, but she discounted it. She'd always heard that heart attack pain radiated down one arm or up into the jaw, and her discomfort was staying put; and so did she.

After a half-hour or so, she took an antacid, but the unpleasant sensation remained, along with some nausea and a little shortness of breath—as if she'd just climbed a flight of stairs. Later that evening, after the eleven-o'clock news began and the symptoms hadn't gone away, she phoned her nearby daughter, who arrived a few minutes later.

"You don't look so good, Ma," her daughter said, regarding her cautiously. She felt her mother's clammy forehead with the back of her hand, the way she herself had been "diagnosed" countless times by that same good-natured woman as she grew up. "We need to go to the hospital."

Annie brushed her hair, and put on a fresh blouse. She had been raised to respect professional people, and wanted to make a good impression on the doctors.

"Ma—come on!" her daughter called, standing by the open front door. "We gotta go *now*!"

They got in the car and arrived at the ER a few minutes after midnight. Annie caught a few minutes of Jay Leno on the waiting room TV while her daughter talked to the triage nurse.

When people think of ERs, they imagine doctors and nurses converging like locusts on a bleeding car wreck or gunshot victim. Of course, that happens—particularly in big city trauma centers— but it's more typical of TV shows than of hospitals. In reality, what keeps most ER doctors tossing and turning in their sleep are patients who enter with chest pain—the most common cause of ER-related malpractice suits. The reason for this is simple. Most people with chest pain aren't having heart attacks; but those who are (or might be) need immediate attention. Sorting out the gastritis and reflux and gallbladder cases—not to mention the good, old-fashioned anxiety attacks—from the true heart attacks (known in medicine as myocardial infarctions, or MIs), is where ER physicians really earn—and keep—their pay.

This winnowing process begins with the electrocardiogram, or EKG. Sometimes the EKG alone is sufficient for a complete diagnosis—the characteristic shape of the waves on a strip of paper telling the whole story of a heart muscle starving for blood. These clear-cut MI patients are whisked immediately to the cardiac catheterization lab for angioplasty, or given clot-busting drugs, in an effort to open blocked coronary arteries and forestall additional damage to the heart. At other times, the EKG is stone-cold normal. This markedly lowers the chance that a patient is having a big MI, and usually leads us to bark up other diagnostic trees. In really tough cases, the EKG looks a bit suspicious—the ER doctor regards it the way police in a patrol car notice a broken window or open door late at night in a quiet neighborhood. Alarm bells may not go off, but it pays to take a closer look.

That's how it was for Annie Jackson when they saw her EKG.

Kent Bennett, the ER physician that night, studied the EKG and was underwhelmed. It was not a normal tracing, but it lacked the big ST-segment elevation pattern characteristic of an acute MI—a shape mordantly referred to as "the tombstone" by doctors. Besides, he had examined patients with chest pains all day ("Looks like the bus from the Chest Pain Hotel has arrived again," the staff joked) and he had admitted one definite MI patient and a few others for further tests, so the CCU, or cardiac care unit (the heart patients' equivalent to the ICU) was already packed. Other than a mildly fast heart rate— which could've been due to anxiety—Annie Jackson's vital signs were fine. Her lungs showed no evidence of fluid buildup, which can indicate poor cardiac pumping action. But when he pressed on Annie's chest, right where the ribs meet the breastbone, she winced. *Aha!* Dr. Bennett thought, *she has costochondritis!*—inflammation of the joint.

Relieved that he wasn't faced with another MI, he began formulating a tentative treatment plan: Take some Advil, climb into bed, and stay there until the inflammation subsides—probably no more than a couple of days. Still, Annie was over sixty and had several risk factors for coronary artery disease. So just to be safe, Dr. Bennett ordered a blood test for troponin—a protein that leaks out from damaged heart cells—and asked her to stick around for the results. An hour or so later, the result came back at 1.1—not quite normal, which would be less than 0.5, but not in the diagnostic range for an MI: 1.4 or higher; and certainly not the stratospheric 20 or 30 commonly seen with a big-league heart attack. Because the troponin test was relatively new—having recently supplanted the old MI blood test, creatine kinase—and its results were sometimes mildly elevated in patients without heart damage, the lab helpfully attached a bit of advice to its reports: "Troponin levels of 0.6 –1.3 are not specific for myocardial infarction." This reassured Dr. Bennett even more.

It was now 2:30 A.M. Bennett went into the waiting room. His green scrubs and authoritative air brought everyone in the crowded little room to attention. He called out, "Ann Jackson?" and Annie's sister, who had relieved Annie's daughter during the vigil, raised her hand.

"Good news," he said, giving her a weary smile. "Your sister's pain is from inflammation in the chest wall—it's nothing to worry about." He went on to explain that both the EKG and blood tests were "negative" and she would be fine with some anti-inflammatory pain medicine and bed rest.

Annie's sister sighed and sank back on her heels in relief. Together, they went to the examining room, helped Annie dress and collect her things, then walked slowly and deliberately to the car. During the drive, Annie kept pressing her chest, and after the short climb up the three steps to her front door, appeared to be a little winded.

"Do you want me to stay the night?" her sister asked.

"No, no," Annie waved her away. "I'll be fine."

The next morning, Annie didn't feel fine. She shuffled slowly into the bathroom to take her Advil but didn't make it to the medicine cabinet. Her sister found her later that day, curled up on the fuzzy bathroom rug. The expression on her face—pained and puzzled—was probably the last image she saw in life, reflected in the mirror over the sink.

We can only guess which cognitive error caused Dr. Bennett to release Annie Jackson from the ER. Perhaps because she was a black woman, he underestimated her chance of having a heart attack. He almost certainly relied too heavily on chest wall tenderness for his diagnosis—it's unusual, but not unheard of, in MI patients. He also overemphasized the lack of clear evidence on the EKG and in the cardiac enzyme test. Although they were "nonspecific," they were both clearly abnormal, and thus justified admission, no matter how crowded the CCU. Maybe he was just exhausted from a long day at a difficult job, or had just had an argument with his teenage daughter—heavy rocks that can leave ripples in anyone's psychic pond.

This particular error—sending patients home with heart attacks—is distressingly common and frequently lethal. Nearly one in twenty-five patients with MIs—about twelve thousand people each year in the U.S.—are mistakenly sent home. These turn-aways have a much higher death rate than MI victims who are correctly diagnosed and hospitalized. So, beginning in the 1970s, several physician researchers, led by UCSF's Lee Goldman and Harvard's Tom Lee, set out to understand how these mistakes are made and how they might be prevented.

The first thing they concluded was that many errors were related to patient demographics. Physicians were more likely to send patients home, despite worrisome histories or abnormal data, if the patients were in groups traditionally believed to be at lower risk for MI, such as women and those under age fifty-five. Nonwhites were also sent home in error more often, raising the question of racial bias, conscious or unconscious, among caregivers.

To further explore this latter possibility, one innovative researcher showed physicians videotapes of actors playing patients with chest pain that could have been heart-related. Four actors appeared on each video: a white man, a white woman, a black man, and a black woman. Each spoke from the same script—relayed exactly the same symptoms in exactly the same way. Seven-hundred twenty physicians randomly viewed one of the four versions, then answered a set of questions about what he or she would do with the patient. By a big majority, regardless of their own background, the physicians were far more likely to recommend cardiac catheterization for the white male than for the black female. This is terribly troubling, and major efforts to tackle the problem—known as "racial disparity"—are under way in medicine.

Of course, patients aren't the only variables in a diagnosis—the human being at the other end of the stethoscope counts, too. One study at three university hospitals showed that senior physicians were significantly more likely to correctly hospitalize chest pain patients—those having real heart attacks—than younger residents; a reassuring fact for those of us with graying temples. Did that mean that the graybeards were better diagnosticians than the wunderkinds? Well, perhaps not: The older docs were also more likely to hospitalize patients *without* heart attacks. With experience came risk aversion: The seasoned clinicians seemed to have developed an "admit 'em all and sort it out upstairs" mentality. Perhaps they had been burned once or twice in their careers.

Of course, age has no monopoly on risk aversion, or risk tolerance. Goldman and his colleagues analyzed the chest-pain triage decisions of 119 physicians. These same physicians then completed a questionnaire assessing their attitudes toward risk. A "risk seeking" physician, according to the study, was one who enjoys adventure and is unconcerned with danger—the sky-diving, Alfa-Romeo-driving, black-diamond-skier types. "Risk avoiders," on the other hand, were cautious, hesitant, and security-minded—the kind of people who pack the parachutes, drive Volvos, and enjoy skiing only when watching it every four years in the Olympics. Perhaps unsurprisingly, doctors who scored as risk seekers were four times more likely to send the same chest-pain patient home than the risk avoiders. The study couldn't tell whether risk takers sent home patients who should have been admitted or if risk avoiders admitted too many people who belonged at home—but each group most likely did some of each. The point is, your ER doctor's risk tolerance may have a lot to do with the way you are treated. So you might ask your next ER doctor if he likes to hang glide, particularly if he's a bit wet behind the ears.

One man who knew all about risk was Amos Tversky, a psychologist and decision theorist whose real-life experience, as well as his formal theories, have a profound effect on our understanding of medical errors.

Tversky was born in Haifa, Israel, on March 16, 1937. His father,

Yosef, was a veterinarian; his mother, Genia, a legislator who served in the Israeli Parliament from its founding in 1948 until her death in 1964. Although Tversky went on to pioneer the science of rational decision making under uncertainty—the condition faced by most medical diagnosticians—the crowning achievement of his youth was based on pure instinct. As a nineteen-year-old lieutenant in the Israeli Army, he watched one of his men freeze in terror after planting a timed explosive under a barbed wire fence. Without thinking, Amos ran to the soldier, picked him up, and threw him to safety, severely wounding himself in the process.

A military hero, Tversky immigrated to the United States in the 1960s and later joined the faculty at Stanford University. Decades later, after Tversky received an endowed professorship at Stanford, he returned to Israel to celebrate the honor with his family. His mother met him on the tarmac. "Amos!" she cried, glancing down as he bolted from the stairway, arms open to embrace her. "Blue socks, brown shoes! What *were* you thinking?"

Tversky's mind, it turned out, was busy figuring out how people make decisions in situations clouded by ambiguity. Through a series of insightful experiments, many reported with an impish humor that added sparkle to the driest concept, Tversky demonstrated that our limited cognitive capacity forces human beings to simplify things—and in simplifying them, distort them to match a preferred way of thinking. Like his fellow psychologist James Reason, Tversky spent most of his career studying nearly everything *but* medicine. Yet his insights are crucial to understanding how doctors think, and how they err.

For example, Tversky proved that, after observing a long run of red in roulette, most people mistakenly expect the next spin of the wheel to come up black—the "gambler's fallacy." In truth, each spin of the wheel, roll of the dice, or flip of the coin contains within itself exactly the same odds as any other; there is no self-correcting process that counteracts random chance. Similarly, Tversky found that people tend to feel worse about losing a given sum of money than they feel good when winning the same amount. These feelings make them risk averse when it comes to gambling for gain, but risk seeking when trying to minimize their potential losses. To illustrate: People prefer a guaranteed gain of $40 over a 50–50 chance of winning $100—an "irrational choice," since the average expected gain in the 50–50 bet is $50. Similarly, faced with a choice between a guaranteed loss of $40 and the prospect of losing $100—or owing nothing—based on the flip of a coin, most people prefer to toss the coin, although this choice, too, is irrational.

When the loss has already occurred, Tversky found, we tend to take risks to recoup it that we would otherwise avoid, since breaking even, at that point, feels like victory. This is one reason golfers feel better shooting a birdie (one stroke below par) after shooting a bogie (one stroke over par) than they do after shooting two pars in a row, even though the score is the same. It also explains why long shots are most popular at racetracks in the last race of the day: You can't lose any more money if there are no more races to bet on, so you might as well go for broke.

"Illusions, not delusions," Tversky wrote, explaining our penchant for irrationality. Rather than weighing the odds of a particular outcome when we choose among uncertain options, we are unduly biased by the way the problem is presented: the so-called framing effect. We guess how a given outcome might change the status quo (most people don't like change) and compare the situation to others we've experienced—usually the most recent—in which the outcome is known: the "availability effect." Subliminally, our minds mix all of this together to invent personal or professional rules-of-thumb to rely on when the available facts don't support an obvious decision. Like carpenters without a tape measure, we base our decisions on past experience, whether that experience fits the facts or not.

This behavior, although irrational, is eminently practical. If we didn't make mental models—even faulty ones—to aid us in making fuzzy decisions, we might make no decisions at all. We would carry umbrellas only when it was actually raining. We would invest money only at the top of the market. As doctors, we would administer treatment only when the patient was either dead or already on the mend. As Tversky himself admitted, "Even after studying rationality for years, I still overeat at buffet restaurants."

The problem is we get so used to cloaking our irrational decisions in the guise of wisdom and experience, we confuse good luck with good judgment, and that's where diagnostic errors often begin.

Tversky's interest in medicine, late in his career, was a natural outgrowth of his investigations into human decisions. To one of his disciples, Dr. Donald Redelmeier, now at the University of Toronto, his opinions about clinical reasoning were as insightful as his conclusions about other forms of psychology. "Decisions about war are infrequent and are usually made by committees," Redelmeier—a quirky, iconoclastic, and brilliant thinker himself—once said. "Psychology experiments using college student volunteers are easy but trivial. In medicine, the stakes are high and the outcomes may be irreparable. So Amos had a field day thinking about the role of individual judgment and decision-making in health care."

Beginning in 1990, Tversky and Redelmeier set out to prove physicians weren't immune from cognitive biases and irrational decision making. For example, they found that framing a clinical decision as being about an individual patient versus a group of the same patients led to different results. A problem described as "a young woman has a fever that is not getting better" generates far different responses than when the problem becomes "consider young women with fever..." And, notwithstanding the centuries-old belief—shared by patients and doctors—that arthritis is influenced by weather, they compared a year's worth of patient "pain scores" with daily weather reports and found that no such correlation existed. Instead, people "look for changes in the weather when they experience increased pain, and pay little attention to the weather when their pain is stable...." They concluded that, "People's beliefs about arthritis pain and the weather may tell more about the workings of the mind than of the body."

Much of the training physicians and other scientists receive in epidemiology and statistics is designed to teach us how to correctly interpret limited observations without being misled by all of these biases. For doctors, the training recognizes that we make scores of decisions each day based on inadequate information. We can't "stop the clock" and perform a controlled experiment to find the right answer, especially when we have a sick patient staring at us, his illness demanding a decision.

One important part of this training is learning to guard against overconfidence—to recognize when intuition and rules-of-thumb may be leading us down blind alleys instead of upward toward the light. But this caution and introspection doesn't come naturally to physicians. We are admitted to medical schools partly because of our self-confidence (or ability to fake it convincingly during interviews) and society places us on a pedestal, in part, because of it. And our confident bearing is reinforced over time: It's easier for patients to trust someone who appears self-assured than someone who is always equivocating and lamenting his uncertainty. We share the struggle of trying to calibrate our confidence with other high-trust, highly uncertain professionals, from economists and investment advisers to demographers and particle physicists. We're all spring-loaded to the confident position; partly because we rely so heavily on our homegrown rules-of-thumb—remembering when they worked and forgetting when they failed—and partly because our professions reward those who can appear certain in a most uncertain world.

Some argue that overconfidence, like optimism, is an adaptive behavior that advances the human race. They may be right. Confidence feels good and empowers people to do things they might never try if they knew the true odds against success. But Tversky reminds us that this warm feeling comes at a high price—like the hot fudge sundae that feels so natural after a big prime rib dinner. "Overconfidence in the diagnosis of a patient, the outcome of a trial, or the projected interest rate could lead to inappropriate medical treatment, bad legal advice, and regrettable financial investments," Tversky wrote. "It can be argued that people's willingness to engage in military, legal, and other costly battles would be reduced if they had a more realistic assessment of their chances of success."

So Tversky and Redelmeier taught us that, as doctors—even well trained doctors—our thinking could be faulty because our brains are programmed to take cognitive shortcuts, reinforced by a professional culture that rewards the appearance of certainty over its reality. Both men realized that to improve the quality of medical decisions, we needed to develop strategies to promote more rational, less intuitive decision making. And to do *that*, we first had to gain a deeper understanding of how great diagnosticians really think.

The media worships dynamic, innovative surgeons like heart transplant pioneers Michael DeBakey and Christiaan Barnard; and passionate, insightful researchers like Jonas Salk and Linus Pauling. But we seldom hear about those doctors whom other physicians tend to hold in highest esteem: the great medical diagnosticians.

These sages, like the legendary Johns Hopkins professors William Osler and A. McGhee Harvey, had the uncanny ability to deduce the truth from what others found to be a jumble of symptoms, signs, and lab results. In fact, Sir Arthur Conan Doyle, a physician by training, confessed he modeled Sherlock Holmes on one of his old professors, Dr. Joseph Bell, a renowned diagnostician at Edinburgh's medical school. For most doctors, diagnosis forms the essence of their practice—and of their professional souls. Yale physician Sherwin Nuland calls the elusive diagnosis "The Riddle" and, in *How We Die*, writes of it with almost religious reverence:

> I capitalize it so there will be no mistaking its dominance over every other consideration. The satisfaction of solving The Riddle is its own reward, and the fuel that drives the clinical engines of

medicine's most highly trained specialists. It is every doctor's measure of his own abilities; it is the most important ingredient in his professional self-image.

For much of the twentieth century, these diagnostic giants seemed to have magical, even mystical powers. In the 1970s, a Tufts kidney specialist named Jerome Kassirer (who would later become editor of the *New England Journal of Medicine*) decided to try to unlock their secrets. If he succeeded, the rewards could be great. The insights, problem-solving strategies, and patterns of reasoning of these medical geniuses might be teachable to other physicians, or even programmed into computers.

One reason this study held such promise is that doctors already learn a structured method to inventory their patients' possible problems, called *differential diagnosis*. Basically, this method treats patients' clinical problems as a tree, with roots and branches; or a flow chart, with intersections and connections. For example, if a female patient complains of "right lower abdominal pain and fever," we automatically begin to generate a differential diagnosis. The immediate possibilities are appendicitis, pelvic inflammatory disease, kidney infection, and a host of more obscure disorders—some quite serious. The physician's job is to follow each root symptom up the trunk and into the branches where—when the right combination of qualitative symptoms and quantitative evidence coincides—you are likely to find the diagnosis. Obviously, there is a systematic (if not mechanistic) aspect to this process, but the great diagnosticians seem to pursue such reasoning not just automatically, but like artists. They seem to know instinctively which sparkling bits of data add up to a meaningful constellation: the coherent picture of a disease, and—even more important—which seemingly important signs are diagnostic dead ends. Their special gift is sorting rainbows into black and white. But how do they do it?

Kassirer and his colleagues observed the diagnostic reasoning of dozens of clinicians. They found that the good ones naturally engaged in a process called *iterative hypothesis testing*. This means they heard the initial portion of a case, then began drawing possible scenarios to explain it, modifying their opinions as they went along and more information became available. For example, when the physician was presented with a mini-case such as, "This fifty-seven-year-old man has three days of chest pain, shortness of breath, and light-headedness," she responded by thinking, "The worst thing this could be is a heart attack or blood clot to the lungs. I need to ask a few more questions to see if the chest pain bores through to the back, which would make me worry about a rip in the aorta, or *aortic dissection* (the disease that killed actor John Ritter). I'll also ask about typical cardiac symptoms, such as sweating and nausea, and see if the pain is squeezing or radiates to the left arm or jaw. But even if it doesn't, I'll certainly get an EKG to be sure no cardiac event has occurred. If he also reports a fever or cough, I might begin to suspect pneumonia or pleurisy. The chest X-ray should help sort that out."

Every answer the patient gives, and each positive or negative finding on the physical examination ("yes, there is a heart murmur; no, the liver is not enlarged") triggers an automatic, almost intuitive recalibration of most-likely alternatives. Such possibilities are written in sand, of course, but good diagnosticians know when to let the wind blow, wiping some alternatives away, and which to shelter for further study.

We recall seeing master diagnosticians—such as UCSF's Lawrence Tierney and Harvard's Marshall Wolf—plying their craft during our training years. We were awed and mystified and knew that, although these experts were performing "iterative hypothesis testing," something more extraordinary was probably happening. Information we thought crucial, they sometimes discarded with a shrug or shake of the head. Other nuggets—useless to us, but gold to them—were snatched up and held out before us as glistening clues that solved the case. What the hell was going on?

We now recognize that much of their art consisted of applying an unconscious, intuitive version of Bayes' theorem, developed by the eighteenth-century British theologian-turned-mathematician, Thomas Bayes. This theorem—often ignored by medical students because it is taught to them with the dryness of a saltine cracker—is really the Rosetta Stone of clinical reasoning, and thus the Holy Grail for avoiding diagnostic mistakes.

In essence, Bayes' theorem says that any medical test must be interpreted from two perspectives. The first: How accurate is the test—that is, how often does it give right or wrong answers? The second: How likely is it that this patient has the disease the test is looking for?

These deceptively simple questions turn out to have enormous implications for both individual and community health. They explain why, in the early days of the AIDS epidemic (when HIV testing was far less accurate than it is today), it was silly to HIV-test heterosexual couples applying for a marriage license, since the vast majority of positive tests would be wrong in this very-low-risk group. Similarly, they show why it is foolish to screen apparently healthy thirty-five-year-old executives with a cardiac treadmill test (or, for that matter, a "heart scan"), since positive results will mostly be false positives, serving only to scare the bejesus out of the patients and run up bills for unnecessary follow-up tests. Conversely, a sixty-five-year-old smoker with high cholesterol who develops squeezing chest pain when shoveling snow has about a 95 percent chance that those pains are from coronary artery disease. In this case, a negative treadmill test only lowers this probability to about 80 percent, so the clinician who reassures the patient that his treadmill means his heart is fine—"take some antacids; it's OK to keep jogging"—is making a terrible, and potentially fatal, mistake.

Good doctors apply Bayesian reasoning every time they ask you a question, or give you a physical examination. Say you are a thirty-year-old woman who comes into the ER with severe back pain that has no obvious, traumatic origin. The doctor knows that the vast majority of back pains are caused by musculoskeletal injury—pulled muscles, strained ligaments and the like. These will get better on their own, although some analgesics, special exercises, or physical therapy might help. But lurking in this sea of ho-hum patients are a few with serious spinal infections, or even one or two with cancer that has metastasized to the back. Some might even have slipped disks that are compressing nerves, and this type of compression can lead to permanent spinal damage unless it is promptly relieved. Still others may have abdominal problems, such as pancreatitis or a kidney infection, that can manifest themselves in the back.

If you could read your doctor's mind during the examination, this is the sort of thing he or she is thinking. You'd have to be a mind reader, because good physicians say nothing until they pretty much know what they're talking about—to do otherwise would be pointless and inhumane. It's one reason the famed physician Sir William Osler said, "A patient has no more right to all the facts in my head than he does to all the medications in my bag."

Thus, your doctor asks you to describe the pain in your own words. You say, "Well, the pain began a couple of days ago—gradually at first, but now it hurts like hell. It's in my lower back, but it sometimes shoots a bit down my right leg."

The iterative hypothesis testing ratchets up a notch. The presence of sciatica now gives your doctor cause to worry about nerve compression, which could still be nothing serious, but might also indicate a bulging disk, a tumor, or a blossoming infection. "Tell me," she says, poker-faced, "have you had any fever? Weight loss? Night sweats?" All could indicate infection; the second might suggest a tumor.

You answer, "Oh, I guess I lost maybe five pounds over the last few months. I'm not on a diet or anything, but I was happy to see it go."

Now your doctor is concerned about cancer. This doesn't mean she *thinks* you have cancer, only that the chance your back pain may be related to cancer has risen above a certain probability. Actually, that probability is quite low—in the range of 2–3 percent. But if you have a 2–3 percent chance of a deadly tornado in the area, the weather forecaster is going to keep an eye on those conditions. "OK," she says matter-of-factly, "let's do a couple of tests."

She goes to the charting room and tells a colleague, "The lady in room six just bought a spine MRI." Of course, she'll complete the exam by checking for leg weakness or reflex changes (how your knee jerks in response to that little rubber mallet) and if those signs are bad, you'll probably leapfrog over less worrisome cases and get your MRI sooner, rather than later. She may even order a conventional X-ray of your back; but in Bayesian terms, your chance of a tumor is now high enough that even negative results on these older, less accurate images are incapable of being sufficiently reassuring.

Keep in mind, though, that even in these circumstances, your "health glass" is still 97 percent full—that's the statistical chance that you *don't* have cancer; but only an MRI will erase 2.999 of that remaining 3 percent.

This brings us back to Annie Jackson. One could easily look at cases like hers—errors in the diagnosis of chest pain—and see careless doctoring, a blown diagnosis, and a fatal mistake. But by now, you're thinking about the second story: How can we improve our ability to diagnose patients who come to the ER with a constellation of symptoms, findings, and risk factors that often yield ambiguous results but can be life-threatening? Too often, without a more systematic approach, the clinical decision—the diagnosis that either admits or discharges the patient—is based on the physician's faulty reasoning, which may be traced to poor training, inadequate experience, personal and professional bias, fuzzy thinking brought on by overwork and fatigue, or even the physician's own tolerance for risk.

As educators struggled to improve diagnosis by getting rank-and-file doctors to channel the Reverend Bayes, information technology (IT) experts saw a perfect example of a problem that would yield well to computerized solutions. By the end of the 1970s, the medical literature was gushing with enthusiastic articles about how microprocessors—programmed to think like experts—would replace the brains of harried human doctors for those tough diagnostic calls. As Harvard's Howard Bleich wrote in an ecstatic paean to his computer, "It is immune from fatigue and carelessness; and it works day and night, weekends and holidays, without coffee breaks, overtime, fringe benefits or human courtesy."

Such thinking was rife in that brave new age of supercomputers and desktop PCs. As long ago as 1957, Nobel laureate and economist Herbert Simon predicted that a chess-playing computer would defeat a human grandmaster within a decade. His assumption was that chess mastery was a simple matter of computational muscle. Although machines might not "think" like humans, they could arrive at the same results by making billions of calculations in a handful of seconds. In fact, it was not until forty years later, 1997, that a supercomputer—IBM's "Deep Blue," a 1.4-ton behemoth capable of pondering 200 million chess moves each second—was able to defeat the Russian grandmaster Garry Kasparov.

But Deep Blue didn't win just by "brute-forcing" a mind-numbing sequence of possible moves and countermoves—most of which would have been nonsensical. It differed from earlier, less successful models because it was taught to recognize *patterns*, not just moves, and analyze their implications and possibilities—the way Kasparov and other masters actually played chess. Like any other successful competitor, Big Blue won because it learned to see the situation as it was, not the way some theory predicted.

Doctors grappling with diagnoses have a tougher time. After all, there are *only* 85 billion possible chess openings—played through the first four moves; while the human body's response to illness—at the psychic, macroscopic, microscopic, and molecular levels—is virtually limitless. But the principles are the same. Although some of the best artificial intelligence (AI) medical programs approach the clinical accuracy of a good physician, none has the capacity to "roll with the punches"—handle unexpected or extraneous data—like an expert. All have a tendency to spew out lists of possible diagnoses that include a few surprising but plausible choices—plus a pile of unusable garbage. Efforts to create computerized substitutes for real physicians—like the wry-humored, digital, holographic doctor on *Star Trek*'s *Voyager*—have been put on hold, replaced by a more realistic goal of using computers to supplement, not supplant, the human diagnostic process. Even in the narrow area of chest pain diagnosis in the ER, where computerized decision making would seem to be ideal (and where some AI programs have demonstrated reasonable accuracy), the computerized solutions have been largely ignored.

Clearly, some of our reluctance to pledge our diagnostic allegiance to a microchip owes to the disappointing track record of most medical AI programs. But there is something deeper going on… and not just for doctors. Moments before a planeload of Russian schoolchildren collided with a DHL cargo jet over Switzerland in early 2002, the Russian pilot received conflicting orders from two sources: one human, the other a machine. The human was a befuddled Swiss air traffic controller whose backup collision alarm system was on the fritz and whose colleague was on a break. The machine was the collision-avoidance system, or CAS, aboard the doomed plane. When the human controller noticed an apparent collision course between the school kids and the cargo flight, he ordered the Russian airliner to "Dive!" The Russian's on-board CAS, on the other hand, detecting an obstacle hurtling toward it, instructed the pilot (in that distinctive, attention-getting, but less-than-confidence-inspiring computer voice), to "Pull up!" With only seconds to react, the pilot chose to obey the human voice, and the result was catastrophic.

"Pilots tend to listen to the air traffic controller because they trust a human being and know that a person wants to keep them safe," said an airport safety consultant soon after the heartbreaking crash. Physicians harbor the same mistrust when it comes to having their decisions guided—or overruled—by computers.

Despite the disappointing history of medical AI, we predict an explosion in computerized decision support that will really make a difference. In the next five to ten years, computers will routinely present your doctor with short lists of probable diagnoses, help her choose the right antibiotic to conquer the hospital's superbugs, and even handle your HMO's often-Byzantine insurance rules—in real time. Computers will also give your doctor bite-sized, easily digestible synopses of the latest research on your condition, targeted to your individual needs, including allergies and coexisting conditions. Given the explosive growth of medical knowledge over the last thirty years—the number of clinical trials published annually has grown from 100 to nearly 10,000—this is the kind of decision support most physicians really need, but rarely get.

All of this support will help us make more accurate diagnoses. But if the last twenty years has taught us anything, it is that while computers may help improve our diagnostic abilities, they are not the complete answer. (To paraphrase one informatics expert: Any doctor who could be replaced by a computer should be.) As far as the chest pain decision—the Tour de France of decision making under uncertainty—most doctors have concluded that the quest for diagnostic certainty is futile. Even the best algorithms could not reliably identify patients whose actual risk was so low that it was safe to send them home—especially when the penalty for even occasional failure can be a tragic death and a multimillion-dollar lawsuit. So the real progress in ER chest pain triage has come *not* from honing our diagnostic abilities, but rather from developing new ways to "rule out MI" inexpensively over a reasonably short (six to twelve hour) observational period. Usually, this involves repeated cardiac enzyme blood tests and a treadmill test prior to discharge from the ER. Before these techniques were employed, ruling out MI meant a three-day hospitalization costing many thousands of dollars. In essence, we have abandoned our quest for the perfect diagnostician—the ultimate "solver of riddles"—and accepted instead the more mundane task of managing our uncertainty more safely by resolving it quickly and inexpensively.

We now know a lot more about how clinicians think, what rules they apply when coming to their decisions, and how their thinking can go awry. Some give in to their instincts when a little more cogitation would serve them better. Some ignore Bayesian reasoning, or use it improperly. Some are simply too quick to pronounce judgment, then defend that turf too vigorously when contradictory evidence emerges.

This last shortcoming is a potent source of medical mistakes. We tend to see what we expect to see rather than than what's actually in front of our eyes. Did you notice the word "than" used twice in a row in the previous sentence? That's what we mean. Even when we don't intend to do it, our brains can take cognitive shortcuts to get us to our goal—whether it's finishing a sentence or discharging a marginal patient.

This problem was illustrated in the early 1970s in an elegant experiment by Stanford psychologist David Rosenhan. Rosenhan recruited two physicians, a housewife, a painter, a graduate student, and three psychologists to check themselves into various psychiatric hospitals under aliases, all claiming to hear voices inside their heads speaking words like "thud" and "empty." After admission, the phony patients were instructed to act in a perfectly normal manner, to answer all questions truthfully, and to tell hospital staff that the voices in their head were gone and they were feeling fine. Rosenhan's goal was to see how well the psychiatric staffs were able to revise their initial diagnoses once new and conflicting data arose. The results were terrifying—*One Flew Over the Cuckoo's Nest* meets the *Twilight Zone*.

The eight participants were hospitalized for an average of nineteen days. One was confined for almost two months. They were fed a total of 2,100 pills. Their normal activities were interpreted as psychopathology. One nurse wrote portentously in her observational log, "Patient engaging in writing behavior." He was probably writing to Dr. Rosenhan, begging him to "Get me the hell out of here!"

Of course, the experiment was eventually revealed, leaving egg on a lot of faces. To gather follow-up data on how the institutions learned from the experience, Rosenhan told one academic hospital he would send one—and perhaps more—bogus patients to them sometime over the next three months. During this period, 193 patients were admitted to the hospital and more than 20 percent of them were identified by at least one staff member as being part of Rosenhan's hoax, Part Deux. The problem? Rosenhan had not sent anyone else to the hospital. The staff had simply recalibrated their expectations and continued to operate on preconceived notions.

What happened to Rosenhan's phony patients in both instances vividly illustrates what happens to hundreds of thousands of patients each year in other clinical settings. Doctors and nurses get caught in their own procedural and cognitive quicksand, put on blinders, and see nothing but those things that reinforce their previous judgments and beliefs.

Perhaps more than any area in clinical medicine, when diagnosing patients we need to learn from our mistakes and to deepen our understanding of clinical reasoning. As with most errors, the answer will come through systems thinking, but here this means better systems for training the doctors of tomorrow. All medical students study Watson and Crick, but few study Bayes and Tversky. They should. As Canadian safety expert and ER doctor Pat Croskerry puts it:

> One uniquely distinguishing characteristic of those who make high-quality decisions is that they can largely free themselves from the common pitfalls to which novices are vulnerable. A rite of passage in all disciplines of medicine is learning about clinical pitfalls that have been identified by the discipline's experts. This [says] in effect, "Here is a typical error

that will be made, and here is how to avoid it."

For Annie Jackson, the "typical error" came when her chest wall tenderness led an experienced doctor to ignore conflicting and suspicious information from the EKG and cardiac blood tests in favor of a simpler diagnosis that seemed to make sense in the heat of the moment. Had he taken the time—or perhaps had the training—to employ a more systematic, methodical approach, he would have correctly diagnosed *his own* uncertainty, and admitted Annie for observation. She'd probably be alive today, singing in her choir.

To put it simply, Annie Jackson died in Dr. Bennett's cognitive quicksand.

CHAPTER 7: OF LIFE AND LIMB

I would like to see the day when somebody would be appointed surgeon somewhere who had no hands, for the operative part is the least part of the work.

— Dr. Harvey Cushing (1869–1936), the pioneer of modern neurosurgery

Bad things happen to good people. Take, for example, the sad case of Willie King.

King, a fifty-one-year-old Florida man with three kids, was the kind of sweet, quiet American soul Frank Capra loved to celebrate in his movies. With his close-cropped, graying hair and thick-rimmed glasses, he looked like a Main Street barber. His warm smile and kind words were well-loved in his small town.

For years Willie King had suffered from diabetes and, despite his proper and conscientious use of insulin, the disease appeared to be winning. The nerves in his legs were beginning to deteriorate like the frayed wiring in an old house. Now when he bruised a toe or nicked his shin, his body's alarm system—the one that normally prompts us to unwrinkle our socks and remove pebbles from our shoes—stayed silent. The seeds of infection were planted.

Compounding the nerve deterioration was the gradual clogging of the arteries servicing King's legs. This peripheral vascular disease, as it's called, blocks white blood cells and other inflammatory agents from getting to wound sites and fighting infection. Even when the white cells do reach the injury, they're too "drunk" from swimming in the sugary soup of the diabetic's blood to remember what they were supposed to do. Protected from the armies of inflammation, a minor infection—which a nondiabetic could have conquered without breaking a sweat—can begin to rage.

When it does, a tiny scrape can blossom into a small ulcer, and even into an abscess. If a diabetic's blood-starved, poisonous abscess isn't treated—and sometimes even if it is—it can become a fetid island of gangrene, which can spread not only to nearby tissues, but to vital organs as well. At this point, even our most powerful antibiotics are all but worthless. The diseased foot, or diseased portion of the leg, must come off—or the patient will die.

This was Willie King's dilemma when, in early 1995, he noticed the first inky stain of gangrene spreading across his right foot. Both feet were already numb, and, because of poor circulation, felt like ice sculptures to the touch. In a cruel trick of physiology, the same diabetic nerve damage that deadens the legs can sometimes cross-circuit, causing intense, unremitting pain; and so it was with Willie, at least in his right foot. The pain had become so bad, in fact, that he was virtually a one-legged man, depending on his left leg for strength and balance. He saw his doctor promptly but was told that, unfortunately, his right foot and lower leg were too far gone to be saved. On February 17, King agreed to amputation of his right leg below the knee.

This procedure is not uncommon for advanced diabetics and others in Willie's condition. Surgeons refer to it as a "BKA" (below-the-knee amputation)—which is preferable to an "AKA" (above-the-knee amputation) because it saves enough tissue and bone below the joint to mount a prosthetic limb, which allows for reasonably fluid ambulation. Sadly, many BKAs become AKAs after a few years, in the same way that the small remodeling job on your kitchen becomes a budget-buster when the contractor unexpectedly discovers dry rot.

Full of his characteristic optimism, King checked into a midsized local hospital called University Community Hospital (though it lacked any discernible connection to a university) on a warmish winter day in Tampa, Florida. The admitting clerk entered his clinical and demographic information into the computer, and King was put on the surgical schedule. Like most of its kind, UCH's information system had no mandatory double-checks and the staff frequently complained of errors. So the first snowball in what was to become a destructive avalanche began with a couple of misplaced keystrokes. The schedule printed out that patient Willie King was to receive a *left* BKA.

Fortunately, a heads-up floor nurse caring for Willie in the surgical ward spotted the left-right mix-up and called the operating room. The nurse answering the phone made a handwritten correction to the computer-generated printout and put it onto the surgical clipboard, which another scrub nurse took into the operation. Unfortunately, there was no system to ensure that the *computer's* record was amended.

Another OR nurse spoke briefly with King about the surgery, and he correctly identified his right leg as the bad one, which she noted in her record. With characteristic good humor, Willie joked, "You know which one it is, don't you? I don't want to wake up and find the wrong one gone!"

She smiled, and then rolled him off toward surgery.

Although the hand-corrected copy of the OR schedule was on the nurse's clipboard, the computer continued to churn out defective copies like an electronic Hydra. The original, erroneous copy of the OR schedule had been printed and was posted, per standard practice, in the OR suite. Another faulty copy was sent to the main OR desk's blackboard, which served as the master schedule-at-a-glance for physicians, surgeons, and visitors. King's surgeon, Dr. Rolando Sanchez, probably saw it as he arrived for the morning's first operation. Its information did not surprise him. It only confirmed what he'd already seen on the original printout. He was mentally— at least subliminally—primed to saw off the patient's *left* leg.

And that's exactly what he did. At one point, as the operation progressed, a circulating nurse began to review King's chart and was surprised to see the hand-corrected sheet showing the amputation was to be of the patient's *right* leg. She immediately told the surgical team, but the operation was too far along to "glue" the leg back on. And of course, the right leg—the one that was supposed to come off—still had all the life-threatening problems that originally brought King to the hospital. Later, that leg too would have to go, leaving King a double amputee, bound to a wheelchair for life.

Naturally, the horrific mistake made big waves when the news hit the media. Everyone called a lawyer and an investigation followed.

The investigators' first story starred the sharp-end caregiver—Dr. Sanchez, the surgeon wielding the knife. Sanchez didn't bolster his defense, or win many points for diplomacy, when he later testified that the "wrong leg" needed to come off anyway—both appeared to be substantially diseased, which may have added to the OR's confusion when they "prepped" it for surgery. This foot-in-mouth performance produced a memorable headline in the *Wall Street Journal*: "A story that doesn't have a leg to stand on: amputation of man's left leg rather than right one may have been medically justified."

Ultimately, Dr. Sanchez was fined $10,000 and suspended from practice by the Florida Board of Medicine. But this was small consolation for Willie King; nor did it do anything to fix the error-prone hospital system that helped put him in his wheelchair.

Wrong-site surgery cases are so shocking that our instinct is to assume that the caregiver involved is truly a "bad apple" who deserves to be removed from the barrel. (In fact, Sanchez would later go on to place a large intravenous line in a "wrong patient," and to remove another patient's toe without informed consent.) Yet even in these cases—and perhaps *especially* in these cases—the second story remains important, since it is the only way to fairly assess both the role of the negligent provider and of the system that allowed the errors to reach the patient.

The second story of the Willie King case revolves around the challenges of correctly operating on body parts, such as arms and legs, hip joints and eyes, that exhibit what biologists call *bilateral symmetry*: mirror-image anatomical features. Adding to the trickiness of operating on diseased organs that are one of a bilaterally symmetrical pair is the fact that all of these body parts are subject to the same diseases, and surgeries, though not always at the same time. Many physicians—vascular surgeons for diabetic complications, orthopedic surgeons for hip replacements, and ophthalmologists for cataracts—spend most of their days operating on one of these paired organs, often on patients they meet only once during a brief office visit weeks, or sometimes months, prior to surgery. Even if the surgeon recalls the case well enough to question the scheduled procedure ("I could've *sworn* it was the right foot!"), a quick reexamination of the patient in the operating room may reveal enough abnormalities on the wrong side to reassure him the questionable data are correct, as appears to have happened to Willie King. In fact, as absurd as Dr. Sanchez's defense may sound, many diabetic "vasculopaths" *do* eventually require double amputation.

Another instance of bad systems complicated by bad doctoring (and bad karma, if you believe in such things) occurred in New York. There, Dr. Ehud Arbit, chief of neurosurgery at the world-famous Memorial Sloan-Kettering Cancer Center, operated on the wrong side of a patient's brain—not just once, but twice in five years!

The first time: Three months after Willie King lost his wrong leg, Dr. Arbit consulted on a case concerning a fifty-nine-year-old woman with a malignant glioma—a particularly terrible form of brain cancer. (Some readers will recognize this as the disease that killed "Dr. Mark Green," the character played by Anthony Edwards on the popular TV series *ER*.) The patient, Rajeswari Ayyappan, was the mother and business manager of a prominent "Bollywood" film star who traveled from India to Sloan-Kettering because of its reputation for excellence in oncology and cancer surgery. Her tumor had already infiltrated the left frontal lobe of her brain, compressing and displacing normal brain tissue as it grew, the way tree roots can warp and crack a sidewalk.

On May 26, 1995, Dr. Arbit spent two hours patiently chiseling through the *right* side of Mrs. Ayyappan's skull and carefully poking at the gray matter inside, searching with growing frustration for the tumor he expected to find. Sadly, as can happen in surgeries like this (even when no error is involved), Mrs. Ayyappan recovered with all feeling on her left side gone and her vision severely diminished. Most tragic of all, the tumor sat untouched, mere centimeters away from the area Dr. Arbit had probed so thoroughly. The patient subsequently underwent tumor resection at New York Hospital, a stone's throw from Sloan-Kettering on Manhattan's posh Upper East Side, but she later died in India.

Dr. Arbit was promptly suspended and later dismissed—not just from his post as chief neurosurgeon, but from the hospital. In his defense, he pointed to various deficiencies in the hospital's organization and testified that he genuinely believed that a *different* fifty-nine-year-old East Indian patient—a man named Gupta from New Delhi, whose tumor really was on the right side—was actually on the table.

After a year on probation, Dr. Arbit was hired by Staten Island University Hospital as chief of neurosurgery. This job was a big step down for Arbit, but the hospital must have felt like a minor league team signing Reggie Jackson. Instead of traveling to the Big Houses across the East River, local cancer patients could now seek world-class treatment in their own backyard. Amazingly, five years after the Ayyappan case, the unthinkable happened again, during an emergency operation on one Johnnie Artis, a fifty-four-year-old security supervisor with a metastatic brain tumor. Dr. Arbit was performing a procedure known as "debulking" the tumor, which wouldn't cure the already advanced disease, but would prolong the patient's life, which was at immediate risk. Arbit incised the skull overlying the left cerebellum, only to be told by a physician's assistant that, as she recalled, the tumor was on the right. We might imagine Dr. Arbit sinking briefly into his shoes, scalpel bravely poised, wondering what he had done in a previous life to deserve all this. The operation continued, and Arbit later claimed he had intended all along to remove the entire back of the skull, since the tumor was very large and apparently crossed the midline. Nonetheless, after another investigation, Dr. Arbit was obliged to surrender his license, and he hung up his scalpel for good on February 18, 2000.

So, like Dr. Sanchez, Dr. Arbit seemed to display a penchant for certain medical blunders. Both were removed from practice, and perhaps deservedly so. But was there any merit to Arbit's countercomplaint that the Sloan-Kettering "system" (as well as the system at Staten Island) let him down and permitted the mistake? In fact, the Ayyappan tragedy's second story tells a tale that again brings to mind James Reason's mental model of holes aligning in Swiss cheese to let errors through. Let's rewind the tape, to the very beginnings of the Sloan-Kettering case.

In May 1995, Dr. Arbit received a request to operate on an Indian man named Gupta. Around the same time, Mrs. Ayyappan was referred to a very senior Sloan-Kettering neurosurgeon, Joseph Galicich, Jr. Galicich was about to retire, so he turned the case over to his colleague, Dr. Arbit. This referral was made by a phone call to Dr. Arbit's secretary, who left a note for her boss that a patient from India was being sent to him by Dr. Galicich. Although Sloan-Kettering has an international reputation, there aren't *that* many patients referred from India for brain surgery in a given year. So Dr. Arbit, on seeing his secretary's note, reasonably assumed the note pertained to Mr. Gupta, whose records—unbeknownst to his secretary—he had already received.

The note prompted Dr. Arbit to review Gupta's X-rays (and his tumor was indeed on the right). After doing so, he decided that the surgery could be performed in India. This is never an easy call, even for busy specialists at elite institutions. Patients like to know they're being treated by the best of the best, and if you turn down too many requests, future referrals can dry up. However, some referred cases can be handled very well by local talent; sometimes the referring doctors are simply seeking reassurance from the Mecca that they can do the job themselves. At other times, the "thanks but no thanks" cases are situations in which the prognosis is so grim that not even a team of All-Stars can likely save the patient. Sadly, Gupta appeared to fit into this latter category.

Having decided to turn down the referral, Dr. Arbit asked his secretary to get the family of the "referral from India" on the phone. Thinking he meant the recent request from Dr. Galicich, she placed a call to the Ayyappans. Arbit picked up the line and, assuming he was talking to the Gupta family, discouraged them from making the trip. The Ayyappans, of course, were shocked, given their family's prominence, and insisted that the operation be performed at Sloan-Kettering. Somehow, the name and gender of the patient never came up; or if it did, it slid across the phone lines unabsorbed. Given our own experience with cross-cultural conversations, we are anything but shocked by this; by this point in the book, perhaps you are equally unsurprised.

In any event, by the end of the call, Arbit had been talked into doing the surgery. The Ayyappans appeared days later on the cushioned chairs of Sloan-Kettering's impressive lobby. Dr. Arbit received a call that "the family from India" was waiting. Still thinking it was the Guptas, Arbit went to meet them at the admitting desk. Speaking to a young man who identified himself as the patient's son-in-law, Arbit described in general his strategy for removing the right-sided brain tumor. The son-in-law questioned the location of the tumor (he thought he recalled that it was on the left), but Arbit played the "doctor knows best" card and moved on to other matters.

At this point, it's easy to criticize Arbit for not catching the son-in-law's assertion as a red flag. But while it's legitimate to chastise physicians for ignoring the questions or concerns of a patient or family member (and we'll return to the matter of physician hubris later), it is sadly true that many patients arrive for procedures without knowing basic details about the nature of the procedure. Although much of the fault for this lies with doctors who fail to provide easily understood descriptions of important aspects of patients' medical care, the point remains that a consultant like Dr. Arbit would routinely encounter patients referred to him by other physicians for procedures that the patients—even educated and alert ones—could not completely describe.

So Arbit, confident that the brain tumor was on the right, not the left, overruled the family's objections. It takes self-confidence, after all, to slice into a living human brain or hold a patient's beating heart in your hands, and few surgeons worth their salt will admit to being wrong about so simple a thing as the surgical site. In fact, there's an old saying in medicine: "A surgeon is sometimes wrong, but never in doubt." It surely never crossed Arbit's mind that there just *might* be two patients from India, and that he just *might* be confusing one for the other.

Later, when the recriminations really started, Dr. Arbit claimed the Ayyappans at one point identified themselves as the Guptas. The Ayyappans dismiss this claim as ridiculous, and it sounds that way to us. Nobody knows what really transpired between the doctor and the patient's family—but, to a certain degree, it doesn't matter, since the system to ensure the correct surgery needs to be more robust than a rushed conversation with a family in a hospital lobby. What of the others on the Sloan-Kettering team? Where were the backups, the checks and double-checks, the *systems* a world-class hospital needs to make sure the technological marvels of modern surgery are being applied to the right body part and the right patient?

One part of the systems-oriented explanation for the error is that the usual protocols for surgery ID, such as verifying the patient's name and matching it to the existing OR schedule, were bypassed because the procedure was arranged on such short notice. Last-minute scheduling occurs often with VIP patients—it's simply a fact of medical life. But it wasn't the celebrity of the Indian family that lifted the velvet rope. The family in the lobby had arrived with $35,000 in cash for the Sloan Kettering cashier. In the modern American hospital—which has learned to live on a diet of fifty-cent-on-the-dollar payments from Medicare and HMOs—no celebrity gets treated better than Ben Franklin staring out from a C-note.

How can we be so confident it was the money, and not the prominence of the Ayyappans, that set heels a-clicking and bypassed standard operating procedures? Well, as you no doubt recall, Dr. Arbit still *thought* he was operating on Mr. Gupta, who (as far as we know) was no celebrity in India or anywhere else.

Both the Willie King and Ayyappan cases involved ID problems: In the first, it was the wrong site; in the second, it was partly the wrong site but also the wrong patient. Many of the wrong-site errors are in fact linked to the "sidedness" of X-rays and other imagery.

Every operating room has a light box, or a computer screen, which projects an X-ray (which resembles a photo negative) or other diagnostic image. These images show the brain tumor, or arthritic hip, or diseased kidney, or whatever else the surgeon is interested in. Unfortunately, X-rays are see-through and can be inadvertently reversed. As with your vacation pictures, you may not notice a flip-flop until you realize that Jimmy's hair is parted on the wrong side, or "Disneyland" is spelled backward. Similarly, a CAT scan of the brain, flipped over, looks precisely the same except the tumor, if there is one, has moved to the other side. Every now and then, a person's peculiar anatomy gives a clue about sidedness—a blood vessel is a bit more prominent on one side than the other, or a previously broken bone declares its position by a characteristic thickening at the break.

Radiology technicians now carefully mark all X-rays with an opaque "L" or "R," but—since human beings are involved—we sometimes still muck it up. The technician may accidentally reverse the markers, or the OR team may fail to notice an image hung backward; as long as an "L" or an "R" appears in their peripheral vision, their brains—in the heat of the moment—are focused on the lesion, or injury, they're getting ready to repair.

Even after taking the time to understand all the blunt-end explanations for wrong-site surgery, from an individual patient's perspective the real question is: What are the chances that *my* surgeon is going to make such an error during *my* operation?

A recent survey of hand surgeons revealed that 20 percent of the roughly one thousand respondents had operated on the wrong site at least once in their career. An additional 16 percent had prepared to operate on the wrong site but were caught at the last minute by a sharp-eyed or less-distracted colleague, or a final check of the data. This doesn't mean hand surgeons are a flakier-than-usual bunch; only that in their particular specialty, the problem of bilateral symmetry is multiplied not just by two (hands) but by ten (fingers). Interestingly, surgeons with the highest workloads also reported the highest incidence of operating on the wrong site. In other words, while practice may make perfect when it comes to technical skill, there are some cases where doing something more often simply translates into a greater opportunity for error.

Since most surgeons do hundreds of operations a year, even this surprisingly high rate of wrong-site cases by surgeons *over a career* translates into a reassuringly low risk for patients in any individual procedure. But let's look at the odds yet another way: What are the chances that any one surgeon, like Dr. Arbit, could be the perpetrator of *two* wrong-sited surgery cases over a career?

As it happens, rolling "snake-eyes" in this case is not as shocking or unusual as we might guess, even if the surgeon is not congenitally careless or incompetent. Recall the New Jersey woman who, in the 1980s, won a huge lottery jackpot on two different occasions. This apparently trillion-to-one shot left most of us incredulous (and jealous) until two Harvard statisticians pointed out that, from the perspective of the national population (as opposed to a specific individual), the chances of one person winning two large lotteries is nearly one in thirty! As they explained in *The New York Times*, this counterintuitive fact results from the Law of Very Large Numbers, a Law that can create some awfully strange results. One clichéd example is the old saying that, left to themselves, an infinite number of monkeys with an infinite number of typewriters will eventually produce *Hamlet*.

Another example is the fact that, in any group of at least fifty people, it's almost certain that two of them will share the same birthday. So, although few would be faulted for avoiding a surgeon with two black marks, the odds are that someone—even a conscientious surgeon—may hit this hellish jackpot from time to time.

All of these probabilistic parlor tricks shouldn't blind us to the fact that many patients are harmed or killed by wrong-site surgery every year, and they certainly shouldn't detour us from trying to do something about it.

Since orthopedic surgeons are most likely to perform wrong-site procedures, that field has led the fight against this most egregious of errors. In 1994, the Canadian Orthopaedic Association launched a campaign to "Operate Through Your Initials," followed four years later by a program called "Sign Your Site," sponsored by the American Academy of Orthopedic Surgeons. Both organizations urged surgeons to initial the intended operative site, using a permanent marker, during a scheduled preoperative visit.

Before these academies entered the debate, many surgeons had already developed homegrown answers to the problem. Unfortunately but predictably, this medley of solo solutions just added to the cacophony, and may have created a few more Willie Kings. Many surgeons put an "X" on the surgical site (like marking a map with buried treasure); but others placed an "X" on the limb to be *avoided*. More than a few befuddled surgical technicians, unclear whether this surgeon was a "good leg" or "bad leg" marker (in the early days, few hospitals standardized this practice), wound up inadvertently abetting the error by misinterpreting the "X" (or the "NO" some surgeons used) and scrubbing and prepping the wrong limb before the surgeon entered the OR suite.

We are enthusiastic about "Sign Your Site" programs, but they will only work with standardization, training, and practice. If a harried surgeon dashes into the room of a nervous patient to "sign the site" moments before the operation, there will be no gain in safety.

But where "Sign the Site" programs have been systematically applied and consistently enforced, the results have been good and promise to get better. Thankfully, "Sign Your Site" is now required by the main hospital regulatory body, the Joint Commission on Accreditation of Healthcare Organizations (JCAHO). Implementing this requirement has been, and must remain, a high priority, since wrong-site surgery resonates so deeply with patients and the media as a mistake for which there is simply no excuse.

Wrong-patient and wrong-limb errors, while horrifying and unacceptable, are to some extent understandable given the chaos of the health care universe. The misunderstood call from India, the reversed X-ray, the typo on the computer printout—outside the operating room, all kinds of mischief can conspire to create an awful mistake. But inside the OR—once the hands are scrubbed, the doors are closed, the surgeon's favorite CD is spinning, and the team members have assumed their positions—one would think that this cloistered world would be relatively immune to the blocking-and-tackling errors we see elsewhere.

But, as we'll see in the next chapter, one would be wrong.

CHAPTER 8: DID WE FORGET SOMETHING?

You have learned something. That always feels at first as if you had lost something.

— H. G. Wells (1866–1946)

In October 2002, a Canadian woman was astonished when she repeatedly tripped the alarm on a metal detector as she attempted to board a flight at the airport in Regina, Saskatchewan. This despite her care to remove all her keys and pocket change, jewelry and hairclips, before entering the queue, per the post-9/11 protocol. Airport security descended on her en masse. Finding nothing in her clothing, they escorted her to the security room for a more comprehensive search. Forty minutes later, she emerged straightening her garments, followed by a half-dozen red-faced officers. They had gone over her with a fine-tooth comb, but the metal-detecting rod continued to *bleep* whenever it passed over her abdomen. Whatever was going on in there, they decided, it wasn't enough to keep her off the plane. She boarded her flight to Calgary and pondered what had just happened, and how it might be related to the equally odd events she'd been experiencing all summer.

It seems this wasn't the first time her belly had caused problems. Ever since her surgery at Regina General Hospital four months earlier, she had suffered recurring stomach pain. Her doctor offered no satisfactory explanation, just the usual bromides about "postoperative stress" and possible sensitivity to follow-up medicine. Time passed, but not the discomfort.

The events at airport security convinced her to push the physicians to find an explanation for her stomach pain. After her trip, she scheduled another appointment with her doctor, who ordered an abdominal X-ray. Shockingly, it showed in dense, white detail the outline of a metal retractor, a tool used by the surgical team months earlier to wedge open the incision in her side. The surgeons had inadvertently left the object behind when they "closed up," which was no small feat—the retractor was a foot long and two inches wide: practically the size of a crowbar.

Like wrong-patient and wrong-limb horror stories, the medical literature is replete with all kinds of cases of recurrent pain and intestinal blockages that turn out to be from instruments, sponges, or needles left behind by previous operations—sometimes months and years earlier. The term "retained sponge" is often used as a catchall phrase for all manner of surgical paraphernalia left behind by absentminded doctors and the nurses who are supposed to assist them.

Perhaps because they are somewhat less horrendous and mediagenic than wrong-limb and wrong-patient surgeries, "retained sponges" have received little systematic study. But recently, Dr. Atul Gawande and his Harvard colleagues reviewed fifty-four patients with retained foreign bodies from 1985 through 2001. Roughly two-thirds were actual sponges—square or rectangular bits of absorbent gauze designed to soak up blood in the operative field—while the remaining third were surgical instruments. The number of cases they identified corresponds to an overall "retained sponge" rate of about one per ten thousand surgeries. Given the number of procedures performed in the U.S. each year, that works out to at least one case each year for a typical large hospital. In fact, a prominent physician-executive at the University of Washington Medical Center candidly told *The New York Times* that instruments were left in patients two or three times a year at his hospital. Since Gawande drew his sample from malpractice claims, and many instances go unprosecuted or unreported, the problem is undoubtedly more common than even this published estimate.

You would think that this particular kind of error would yield to systematic, mechanical solutions. In the 1940s, manufacturers produced sponges with loops that allowed the scrub nurse to attach them to a two-inch metal ring. The ring then hung outside the operative field while the sponges soaked up whatever needed mopping up inside. When the operation was over, the nurse simply harvested the sponges by gathering the rings—the way a trail of fishing hooks is pulled out of the water merely by reeling in the line.

Clever as this sounds, surgeons didn't like the ring system much. The rings were often in the way, so the surgeons frequently cut them off: a classic example of the "routine rule violations" we saw earlier. By the 1960s, manufacturers tried another approach, producing surgical sponges infused with radiopaque dye so they would show up on X-rays (soggy gauze cannot be distinguished from human tissue on an X-ray without this aid). But obtaining a postoperative X-ray on *every* patient is impractical (we'll explore why shortly), so the X-ray solution usually comes into play months later, when a patient has persistent postoperative pain and the doctors are trying to figure out why.

Leaving a sponge or tool behind may seem like a particularly boneheaded error—after all, some sponges are the size of dish towels—until you remember that complex or emergency surgeries often require hundreds of sponges. Some of these are placed delicately, when time permits and the situation demands it; but more frequently they are just jammed frantically into a bleeding wound. In these major surgeries—and in some minor ones, too—the number of sponges, instruments, and needles used becomes too great to track. This is one reason surgical teams have for decades used "sponge, sharp, and instrument counts."

The Association of Operative Registered Nurses recommends a standard protocol of four separate counts. The first is when the instruments are set up and the sponges are unpacked. The second is when the surgery begins and the items are called for and used. The third begins with closure, so that what went in, theoretically, is counted as it comes out. The fourth is during external suturing—the last chance to retrieve something if the previous counts were short. No matter how many counts a team uses (few actually do all four), the idea is to find discrepancies and reconcile them by repeated counts. When the discrepancy recurs, the surgical Easter Egg Hunt begins. The doctor pokes around in the surgical field (you'd be surprised what can hide between loops of bowel) while other OR personnel glance around the operating table, the floor, and, when all else fails, the used linen hamper and waste basket. If the count still doesn't tally, the hospital's protocol typically requires an X-ray to confirm (or, hopefully, eliminate the possibility) that the forgotten item is still in the patient's body.

If this procedure sounds painless and simple, try checking your living room couch for loose change, your office for errant paper clips, or your laundry basket for a particular sock or handkerchief—especially if you have a big family. Now turn on the radio and TV, open and close your cupboard doors, and try to hold an intelligible conversation on the phone—all at the same time as you conduct your search—and you approximate the conditions in a busy OR. Couple this with the reluctance of the players to admit (consciously or not) to the fallacy of an earlier count, and you'll begin to see why so many people take unwanted souvenirs home from the hospital. "Let's see here, I got eighty-nine...plus six more there and five over here and that makes a hundred. Yep, got 'em all."

This leads us back to the nature of systems and statistics. As a rule, counts are frequently off—by a little or a lot, depending on who's doing the counting and the method of keeping score. For any count of objects or events—surgical sponges, marbles in a jar, stars in the sky—it is vital to consider the *margin of error*. Say a nurse counts 100 sponges at the start of an operation. Let's say he's human, and thus has an entirely human 1-in-1,000 chance of counting any individual sponge incorrectly—as when he's distracted or two sponges stick together. Even with this very low error rate per sponge, probability theory tells us that there is a 10 percent chance that his recount will *not* tally 100, no matter how hard he tries. Moreover, even if every sponge has been removed from the patient, four counts will fail to match one time out of every three. No wonder surgical teams often fudge the counts, or simply go without them.

In many cases, the absolute count can't really be interpreted without knowing the error margin. When a Gallup poll tells us that 42 percent of voters favor a tax cut, and 45 percent oppose it, with an error margin of plus or minus 3 percent, what they're really saying is that it's entirely possible that 42 percent oppose the cut and 45 percent support it—an entirely opposite result.

But in a surgical setting, we don't want an *estimate* of how many sponges we may have left behind—even one is too many. As with airport security in the post-9/11 era, the only acceptable outcome is zero mistakes.

One way to make multiple counts more reliable is to conduct them independently; that is, have different nurses conduct different counts, each of them ignorant of what the previous nurse concluded. Of course, assembling special "counting teams" uses up valuable OR resources, so few hospitals indulge in the practice. Moreover, independent counts don't address the fundamental problem caused by the intersection of probability theory and human nature: Counts will often disagree because of the laws of statistics, most of these disagreements will be false alarms, and over time teams will be inclined to "cheat" on the counts to make everybody happy.

Gawande's *New England Journal* paper bears this out. In the study's most startling finding, while one-third of the retained sponge cases had not been subject to a documented count, two-thirds of the cases were. And in about half the cases, there were actually *multiple counts documented to be in agreement*. This means that every last sponge and instrument was thought to be accounted for, despite the fact that one would turn up later—rather inconveniently—in the belly of a patient.

The real lesson from all of this is that what appears on the surface to be a perfectly logical safety practice often turns out to be full of holes. Because sponge counts of any kind are inherently unreliable, some experts have recommended taking an X-ray of every surgical site before the field is sutured. Even if X-rays were free and patients and staff were willing to put up with the procedure, keeping anesthetized OR patients on the table any longer than strictly necessary is like holding airliners—each low on fuel—circling over a runway. Eventually, the new risks you create (post-op complications, other patients waiting too long for their procedures, and so on) make the marginal gains too expensive.

Partly for this reason, Gawande and his colleagues recommend taking X-rays only in high-risk cases: those involving emergency surgery, prolonged surgeries, surgeries involving a real-time change in clinical strategy, and surgeries on obese patients (in these cases, there are simply more places to lose things). Even if these were the only cases subjected to extra scrutiny, we would still need three hundred extra radiographs to prevent one retained foreign object. At $100 per X-ray, this would amount to $30,000 to prevent one case, which sounds high until you consider that the malpractice awards in these cases are usually many times higher. The real gremlin in this plan, however, is that radiopaque markers are subtle and can be overlooked on X-rays, even by skilled radiologists.

So, in the end, the best solution to the retained sponge problem probably lies in new technology. Some companies are working on sponges that cause a detecto-wand to *beep* when the surgeon waves it over the body before closure. Others envision automatic "sponge counters," like toll booth collection machines or casino money counters, that can be loaded up and checked after every surgery.

Creating systems and technologies that relegate retained sponges (and wrong-site operations) to the surgical history books cannot come soon enough for surgeons. They'd much rather be focusing their energies on mastering the technical art of surgery, an ongoing challenge we'll turn to in the next chapter.

CHAPTER 9: PRACTICE MAKES PERFECT

They say that "practice makes perfect." Of course, it doesn't. For the vast majority
of golfers it merely consolidates imperfection.

— Henry Longhurst (1909–1978), legendary golf commentator

Fortunately, bad as they are, errors involving retained objects and wrong-site surgeries are not common. What is faced in every operation, however, are issues regarding each caregiver's judgment and technique. System, schmystem, patients may say as they approach the scalpel. At those anxious moments right before surgery, a patient's main concerns are that her surgeon is technically skilled and that her recovery is free of infection, bleeding, heart attack, or stroke. Figuring out which surgical complications can be attributed to error and which to unfortunate inevitability is far from simple, but it's essential if we are to try and shape a safer medical system.

One of the things that makes it hard to sort all this out is that complications are common, even with perfect technique. In fact, because postoperative infections and bleeding occur so frequently (enough to be listed on your pre-op consent form, so you won't feel too surprised—or litigious—when one happens), a single complication does not automatically suggest poor quality or a safety problem. But, of course, good doctors don't want them to happen at all. Beginning in the late 1800s, surgeons established a tradition of reviewing every case that resulted in a life-threatening or unexpected complication. Was the surgical procedure or the surgeon's technique to blame? Were the nursing protocols adequate? Did the hospital's systems let the sharp-end caregivers down?

These (sometimes literal) "postmortem" meetings became known as *Morbidity and Mortality Conferences*, or M&Ms for short. We'll say more about these useful and cathartic sessions later, but for now it's enough to realize that the quest for safety and excellence in health care is very old and the vast majority of doctors, the vast majority of the time, take it very seriously. The main problem is that while good information is often exchanged at M&Ms, single-case war stories raise all of the usual issues about hindsight bias. Moreover, even when the conference points the way to an important change in practice or system, there is no easy mechanism to make sure it finds its way into the day-to-day habits of the institution, let alone to other hospitals, independent practitioners, or medical and nursing schools.

Another challenge in preventing postoperative complications is that most are, strictly speaking, nonsurgical. They involve administration of antibiotics at the right time; careful assessment and treatment of risk factors to prevent post-op heart attacks; preventing blood clots and adverse reactions to medications; and so on—all problems that are more in the internist's court than the surgeon's. It's not that surgeons are completely disinterested in such matters, only that their training and experience is not specifically geared toward anticipating and treating them. As some surgeons like to say, "Nothing heals like cold, hard steel," and for many human maladies, they're right. But for everything else, other ways of thinking serve the patient better.

Even if we confine our lens to the technical skills of the surgeon, it is often tricky to attribute a bad outcome to poor technique. Aside from the obviously egregious, and therefore uncommon, instances when a particular surgeon's sutures keep coming undone or his scalpel repeatedly slices through major blood vessels, second-guessing the real-time actions of highly trained professionals is very difficult. Like race drivers, test pilots, Olympic gymnasts, and symphony musicians, good surgeons are virtuosos whose results speak for themselves, and whose flaws are often subtle enough to escape notice by everyone except other experts. Of course, in sports and music, life and limb are seldom on the line, with the possible exception of a boxer's financial backers or the folks sitting in the first few rows at Daytona. However, the surgeon who fails to achieve technical mastery may be a public menace.

In 1979, Harold Luft, then a cerebral young health economist at Stanford, published what turned out to be a seminal paper in the *New England Journal of Medicine*. Recognizing the difficulty of judging the technical skills of individual surgeons, Luft and his coauthors turned to the deceptively simple premise that practice might just make perfect when it comes to surgery. Nobody had thought to relate the outcomes of surgeons and hospitals as a function of "volume," and the result was revolutionary. Centers that performed more operations of a specific type—from coronary bypasses and other vascular surgeries to prostate resections and hip replacements—enjoyed better outcomes.

Luft's study spawned an entire branch of medical research. At last count, over 250 studies have examined the "volume-outcome" relationship for more than twenty-five different procedures, and in most cases, the results are the same. Clinical outcomes are better and complications fewer when the surgeon or the hospital (or both) do a lot of what they do best.

This relation seems so logical, and applies to so many other professions and life activities outside of medicine, it's astonishing that nobody'd thought of it before. Since surgery seems so individualistic—the surgeon as the megastar with a large but unknown supporting cast—it may surprise you to learn that the relationship between volume and outcomes is more tightly linked to the number of procedures performed in a particular *hospital* than by a specific doctor. The practical significance of this is that the cardiac surgeon who performs hundreds of coronary bypass operations each year at a major hospital but occasionally performs "cabbages" (professional slang for "coronary artery bypass graft," or CABG) at smaller hospitals as well will probably have a less successful record at the smaller facilities—he's the same doctor, but the infrastructure just isn't there to support him, or the patient, at these places.

It would be useful to know which way the relationship between volume and outcome works: Is the outcome better *because* of the high volume of surgeries ("practice makes perfect"), or does the volume increase because word-of-mouth spreads the news about better outcomes? In other words, there's a chicken-and-egg problem in interpreting the volume-outcomes relationship. If practice really does make perfect, the answer might well be to regionalize procedures: Have one of the Big Houses do *all* of the CABGs for a city, for example, and close down the cardiac operating rooms of the smaller shops. If not, then perhaps a high volume hospital's successes might be portable. That is, if smaller hospitals just copied more effectively what the Big Houses were doing, their results might be just as good.

Although this might seem fairly straightforward (practice does make perfect, after all), consider a more familiar analogy. Here in San Francisco, we often see long lines spilling out of neighborhood bistros. If the packed restaurant serves great food and has attentive service, one would hardly make the point that the place was good *because* of the queues. The restaurant's excellence doesn't derive from having "practiced" on many customers; rather, it's crowded because word has gotten out that the place is happening.

In medicine, this effect has been dubbed "selective referral," capturing the possibility that the hospital is crowded *because* word has gotten out that the place is good, rather than the opposite. Once that happens, the crowds might make the outcomes better (if practice truly does make perfect), but they can also make them worse—overloading the system to the point that quality begins to suffer. Urban freeways were designed to move a lot of cars very quickly, which they used to do—until everybody started using them. Now, nobody takes the freeway if they're in a hurry, especially at peak travel times, bringing to mind Yogi Berra's great line, "Nobody goes there anymore, it's too crowded."

After publication of his seminal article, Luft (who is now a colleague of ours at UCSF) found that selective referral did, in fact, partly explain the volume-outcome relationship—mostly for highly elective surgeries that patients could research themselves, the way they shopped as consumers for luxury cars and vacations. But even in settings that did not allow for comparison shopping, such as for heart attack patients who need a CABG and need it *now*, the volume-outcomes relationship still held true. Practice *does* make perfect, but only if the practitioners start out knowing what they're doing.

So high-volume and good outcomes tend to go hand-in-hand if the providers are already skilled. How can you use this information to make better health care decisions for you and your family?

First, ask about volume, but make sure it's for the procedure you're getting. There doesn't seem to be too much crossover between excellence in cardiac surgery and in liver transplantation, particularly for the hospital that does lots of cases of one but few of the other. And of course, high volume coupled with low resources is a prescription for overwhelmed providers and high complication rates, as a trip through many of the nation's underfunded municipal hospitals quickly demonstrates.

But why should *you* have to do the comparison shopping? Since high-volume institutions enjoy better outcomes, why don't insurers or regulators push to close down the smaller facilities and regionalize procedures in high-tech "Centers of Excellence?"

The answer, in short, is that patients don't seem to want this, for reasons that appear to be part economic, part emotional. Few people would opt for surgery at a medical megaplex forty miles away, in another city (where pre-op and follow-up visits are a ninety-minute drive, and friends and relatives would have a hard time stopping by), just because its mortality rate for the procedure they're having is 3 percent, versus 4 percent at their neighborhood hospital (where, incidentally, they had their tonsils out and all of their children were born). When quality rankings are that close (and they often are), people pick the nearer facility most of the time.

But let's assume human nature changes overnight, and people in significant numbers begin clamoring for Centers of Excellence.

If we've learned anything so far in our tour of medical mistakes, it's that problems jump out when you least expect them. If outcomes are better at well-managed, high-volume facilities, what's wrong with such a policy?

First, local hospitals might not survive if they lose too many of their big-ticket patients to bigger hospitals. Remember, hospitals do lots of things besides complex brain surgeries and bypass operations. When you need an ER after a car accident or have a serious allergic reaction to a new prescription, you usually can't afford to drive forty minutes to find a hospital. Although forced regionalization is unusual in the U.S., market-driven regionalization is beginning to occur with the advent of so-called boutique hospitals (such as "heart centers"), which specialize in just one kind of medicine or procedure. These hyper-specialized and often very expensive facilities may, in fact, improve outcomes for a narrow range of patients, but, by removing profitable services from local hospitals, they have already caused some general hospitals to close departments or shut down entirely. This has left many patients—including the uninsured—without adequate care.

Another unintended consequence of regionalization may be the dark side of high volume itself: A too-crowded hospital eventually creates an error-prone, overworked staff. While studies looking for this effect have generally not found it yet, a wholesale policy shift designed to shunt patients to high-volume centers (or a major uptick in patients voting with their feet to go to these centers) could ultimately cause problems, especially if the increased volume isn't anticipated and budgeted. Although their bad outcomes would eventually catch up to the hospitals, in medicine, as in other industries, it takes a while before the truth trumps a marquee reputation.

All this talk of hospital volumes can obscure the plain fact that the skills of the individual surgeon matter too. Sure, volume and experience seem to be important, but how do we know whether a surgeon—or anyone else performing complex technical procedures—has the aptitude to succeed, even if he has a work ethic like Cal Ripken, Jr.? Like the tongue-in-cheek adage about the failing business —it loses money on every transaction but makes it up in volume—the surgeon lacking technical aptitude at the start may well be unable to "make it up in volume."

In the field of medicine, physicians traditionally get jobs like surgical residencies by answering such questions as, "Did you pass the Boards?" and "What were your grades in organic chemistry?" In the early days of aviation, the British Royal Air Force used a similarly bland system for selecting potential pilots. A few senior officers interviewed the candidates, chatted a bit and asked a few questions, then put their heads together and made a selection. This unstructured assessment of unspecified abilities may have worked well to ensure congenial company at the Officers' Club, but it didn't do much to put the best candidates into RAF cockpits. During World War II, the RAF began to employ a battery of objective tests targeting mental agility, physical stamina, coordination, and a host of relevant characteristics. These tests are now taken for granted not only in aviation and the space program, but in a variety of other physically and mentally demanding careers where lives are on the line, such as firefighting and law enforcement. Interestingly, many of the same physical and mental tests used by the Air Force would be completely relevant to surgical training without changing them one iota.

Still, senior physicians and hospital administrators usually settle for checking grades and Board scores, assessing a candidate's demeanor (call it professional bearing or bedside manner) and looking at the cut of his suit. No joke—in some cases, the clothes make (or unmake) the doctor. For his first medical school interview, Bob—hoping to make a good impression—wore a new corduroy suit (a fact that gives away both the era and Bob's fashion sense), right off the rack. During the otherwise amiable discussion, the interviewer (a highly qualified surgeon) began staring at the left cuff of Bob's jacket.

"Is time up?" Bob asked, thinking the surgeon was trying to see his watch.

"Turn your arm over," came the surgeon's stern reply. There, on the underside of the cuff, was one of those big cardboard tags retailers sew onto every garment. "OK," the doctor continued, handing Bob a pair of scissors from his desk, "let's see your surgical technique."

Bob nervously began snipping at the tag, taking off some threads along with a good bit of corduroy. Chuckling, the surgeon got up, took the scissors, and completed the excision in a few deft strokes. Perhaps this serendipitous test should be formally integrated into interviews for surgical programs; you'll be comforted to know that Bob does no surgical procedures in his present-day work.

Even if, like the military, we tested for procedural aptitude, and accepted only those candidates with the most promise, novices' first few operations would still be hazardous to patients' health. Recognizing this, a new surgeon traditionally performs under the close supervision of a veteran—but not for very long. The old academic adage of "See one, do one, teach one" isn't too far off the mark in real life: After a couple of years of training, apprentice surgeons are largely on their own for all but the most complex cases.

And—once residency is over—practicing surgeons are essentially left on their own to acquire new skills or keep up with the latest techniques. In *Complications*, Atul Gawande, himself a newly minted surgeon, writes that his father, a senior urologist in private practice, estimated that three-quarters of the procedures he now performs routinely did not exist at the time he was trained. While most surgeons make a conscientious effort to stay on top of their fields, some don't—and quality can suffer.

A case in point is laparoscopic gallbladder removal, or *cholecystectomy*—known as "lap choley" in scrub-room vernacular. This procedure involves removing the small, pear-shaped organ that sits beneath the liver, usually because it's filled with stones and has caused pain or infection. The surgeon makes a few inch-long slits in the abdomen, then inserts narrow mechanical arms that can cut and sew while monitoring events inside with a tiny camera. This revolutionary technique has almost entirely replaced the much more invasive and traumatic "open choley"—a conventional "up to the elbows" operation that has far more complications and deaths. With lap choley, patients have shorter hospital stays (cutting costs and reducing the chance of hospital-acquired infections), and a much shorter convalescence. (Interestingly, despite the fact that the procedure is far less expensive than open choley, as a nation we now spend much *more* money on cholecystectomies than before, since doctors are more apt to recommend the safer and more user-friendly laparoscopic procedure in situations where, in the old days, we would have bided our time—a telling example of why technological innovation in health care, unlike in most other industries, often raises costs.)

Laparoscopic surgery has revolutionized procedures in other medical fields, including gynecology (hysterectomies), orthopedics (joint repair), and even cardiology—where laparoscopic heart bypass surgeries (sometimes called "keyhole coronary surgeries") are showing great promise. This puts pressure on surgeons to keep up with new techniques and to continuously build their skills: Most new procedures have steep learning curves that novices need to traverse. One early study of lap choleys showed that injuries to the common bile duct—not fatal, but often a painful source of jaundice and infections—dropped almost twentyfold once surgeons had at least a dozen cases under their belts. After that, the learning curve shallowed, but not by much: The rate of common bile duct injury on the thirtieth case was still ten times higher than the rate seen after fifty cases.

This mismatch between what new surgical methods offer and how "the system" supports practicing surgeons in acquiring the skills needed to perform them highlights a big gap in health care quality. This doesn't mean that most surgeons aren't safe when undertaking these new techniques, only that there is no system in place *requiring* them to be so, or to boost them past those early, error-prone cases with minimal risk to patients. This is the opposite of how aviation—both commercial and military—handles a similar problem: How to make otherwise experienced professionals competent, as quickly as possible, in high-risk situations using new equipment and procedures.

In both the airline industry and the military's flying branches, pilots are prepared to fly new planes by first undergoing considerable formal training—in classrooms and in simulators (some of which are astoundingly realistic)—followed by extensive, hands-on experience in the real thing, with an instructor pilot seated beside the pilots (or, in the case of military fighters, in the backseat), with his own set of controls. After that, the pilot must pass both written and flight tests to qualify in the new machine; and he is continually evaluated with annual "check rides" administered by senior instructors. If a pilot flunks a check ride, he or she is put back on training status until the deficiencies are eradicated. When pilots fail these checks continuously, or are involved in a serious incident or accident, they are evaluated by what the Air Force calls a "Flight Evaluation Board," which has the power to permanently clip their wings.

Contrast this with medicine's laissez-faire attitude toward recertification, which in most fields involves attending a certain number of continuing education courses for a certain number of hours each year. There is no testing (although some fields are beginning to require general recertification every five to ten years), no demonstration of competency, no apprenticeship in new techniques—no evidence that the doctor even stayed awake during the continuing education lectures or wasn't daydreaming about an afternoon tee time.

Modern medicine does have one thing on its side: Even if requirements to demonstrate ongoing proficiency are skimpy, proceduralists of all kinds—from surgeons who perform CABGs to cardiologists who do angioplasties and gastroenterologists who probe bowels with colonoscopes—learned their basic techniques well during their residencies and fellowships. Their training period is far longer (at least five to seven post–medical school years) and more rigorous than that of pilots or those in other skill-intensive professions.

But our continued reliance on drive-through training—the medical version of the "weekend warrior"—for new and complex procedures is cause for alarm. A 1991 survey found that more than half (55 percent) of 165 practicing surgeons who had participated in a two-day practical course on laparoscopic cholecystectomy felt the workshop had left them inadequately trained to start performing the procedure. Yet 74 percent of these same surgeons began churning out lap choleys immediately afterward.

Even worse, laparoscopic techniques represent such a radical change from traditional surgical practice (where tactile feedback is key; in laparoscopic procedures, the surgeon does virtually everything by remote control) that surgeons, believing they have mastered lap choleys over a weekend, may be tempted to apply the technique on other parts of the body. This is rather like a novice skier, who has just learned to "snow plow" and weight-shift, trying those new techniques on the Black Diamond run.

Laparoscopy has become so widespread that new surgeons coming out of formal training are now qualified to perform it, as well as a number of other minimally invasive procedures—it's the direction medicine is taking. But what about the next new thing?

The most promising approach to building surgeons' skills quickly without putting patients at risk involves the use of simulators. As we've mentioned, procedural simulators have been around for decades in other industries. Military fliers used them even before World War II, although these "Link Trainers" were only crude approximations of the real thing. Static aircraft simulators (that is, those in which the cockpit is fixed to the floor while instruments give the impression of flight) became quite sophisticated during the jet age, allowing fledgling pilots not only to learn and practice normal instrument procedures, but also to handle a wide variety of airborne emergencies thrown at them by instructors at electronic consoles. By the age of jumbo jets, supersonic airliners, and space shuttles, "full motion" simulators gave the illusion of true flight and pilots could actually look out the window and take off or land visually at any airport in the world. They can feel the aircraft climb, bank, and dive as they manipulate the controls. And this technology is not confined to the ethereal world of flight.

"Real War," a popular video game, was first developed by the Joint Chiefs of Staff as a training aid for soldiers, Marines, and airmen. The program was so successful that the military may spend up to $50 million over the next few years refining its "Mission Rehearsal Exercise," a five-minute, bone-shaking combat scenario with ten-channel sound effects, voice recognition software (including the foreign languages of potential enemies and allies) and optional smells of battle, such as burnt charcoal pumped into the training room, which is surrounded by a 150-degree movie screen.

These kinds of training and performance evaluation aids— where the trainees interact with other human beings as well as with machinery and virtual displays—may hold the highest potential for medical simulations, which to date have been pretty primitive.

For decades, doctors practiced giving injections to oranges and learned suturing on pig's feet. A somewhat lifelike mannequin (nicknamed "Annie," for obscure reasons) has been used for years to teach CPR to civilians. Although physicians, some nurses, paramedics, and firefighters learn a more advanced method of CPR, their simulator, too, is little more than an anatomically accommodating dummy. Recently, these training mannequins have become more realistic, allowing students to deliver electric shocks with defibrillator paddles and note changes to heart rhythms, insert IV and intra-arterial lines, and perform intubations—inserting an endotracheal tube into dummy "lungs" and connecting the rubber patient to a ventilator—giving the trainee the supremely satisfying opportunity to shout, "I'm in!" like the doctors on *ER*. Although most of these devices are decidedly low-tech, they do a reasonably good job of approximating the clinical environments of emergency physicians, anesthesiologists, and surgeons. And new and better systems are on the way.

Surgical simulators, some computerized, are now emerging that can provide virtual training for complex operations. These would likely be used as standard practice for med school trainees, and as aids for experienced surgeons upgrading to new techniques—letting the surgeon get the steepest part of the learning curve over with before encountering the first real patient. The major hurdle for these systems is accurately simulating the feel of real flesh, but even that obstacle is being overcome.

The "unreal" feel of the procedure is a major challenge in laparoscopy. Instead of looking at the real deal—the patient's innards—directly, the surgeon must probe the murky goo with a little periscope and manipulate a set of metal flex-tubes as a substitute for fingers. In a way, it's like that cheesy arcade game where little kids try to pick up cuddly stuffed animals with a remotely operated "crane" that always seemed to be too weak to lift any of the bigger, cooler toys. Multiply the difficulty of that vexing game by about twenty—and picture trying to play it now that you're no longer eight years old—and you'll have a sense of what it's like to learn even the most basic surgical task, like tying a knot, via the laparoscopic approach. But once you have the knack of it, the new set of skills can be used for all sorts of minimally invasive surgeries and procedures.

For most medical operations, the link between improved dexterity from simulator training and fewer errors remains intuitively attractive but not yet fully proven. In the absence of hard proof, and because they are expensive (some surgical simulators run over $100,000) and sexy, manufacturers will spend lots of money to market them and pressure will mount on administrators either to buy them (or be left in the Stone Age) or reject them (budget, budget, budget...). Since purchasing in medicine, alas, is driven as much by return-on-investment calculations as by clinical effectiveness, it may well be that the ultimate argument in favor of such systems will be their contribution to efficiency, rather than to quality or safety. One study showed that because novice surgeons are slower in the OR and require both supervision and hand-holding by senior physicians, an average of $50,000 in precious OR time is "wasted" during each resident's four-year training period. Cutting this cost may be the only reason some hard-nosed administrators buy into the system. But no matter—it's as good a reason as any so long as physicians get the training they need, and patients don't pay for it with unnecessary complications.

Of course, in some cases, penny-pinching administrators will be right: A fancy new machine just isn't worth the cost. One study tested whether the use of simulators would improve the ability of surgeons to remove kidney stones from one of the patient's ureters, the narrow tubes that connect the kidneys to the bladder. When a stone gets lodged in one, the pain is one of the worst that's known to man (men are fond of saying that it is like labor, as if we know...). Sometimes the stone can be extracted using a scope inserted through the urethra—the small tube through which urine flows from the bladder to the outside world—if the stone won't pass on its own. In the study, one group of students received a series of lectures on performing the technique. Another group used a pricey, high-tech, 3-D simulator that realistically duplicated the pelvic anatomy. Predictably, students training on the simulator did far better than those without hands-on practice. But there was a third group in the study. They, too, trained on a simulator, but theirs was a dime-store mockup in which a Styrofoam cup stood in for the bladder, a plastic straw for the ureter, and a flexible latex tube for the urethra. The whole thing cost less than a dollar. The performance by students in this group, too, was better than the passively trained students, and just as good as those who trained with the fancy anatomical simulator.

Still, like military simulators and everything else in our society, medical simulators are likely to continue on the high-tech track. Modern virtual reality simulators are beginning to input actual human data, such as that drawn from an extraordinarily detailed model known as the "Visible Human," which is based on surgical cross-sections of an actual cadaver converted to digital form. Lockheed Martin, the military contractor, has developed an Endoscopic Sinus Surgery Simulator ("ES3") that allows the operator to explore the nooks and crannies of facial sinuses while the controls feed back tactile signals and the screen shows the location of surgical tools, like forceps, and their surroundings. Take a biopsy from the wrong site, and—oops!— the screen quickly fills with red "blood." Curious about that little bump to the right? Touch a button and its name appears. The computer tracks the operator's economy of motion (how many moves it took to complete a given procedure), time to completion, and error rate—then lets the trainee try again to improve the score. Ultimately, designers hope to build simulators that use not just generic data like that from the Visible Human, but real patients' anatomy fed into the machine from CT or MRI scans. Dr. Marvin Fried, a New York otolaryngologist who is testing the ES3, says that, "eventually it will be standard procedure for a surgeon to do a walk-through of his patient's operation the night before the real surgery, using that patient's actual anatomy."

It's easy to get breathless over all these flashy gizmos, but before we get too excited, we should remember that no hard evidence really exists that the new machinery will reduce medical mistakes. Computerized systems and other high-tech simulators will undoubtedly play a part in future surgical training, but they will likely supplement traditional methods, which are essentially "master and apprentice": a well-prepared young learner observing, then doing, then being corrected by a seasoned veteran. The line between learning and doing will be further blurred as simulations become more realistic and real surgeries become less invasive and more like the simulations. As software and equipment costs come down and the Internet becomes more efficient, rural surgeons will be able to receive the same training as their big-city counterparts without ever getting on the interstate. As Sir William Osler, the father of academic medicine, remarked a century ago, "To study the phenomena of disease without books is to sail an uncharted sea, while to study books without patients is not to go to sea at all." Sophisticated medical simulators may represent the long-awaited medical training breakthrough that allows surgeons to traverse the learning curve without taking it out on their patients.

As we ponder whether practice makes perfect and reflect on training in the Jetsons era, an ultimate question remains: Are great surgeons born or made? And if they *are* made, how can we make them better and less prone to error?

In a 1999 *New Yorker* article called "The Physical Genius: What do Wayne Gretzky, Yo-Yo Ma, and a Brain Surgeon Named Charlie Wilson Have in Common?" *Tipping Point* author Malcolm Gladwell reflected on the traits shared by individuals who excel at tasks involving high-demand perceptual motor abilities: playing sports, making music, and removing brain tumors.

First, he found that all exhibit an incredible dedication to their craft. Studies have shown that exceptionally talented music students are more likely than their peers to spend long hours practicing— and not just rehearsing a difficult piece, but simply playing their scales. And these tendencies show themselves at a very early age. In other words, far from effortlessly producing one masterwork after another (be they concert performances, winning seasons, or delicate surgeries), these geniuses apply greater diligence, not less, to perfecting their crafts.

The second major quality Gladwell found was a unique use of imagery. He says:

When psychologists study people who are expert at motor tasks, they find that almost all of them use their imaginations in a very particular and sophisticated way. Jack Nicklaus, for instance, has said that he has never taken a swing that he didn't first mentally rehearse, frame by frame. Yo-Yo Ma told me that he remembers riding on a bus, at the age of seven, and solving a difficult musical problem by visualizing himself playing the piece on the cello.

In the film *Searching for Bobby Fischer*, Ben Kingsley's character, Bruce Pandolfini—a well-known U.S. chess coach and writer— swipes all the pieces off the board at a particularly difficult moment and tells young Josh Waitzkin to visualize the pieces and not touch them until he sees the entire series of moves in his head. Charlie Wilson, the noted neurosurgeon, also reported that he mentally and visually rehearsed operations scheduled for the day while jogging each morning.

The third trait Gladwell noted was that these remarkable performers were extremely intolerant of their own mistakes, no matter how small. They are perfectionists. Charles Bosk, a University of Pennsylvania sociologist who observed surgical residents for eighteen months as an anthropologist might study an aboriginal tribe, saw a few who either quit or were asked to leave their training program. He told Gladwell that he eventually recognized certain patterns among the surgeons who had failed:

> When I interviewed the surgeons who were fired, I used to leave the interview shaking. I would hear these horrible stories about what they did wrong, but the thing was that they didn't *know* that what they did was wrong. In my interviewing, I began to develop what I thought was an indicator of whether someone was going to be a good surgeon

or not. It was a couple of simple questions: Have you ever made a mistake? And, if so, what was your worst mistake? The people who said, "Gee, I haven't really had one," or "I've had a couple of bad outcomes but they were due to things outside my control"—invariably those were the worst candidates. And the residents who said, "I make mistakes all the time. There was this horrible thing that happened just yesterday and here's what it was." They were the best. They had the ability to rethink everything that they'd done and imagine how they might have done it differently.

The picture of ideal surgeons that emerges is one of people who constantly practice their craft, rehearse their procedures mentally, and are their own worst critics. Are any of these traits transferable to their less gifted counterparts, those who toil in the land of ordinary mortals? We think so, if we combine new insights into the psychology of procedural learning, intelligent adoption of simulators, new and more robust training requirements, and, as ever, thousands of hours of training and an unwavering commitment to excellence.

But achieving true excellence—and freedom from errors—will take much more than the efforts and dedication of individuals, however talented, well-meaning, and committed they may be. For medicine—even the surgical part of medicine—is a team sport, as we'll see in the next chapter.

CHAPTER 10: HANDOFFS AND FUMBLES

Gentlemen, it is better to have died as a small boy than to fumble this football.

— John Heisman (1869–1936),
legendary football coach for whom the Heisman Trophy is named

Tung Jan was a slightly built, taciturn man of seventy-one. Born in Taiwan, he immigrated to the United States to find a better life. The lines on his thin face were a résumé of years of struggle. He seldom displayed emotion—not even irritation at the sometimes maddening bureaucracy of the nursing home where he, like 1.6 million other elderly Americans, was living out his final years. Bound to a bed or wheelchair, he saved what smiles he had left for his grandchildren, who came to visit him regularly. They sat in his lap and ran like puppies behind the wheelchair as his nurse wheeled him from room to room, showing off the bright-eyed legacies he knew he would soon leave behind.

Jan, a lifetime smoker, had end-stage emphysema. His lungs, once fluffy with millions of lacy air pockets, now sagged like a sooty blacksmith's apron inside his sunken chest. With luck he might live to see his grandkids finish grade school.

Jan had always been a careful planner. He'd thought seriously about his care in these final years and put his wishes in writing. When the end came, he wanted no heroic measures—no "Code Blue," no CPR—just a little medication to ease the pain and enough care to keep him clean and comfortable until he drifted off. These advance directives—which appointed his son as surrogate medical decision-maker should he slip into a coma, and made clear his desire to avoid heroic, life-sustaining procedures—were dutifully placed in his nursing home chart. He knew how hard it would be for his family to make these life-and-death decisions when the time came, and, by documenting his preferences in advance, he hoped to spare them this wrenching ordeal. As with everything else in his life, Jan had thought about the needs of others, been realistic and practical, and tried to do the right thing.

Still, it wasn't enough.

One evening, a new nurse came into Jan's room to find him fighting for breath. She questioned him about the problem, but he was too air-hungry and confused to respond. Whether the new nurse simply panicked or was unaware that Jan had specifically asked not to be "Coded" (hospital slang for resuscitated) isn't clear. We do know that she immediately called 911 and, ten minutes later, the EMTs entered Jan's room and found him comatose and straining to breathe. Because nobody had flagged the patient as "DNR" ("do not resuscitate"), they tried to place a breathing tube into Jan's lungs—but didn't succeed. They then put him on oxygen, threw him on the folding gurney, and rushed him—sirens blaring—to the ER at a nearby university hospital. One of the paramedics later recalled, "[Mr. Jan] was laying there exposed; there was no bracelet or necklace letting us know that he might be something other than a full Code. I didn't ask the question, and it was not told to me."

In the emergency room, Jan remained both unresponsive and profoundly short of breath. The ER physician, having no information about the patient's preferences or any existing DNR order, wrote in his chart: "Full Code for now, status unclear." He tried again to thread a thick plastic tube through Jan's vocal cords and into his lungs, this time successfully. They attached the tube to a portable ventilator and transferred him to the ICU, where he was given powerful potions to open up his pencil-thin breathing tubes and combat his pneumonia.

After several hours, a staff member managed to track down Jan's son, who promptly came to the hospital. The son told them that his father had previously stated that if he was ever "in a state where he... needed the extraneous support to be kept alive, he didn't want it." This was the first time anyone at the hospital had heard the patient might be a DNR—the paperwork still remained buried in Jan's chart back at the nursing home. When the son finally came face to face with his father, he felt heartbroken—and ashamed. Despite all their precautions, here was his father—trapped like a fly in the spider's web of tubes and wires he specifically wanted to avoid. As the ICU attending observed: "This was really, really difficult for the son... He saw his dad in the intensive care unit, intubated, with a [nasogastric] tube, with central lines, and a [urinary] catheter and the whole full court press of supportive measures. But again, Mr. Jan was also stabilized and his oxygenation was better. The son was incredibly torn as to what step to take."

Although legal scholars and medical ethicists agree that the decision to withdraw life-sustaining treatment is no different from the decision to initiate it, to a family member tasked with pulling the plug, the two choices feel like night and day. Should the son ask the doctors to disconnect the life support, since that was his father's wish? Or should he leave things the way they were, since the "damage" (in this case, an undesired resuscitation) had already been done? After all, Tung Jan was sedated and seemed relatively comfortable, and other family members would arrive soon and might want to see him while he lived, even if it was for one last time. The decision to pull out the breathing tube now seemed much weightier than the one they made a few months earlier not to put it in at all.

Jan's son said he needed more time to talk with family members and think through the situation, so the doctors continued to aggressively support his father through the night. This was torture for the doctors and nurses, too. Everyone wanted to lighten Mr. Jan's sedation so he could spend some meaningful time with his family, but every time they did he became combative and tried to yank the breathing tube out of his lungs. Finally, the medical team and the son agreed to remove the tube in a careful, controlled manner and see if Jan could breathe on his own. Physicians often compare these trials off the ventilator to test flights; and to everyone's surprise,

Jan "flew" on his own. A few days later, he was discharged back to the nursing home.

Once back in the home, "I made sure the [DNR] documentation was there," Jan's son said, "and that it was sure to be followed thereafter. Even though I was glad that he came back, I didn't want him to have to go through that again."

Soon thereafter, Tung Jan entered hospice care and died, peacefully, two months later.

On the surface, Tung Jan's story might seem to be about life-ending choices: Whether to respect a dying patient's preferences or bring all available medical weapons to bear to keep the grim reaper at bay. Neither choice is as obvious as it seems. As Dr. Joanne Lynn, a national expert in end-of-life care, points out: Many of us will suffer from serious chronic illness at the time of our death, but the suddenness of the end surprises patients, family members, even doctors. In one study, on the day before emphysema patients died, their physicians thought they had a 20 percent chance of surviving another six months. Just one week earlier, the average patient was given a nearly 50–50 chance at six-month survival.

The second story behind Jan's case, however, shows not just the difficulty of life-and-death decisions, but the hidden traps and roadblocks on the road to a smooth and effective transition in patient care.[1] Although every handoff between caregivers takes place over potentially dangerous gaps, the crack through which Tung Jan's DNR instructions fell was wide enough literally to drive an ambulance through. This was doubly distressing to the professionals involved because the error took place while moving a patient from one well-equipped and well-staffed health care facility to another—places where you'd think such things would not and could not happen.

In the late 1980s, researchers in North Carolina designed a program to aggressively promote the use of advance directives, such as Mr. Jan's, in nursing homes. The effort was moderately

---

[1] In the next few chapters, we will return to this issue of advance directives and DNR orders to illustrate several very different types of errors.

successful: 126 mentally competent nursing home residents and forty-nine families representing patients with advanced dementia completed these forms, which were then placed in the nursing home charts. However, when patients from these homes became ill and were transferred to local hospitals, only *one in three* advance directives went with them. This is even worse than it sounds, since the nursing homes involved knew they were part of a study on this very issue, and were more likely to pay attention to such protocols. The real track record for institutions, patients, and families in other, less controlled environments is undoubtedly much poorer—and these fumbles aren't confined to the gaps between institutions, but can occur anywhere, even if a hospitalized patient never leaves the bed.

Joe Silber's chest pain wasn't going away. The forty-three-year-old mechanic, an avid racquetball player, had made it past the ER's gatekeepers and was admitted for observation and further tests. So far, things looked good. His blood work showed no elevation in troponin, the cardiac enzyme released by damaged heart muscles, and each of several EKGs turned out OK. Although his pain persisted through much of his ER stay, he was completely "ruled out for MI," no alternative causes emerged, and he was reassured by the doctors that the pain was nothing to worry about.

Although there was little clinical reason for it, Silber's ER physician also ordered a chest X-ray. While this is important if the chest-pain patient also complains of breathing problems or a cough, it is more of a dot-the-i's and cross-the-t's (and C-your-A!) kind of test for patients who lack lung symptoms. Since nobody expected Silber's X-ray to yield anything exciting, and since there was no checklist or protocol to remind anyone to check it, it was forgotten as soon as it was taken.

Twelve hours later, after all of the heart attack tests proved negative, Silber was prepped for discharge. By now, the hospital shifts had changed, and the new physician overseeing the discharge was unaware that the X-ray even existed. She gave Silber a clean bill of health and told him to schedule a follow-up appointment with his regular doctor. By now, his chest pain had subsided and Silber was anxious to get back to normal life, including his racquetball game.

Meanwhile, the hospital's radiologist had reviewed the X-ray and noticed a small lung nodule. In the old days, radiologists waited to be asked about results. However, after a slew of big malpractice suits involving unreported mammogram abnormalities, radiologists are now proactive in making sure somebody, somewhere gets the word—especially when dealing with biggies, like potential breast and lung cancer. In this case, since the discharging attending was not the patient's regular physician, the report was called in to the primary physician's office and a paper version was sent as backup.

The primary physician's partner received the paper report (the telephone report apparently got lost in the shuffle) and he rerouted it through interoffice mail to his colleague. Somehow, the report got lost in mailroom limbo, and Silber's primary doctor never saw it. Over the next couple of years, Silber came to see Dr. Hewitt half-a-dozen times, for cholesterol, for belly pain, and for a rash. Since neither knew of the chest film's findings, it, of course, was never discussed.

Two years later, Joe Silber developed a chronic cough and a repeat chest X-ray revealed an obvious lung nodule. The radiologist's report read, "the nodule is markedly enlarged compared to the one seen on the X-ray of October 18, 1999." That was the first Dr. Hewitt had heard of the prior X-ray, and it was too late. Eighteen months after that, Joe Silber was dead—another victim of lung cancer. We can't be sure if Silber's life would have been saved by a more timely diagnosis of this terrible disease; but in those cases where cure or remission is possible, it's usually because of early detection, often serendipitously on an X-ray ordered for another purpose.

The Tung Jan and Joe Silber cases, despite their obvious differences, have one big thing in common. Both patients suffered from fumbled handoffs between otherwise competent and caring professionals. These handoffs—between and within institutions—occur millions of times each day in hospitals, doctors' offices, and laboratories all over the country. Each one is like a complex electrical circuit: Push the wrong button, leave a switch open, drop a live wire, or spill a little coffee on the machinery, and a vital record—even a life—can go up in smoke.

Although every handoff carries the potential for information loss, the most worrisome is at hospital discharge. Part of this is because patients are usually left "to their own recognizance," which means it's up to them to obtain and take their meds, observe any physical precautions, and make follow-up appointments with their primary care physicians or recommended specialists. Many patients—particularly the elderly or others with unstable home lives—are incapable of taking these important steps.

This problem has been magnified in the last twenty years by the economic drive to discharge patients promptly— "sicker and quicker." A 2003 study found that nearly one in five patients experienced an adverse event during the transition from hospital to home, two-thirds of which could have been prevented or ameliorated with better care across the divide. In one case, a patient was started on a new heart medicine known to cause major swings in blood potassium, but no post-discharge plans for monitoring blood chemistry were put in place. The patient developed extreme weakness and was eventually found to have a potassium level *double* the normal range—enough to have been fatal. Studies have shown that a simple follow-up call by a doctor, nurse, or pharmacist could prevent many post-discharge errors, but few hospitals have hardwired these protocols into their system, mostly because nobody wants to pay for the service.

Even knowledgeable and well-connected patients aren't immune from handoff fumbles. Bob's dad, seventy-three, now living in a retirement community in Boca Raton, Florida, was diagnosed with prostate cancer in 1998. He received his initial care from a urologist in suburban New Jersey and then from another, quite prominent urologist at a famous Northeastern hospital. His cancer, discovered like so many others after an elevated PSA level was detected in a routine blood test, was small, so the superstar urologist recommended "watchful waiting." This is tough for a lot of men, and it was particularly tough in the Florida retirement community since most of the tennis crowd seemed to have prostate cancer and they had all done *something* (the group had even taken to betting hi-low on each other's PSAs after each other's doctor visits). But Bob reviewed the evidence with his father, and, because the tumor was very small, they agreed that the conservative strategy was sound.

Bob's dad had left the Northeast and was now living in Boca Raton year-round, so it seemed wise to find a new primary caregiver and new set of specialists in Florida. He made an appointment with a Miami urologist, who sensibly asked to see all the records from up north. The patient signed the appropriate releases, then took to the phone to try to gather up the records himself. That's when the fun began.

Three calls to the New Jersey urologist connected him to three different back-office assistants, none of whom could find the appropriate records. His calls to the Northeastern cancer center hit an even bigger wall. The famous urologist referred him to medical records, which referred him back to the specialist's office, which told him to ask the pathology department directly for the slides, then call the radiologist for the X-rays. Three weeks later, no records, slides, or X-rays had been sent. Bob's dad made another round of calls to everyone he had talked to, then placed a final call to his son.

"What the hell kind of system do you have here?" he demanded.

"Welcome to my world" was the only thing Bob could say.

Two weeks after that, a FedEx arrived from the Mecca. Bob's dad tore open the package and began reading. One record said, "Diagnosis: Adenocarcinoma of the prostate, Stage T2 N0 M0." He didn't know what the initials meant, but he had heard the term *adenocarcinoma* before. Another read, "Operation: Radical Retropubic Prostatectomy"—that came as news to his prostate, which was still where it had been placed as original equipment. The chart went on: "The patient wishes to discuss his potency. He grades his potency as approximately 20 percent on Viagra."

That didn't sound familiar at all. So he looked up at the name on the record. Not surprisingly, it read Daniel Levy, not Murray Wachter.

Some analysts think the answer to all our dropped balls is to simply reduce the number of handoffs. As legendary Ohio State football coach Woody Hayes once said of a forward pass, "when you put the ball in the air, three things can happen and two of them are bad." Maybe we'd be better off if medicine just stuck to the "ground game" and did more things with the same team in the same place.

Unfortunately, transitions in health care—whether made on the fly or with plenty of deliberation—are an inevitable by-product of technological and clinical progress. In the old days, Dr. Marcus Welby (or somebody like him) would see you in his office, make housecalls when you were sick, and remove your appendix or deliver your baby in the hospital. From a continuity of care standpoint, this kind of system was ideal; but around the 1960s it bumped heads with a couple of significant trends.

First, techniques in even the most basic treatments and surgeries were becoming so varied and sophisticated that no one doctor could keep up with them, no less perform them all reliably. Physicians began to focus, as organ-based specialists (such as cardiologists for hearts, dermatologists for skin, and so on), disease-based specialists (like oncologists), or procedure-based specialists (like hand or thoracic surgeons). Second, as we saw earlier, practice really does make perfect; those doctors with the best outcomes were those who tended to treat similar patients with similar problems using similar techniques. When you show up at your local ER, you want a doctor experienced in trauma care and acute conditions to greet you—not wait forty minutes until "Dr. Welby" shows up, which is how most emergency care was dispensed forty years ago. One of the newest specialties, in fact, is our own—the *hospitalist*: a physician who focuses his practice on the care, coordination, and safety of hospitalized patients.

Although some people lament this panoply of specialists and the handoffs they make necessary, few would go back to the "good old days" of the one-size-fits-all generalist for every condition. Research has confirmed the benefits of these new hospital-based specialists (both hospitalists and intensivists, physicians who specialize in critical care), because their extra training, professional focus, and experience with complex cases—not to mention their on-site, often around-the-clock availability—is too often simply indispensable.

Another benefit of specialization and centralization is that caregivers—doctors, nurses, pharmacists, and technicians—who work together in a particular department or at a particular function, be it in the OR, the ER, the cath lab, or at Code Blues, will see themselves as a team, train for common or unusual events (from the occasional train wreck to a bioterrorism attack) and implement the latest techniques and safety procedures in their field. This isn't going to happen when such things are left to your favorite folksy family doctor, who—acting as primary caregiver for thousands of patients—must complete his hospital rounds before the sun comes up, then rush back to his office to see patients every fifteen minutes until 5 P.M., then return all his phone calls and, as the afternoon shadows lengthen into night and commuter headlights snap on, spend a few hours catching up on his professional journals. Handoffs are here to stay.

Sadly, fumbles can occur even when your doctor never leaves your bedside.

Gino Cervone, a big, vigorous sixty-four-year-old who loved to play backgammon, fix old cars, and cook vats of gnocchi and marinara sauce for his grandchildren, was in a bad way. Admitted two days earlier to a ward on the seventh floor of a major hospital, he was suffering from a severe urinary tract infection. Initially stabilized, he had rapidly "detuned," as physicians say, and become increasingly confused—perhaps from anoxia or uremic poisoning.

The usual "name the last five presidents" mental status test was now moot: He thought he was in church and no longer knew his name. His blood pressure had plummeted and his breathing was labored.

Tom Rivers, his physician—a conscientious *mensch* in horn-rimmed glasses who looked more like Woody Allen than George Clooney—eyeballed Cervone and quickly decided he would be safer in the hospital's fourth floor ICU, where he could be continuously monitored and, if necessary, hooked up to a mechanical breathing device. Rivers called the ICU, which agreed to the transfer.

Rivers checked his watch—it was 10:18 P.M.—and called over Debbie Lovett, an athletic, experienced floor nurse who towered over the diminutive doctor. Together, they wheeled Mr. Cervone's hospital bed out of his room for the three-minute trip to the fourth floor.

Of course, Gilligan's tour on the S.S. *Minnow* was only supposed to take three hours.

It took them a minute to reach the seventh floor's two wide-doored service elevators, where they punched the down button. Trips to the ICU are often accomplished in an atmosphere of anxiety, if not near-panic, but this situation seemed under control. The patient was quite ill, but not moribund. In the vivid language of hospitals, he was not yet "circling the drain." Still, there was no time to waste. The six passenger elevators around the corner in the floor's main lobby ran a little more often, but the hospital beds were too big to fit in them, so transfers like these had to use the slower and bigger service elevators. They waited.

The hospital had strict policies about who could use these wider elevators: They were reserved for patients on their way to surgeries, X-rays, or the dozens of other services and labs located on other floors. The service elevators were also reserved for emergency response (Code Blue) teams, whose members had their own override keys to summon an elevator and rocket it directly to the destination floor. These policies, of course, were ignored by almost everyone. Maintenance crews, janitors, staff, and even administrators often rode the service elevators when it was convenient, punching the button for their own floors while the paying customers, trembling in their gurneys, anxious to get on with their procedures, went along for the ride. As far as special "Code team" keys went, like the house keys you've given to countless repairmen and housecleaners over the years, nobody really knew how many were out there, and more than a few had been duplicated and were now in the hands of hospital staff who figured their lunch breaks after a hard morning were as big a priority as anything. Rivers and Lovett continued to wait.

To kill time, the doctor made small talk about the endless construction going on in the building. Nurse Lovett agreed, as she drummed her fingers nervously on the patient's bed rail. After a couple of minutes, Rivers looked up and groaned.

"Jesus Friggin Christ!" he swore. A piece of paper was Scotch-taped in the upper right-hand corner of the second elevator. On it was scrawled in barely legible ballpoint pen: *Out of Service for Repair.* Their wait, whatever it was normally, would now be twice as long.

Rivers glanced at his patient. Mr. Cervone looked a bit sweatier, and shifted uncomfortably under the thin hospital sheet. Rivers took his pulse. It was strong, and his labored breathing seemed steady. Still, the unblinking white elevator call light taunted him… He strained to hear the rumble of cables behind the door, but there was nothing.

Rivers checked his watch. It was now almost 10:25. Seven minutes and counting… Nurse Lovett pointed out that the patient had started panting and was getting more restless under the sheet.

"Goddamnit," Rivers said. "I don't know if this sucker's coming."

"Want to put him on a gurney?" Lovett suggested. The narrower gurney would fit into the smaller passenger elevators around the corner, but transferring a 225-pound, almost delirious patient would be a big challenge for the diminutive doctor and a single nurse. Still…

"OK, let's give it a try," Rivers said.

Lovett called to another floor nurse to bring a gurney, but after more minutes wasted in a frantic search of the ward, none was found.

The portable oximeter attached to Cervone's index finger now showed his blood oxygen level starting to fall.

"Forget the gurney," Rivers spat. "Get the ICU Team up here, stat."

Since there was a good chance now that his patient would need a breathing tube before they could get to the ICU, Rivers decided it would be smart to have a qualified acute care team on hand in case his breathing stopped. The "Code Blue" squad was expert in managing critically ill patients, and they came equipped with the required paraphernalia. This time, the mountain would come to Mohammed.

Another nurse was dispatched to the central nursing station to phone the ICU and get the team on its way. Meanwhile, Rivers had a brainstorm.

"Wait a minute," he said. "Forget about *our* service elevators— let's use the ones in the other wing."

"You mean at the other end of the complex?"

Lovett's skepticism was well founded. The huge hospital indeed had another wing—actually, a separate, massive building connected to their wing by a long corridor. It had its own bank of elevators, of course, including four service elevators dedicated to bed-ridden patients. If they hustled, they could get down the long hall, into a service elevator, go to the fourth floor, then backtrack down the corridor on that floor to the ICU while the Crash Team was still packing their gear.

Without further discussion, they set off down the long, polished corridor.

Halfway down the seldom-used corridor, they ran into a wall of plastic sheeting and a row of plywood slabs sealing off the hall. On one of them, however, was cut a flimsy door secured with a small padlock—undoubtedly used by the construction crew and left open during working hours. At 10:30 in the evening, of course, it was locked.

They screeched to a stop and Rivers checked his patient. Cervone's skin tone had gone from mottled pink to an ominous gray-blue. His mouth worked feverishly—saying nothing, just babbling like a baby.

"What the hell—we gotta get this guy to ICU—" Almost comically, Rivers made a run for the plywood door, plowed into it with his shoulder, and bounced back like a Ping-Pong ball.

"Wait a minute—wait a minute!" came a voice behind them in the corridor. It was a heavy-set nurse from the floor's main station trotting toward them with a set of keys on a big steel ring. While Lovett watched the patient, Rivers and the nurse went through five or six keys before finding the one that opened the lock. Rivers flung open the plywood door, and with Lovett on one side and himself on the other, wheeled Cervone from the brightly lit hall into the eerie dark of the construction zone.

They pushed the big bed like a creaky, oversized shopping cart—tentatively first, then like shoppers at a holiday sale. Built neither for speed nor agility, it bounced over power cords and skidded through sawdust, bumped into a sawhorse and knocked a half-finished can of Coke to the concrete floor.

After a minute in the dark, they made out another makeshift door in the plywood panels ahead, the light seeping in from the cracks guiding them like a beacon. They lined the bed up with the door and were gearing up to barrel into it like a battering ram, when they noticed something that took *their* breath away. The door was not as wide as the one they used to enter the construction zone; instead it was six inches too narrow. The bed wouldn't fit. They had to go back.

Meanwhile, the Code Blue team had rushed up in the passenger elevators and swarmed into Cervone's room. Finding it empty, they ran to the nurse's station, where they were told that the patient was on his way to the ICU. Thinking the floor's service elevator had finally come while they were in transit, they rumbled back down the steps so they could meet Cervone when he arrived on the fourth floor.

By this time, Rivers and Lovett had navigated their way from the construction zone and back into the corridor that led to their wing. The nurse with the key ring was astonished to see them come back. Before she could say anything, Rivers barked: "A wheelchair. Get us a wheelchair. There's gotta be a wheelchair somewhere on this goddamned floor!"

Cervone was now nearly comatose and blue from lack of oxygen. By some miracle, a wheelchair was produced and they struggled to get his 225-pound frame off the bed and into the seat. Again, they rushed for the elevator lobby—but this time for the passenger elevators. A wheelchair is not the best place for a patient with low blood pressure, since the upright position limits the already limited amount of oxygen available to the brain. But any port—or mode of transit—in a storm.

Waiting for at least *one* of the red triangles above the shiny steel doors to illuminate and go *ding*, Rivers looked again at his watch. It was 10:42—nearly twenty minutes since he made the first call to "Code" his patient.

The elevator door finally opened and a few startled passengers stepped back as Rivers and Lovett commandeered their car and stabbed the fourth floor button. With Mr. Cervone comatose and Rivers struggling to hold the chair in "wheelie" position to keep at least a few drops of blood in his brain, the door opened again and they dashed into the ICU.

Gino Cervone suffered severe and irreversible brain damage during his odyssey, and died a week later. The death was recorded in hospital records as "cardiac arrest" due to "sepsis," a severe blood infection. A more accurate diagnosis would've been "death by elevator."

The subsequent investigation showed that both service elevators in Cervone's wing were out of commission on that fateful night. One had been shut down for several weeks for a long-scheduled upgrade. The other had broken down late that afternoon. Nobody had thought to put a separate sign on the door of the second elevator. Besides, building maintenance was on top of the problem. They had scheduled a crew to get on it first thing in the morning. And there were other functioning elevators on the floor, and four service elevators down the corridor in the second wing, so where was the big emergency? In this eighteen-story hospital, it never occurred to anyone—medical staff or administrators—that, with the corridor under construction, the downed service elevators had effectively severed the seventh floor's lifeline.

*　*　*

In a major report issued two years after the headline-grabbing IOM report on medical mistakes, the same institute published another finding that was even more damning of American health care. In *Crossing the Quality Chasm: A New Health System for the 21st Century*, the IOM portrayed a chaotic care delivery system that resembles a railroad whose tracks change gauge every few miles:

> Health care is composed of a large set of interacting systems—paramedic, emergency, ambulatory, inpatient, and home health care; testing and imaging laboratories; pharmacies; and so forth—that are connected in loosely coupled but intricate networks of individuals, teams, procedures, regulations, communications, equipment, and devices. These systems function within such diverse and diffuse management, accountability, and information structures that the overall term *health system* is today a misnomer.

Unfortunately, we see nothing on the horizon that promises to align the tracks of U.S. health care anytime soon. So while we wait, we need to focus on designing trains that are less dependent on rails.

One potential failure point in all of these interlocking systems is the basic unit of medical records: the piece of paper. Moving paper from one place to another is always a dicey matter: It can get misrouted, it can get lost, it can get trapped between two other pieces of paper and become invisible, it can be placed in the wrong file and—ultimately—it can contain the wrong information or, even if it's the right information, it can be misinterpreted or ignored. On an individual basis, a patient going from specialist to specialist and hospital to hospital over the years can accumulate records the way signatures pile up in an autograph book. And those autograph books can then become scrapbooks when other forms of records, such as X-rays and lab reports, are thrown in. The resulting ambiguities can be small (did this patient get his morning dose of antibiotics before transfer?), but often aren't. Consider the patient that arrived at our own medical center from a community hospital utterly paralyzed, his records silent about the dose of paralytic medication he erroneously received prior to transfer.

Of course, paperwork errors can go both ways. As Bob's dad's experience shows, big teaching hospitals are often black holes when it comes to getting important records to outside providers, or to patients.

Even "sign-outs" from one doctor to another can create unbridgeable gaps. Hospitalized patients are often cared for by a "covering" physician when their primary attendings or residents go off duty, such as on evenings and weekends. In a study at Brigham and Women's Hospital in Boston, researchers found that being covered, principally at night, by a different physician was a far better predictor of hospital complications and errors than was the severity of the patient's illness. The same researchers devised a standardized, computerized sign-out form and the error rate—from that particular gap, at least—fell by a factor of three.

Computers are an essential part of the answer, but only part. Even the fully wired hospital of the future will require thousands of oral handoffs each day. This is ultimately reduced to one person talking to another: face-to-face, by phone, even shouting unseen from another room. While medicine has largely ignored the errors created by oral handoffs, other industries that rely on unambiguous oral communications have developed some standard protocols to avoid common mistakes. Such protocols generally attack two potential problems—first: Is the information correct? Second: Has the overall message been received and understood?

In civil and military aviation, as well as in other branches of the service, including NATO, voice communication frequently involves use of the so-called phonetic alphabet. This simply substitutes a standardized word for a single letter, such as *Alpha* for "A," *Bravo* for "B," *Charlie* for "C," and so on. This permits one person to clarify a bit of information, such as the spelling of a name, without wasting time thinking of words that might have a common reference—the way 1-800 operators try to spell your name using words that make sense to them but may be Greek to you. ("Now let me get this straight, the name is Kaveh—K as in knight...")

Phonetic alphabets not only decrease the likelihood of miscommunication when pronouncing sound-alike letters such as T, D, P, and B, (which convert to Tango, Delta, Papa, and Bravo) as well as M and N (Mike and November), but create an accurate and efficient shorthand as well. Using this same system in a hospital, "Oscar Romeo" for Operating Room (OR) would never be confused with "Echo Romeo" for ER.

To prevent the second type of error—a message that may not have been properly received—"read-backs" are commonly used. For example, a pilot receiving clearance for a flight plan from Air Traffic Control over the radio *always* reads it back; just as the same pilot is supposed to acknowledge a directed change in altitude or heading by repeating the instructions. In health care, we have long used read-back procedures to verify the identity of blood transfusion recipients—which, if wrong, can be fatal (as witnessed by the 2003 tragedy at Duke University Medical Center, where a young heart-lung transplant patient died after receiving organs of the wrong blood type—a case we'll discuss later in the book). Still, doctors and nurses, technicians and pharmacists rarely take time to read back what they feel is obvious—with the occasional disastrous consequences. Even after the Duke transplant tragedy, you are far more likely to hear the reassuring words, "Let me read your order back to you," when you call your local Chinese takeout restaurant than we would be if we called the nurses' station of virtually any U.S. hospital.

Not surprisingly, integrated systems of care—those in which the same organization owns or runs the doctor's office, the nursing home, and the hospital—seem to manage handoffs better than the rest of us, although we've no reason to believe that their intrahospital or intraoffice fumble rate is any lower. Patients who leave a VA hospital for a nursing home generally go to a VA-owned facility; the same is true for patients in the huge Kaiser Permanente system and the other multi-institutional giants of health care.

The reason these handoffs go better is partly organizational, partly psychological, and partly informational.

Organizationally, when a single system is responsible for care on both sides of the specialty or facility gap, they collaborate on smoothing the transition and bear the consequence of any glitches. It's hard to pass the buck when the left hand knows what the right hand is supposed to be doing.

Psychologically, human beings simply communicate better and more often with people they know than with strangers—particularly if they feel those others are on the same team, have the same interests, and share the same goals.

From an informatics standpoint, large integrated health providers quite naturally devote more resources to constructing, maintaining, and improving the big computer systems that now seem so essential to medical communications. In the parlance of the second IOM report, they have more tracks with the same gauge, and thus fewer derailments.

One monkey wrench in even the best integrated system, however, is concern about patient privacy and the unauthorized use of medical information. These concerns, codified in the Healthcare Insurance Portability and Accountability Act (HIPAA), which went into effect in April 2003, pose a real barrier to developing a national medical database, or even to moving patient information from clinic to hospital and back out again. While abuses are always possible, at some point policymakers will have to balance the desirability of strict control over even trivial patient data with the *necessity* of linking systems to save lives in an increasingly mobile society. Frankly, it's hard to see how the hypothetical harm that might come to people whose EKGs, X-rays, or medication lists fall into unauthorized hands outweighs the tremendous advantages those same people gain when their medical data are available to nurses and doctors who need them. You can be sure that this tension—between privacy and accessibility of medical records—will become even more taut in coming years. As "Bones" McCoy used to say on *Star Trek*, "Damn it, Jim, we're doctors, not lawyers!" so our preference in this matter is clear, mostly because we know from firsthand experience what it's like trying to care for sick patients without critical parts of their medical history.

All in all, while it is important for patients to do all they can to prevent fumbles from happening (we'll make some detailed recommendations in the final section of the book, but they include always carrying your list of current medications and asking what any new medication is for), the burden of making transitions smooth and error-free rests with the professionals and the systems at their disposal. When Marcus Welby did everything, handoffs were no big deal—there just weren't that many to make. Today, no single physician can do everything—or know everything—it takes to keep you and make you well. We can't go back to those good old days of the '50s, and, quite frankly, few patients or caregivers would want to try.

In the past, we have been far too laissez-faire about handoffs and far too resistant to standard procedures. We need stricter protocols and checklists for transitions. We need standard read-backs for critical voice exchanges. We need "bridge the gap" training for caregivers on both sides of a transfer—to make our hypothetical health care system less virtual, more real, and better integrated. We need to talk to each other not just after we make mistakes, but before they happen.

CHAPTER 11: SEE ONE, DO ONE, TEACH ONE

Whatever you do, don't say, "OOPS!"

> — Traditional advice passed down from doctors to their students before they try their first procedure on a patient

Even in retrospect, it was a *very* hot day.

Philadelphia in the summer. Bob cringed at the mere thought of leaving his air-conditioned flat to head for the hospital. As he walked the five blocks, his shirt stuck damply to his chest, and sweat pooled in the small of his back. For some reason, his mind locked onto an image of rows of kielbasa, half-cooking in the heat as they hung from the rafters of the Italian Market, a mile away.

It was 1981. He was a second-year medical student at the University of Pennsylvania and today was the second day of his initial medical rotation. Penn's philosophy, ahead of its time but widely emulated since, was to expose students to patients early in the process. Part of this was to break the drudgery of endless classes in anatomy and biochemistry; the other was to introduce the practice of medical diagnosis and treatment. Its effect was to put a human face on all those facts. Nice idea, but it overlooked one small detail: Second-year students know next to nothing about medicine.

The novices had already spent one afternoon a week in the hospital during their first year, so they weren't completely virginal when it came to patients and their problems. In those sessions, the students were assigned to a single patient and asked to perform an "H&P"—a history and physical. The patients were hand-selected by the chief residents for their saintly patience and stoicism. Bob and his equally green colleagues struggled mightily to prepare, grappling first with the monumental: Do I introduce myself as "doctor," "student doctor," or "medical student"? (Bob settled on "student doctor," the compromise candidate.) That decided, each student bounded into his patient's room like Pooh's friend Tigger with a stethoscope: enthusiastic but a little bit goofy. They asked their questions and wrote on their crisp clean notebooks and tried out the physical exam techniques they'd just seen demonstrated in books and videos.

"Do you have gout?" Bob asked one particular guinea pig who had a flaming red nose and complained of pains in his toe.

"What's gout?" the patient asked.

Bob smiled sheepishly. "To tell you the truth, I don't really know."

That answer seemed to satisfy the patient. At least he knew he had an honest doctor.

But today was the start of the medicine rotation, and it was for real: no games, no handpicked patients, no videos. Each student joined a medical ward team and made real rounds, with real physicians, examining really sick people.

The team's leader is an "attending"—a senior faculty member who, back then, did a bit of teaching, but was mostly around to let patients feel they weren't being left entirely in the hands of amateurs. Many of these attendings spent most of their time doing basic science research; their one-month-per-year stints as team leader were their primary exposure to real patients each year—the way police officers who never draw their weapon still have to qualify at the pistol range. Although the medical residents regarded a truly knowledgeable and involved attending as a nice treat, they mostly fretted about getting stuck with one who would annoy them, step on their toes, or slow them down. The attending assigned to Bob's team was an arthritis specialist—a very pleasant guy in his late fifties who didn't know much about modern hospital care, and worried even less about it. Bob's resident was ecstatic. This meant the attending would mostly leave the team alone.

By now you've probably concluded that it is the resident who really runs the team, and—at least in those days—you'd be right.

The resident is a godlike figure whose mastery of medicine is staggering to a second-year student—despite the fact that most residents are only a couple of years out of medical school themselves. This month, Bob's resident was a brusque, brainy woman with what is known as a "surgical personality": tough as nails and ready to hammer those nails into any problem. "Be wrong, but don't be in doubt" seemed to be her motto. She was the kind of person who either liked you or didn't. Bob was worried.

The team also had two interns. These guys were as green as Bob was, but in a different, scarier way: They had recently finished medical school and so were technically MDs—but just barely. At a good school like Penn, they had probably been honors undergrads and sterling medical students, but now they were "scut dogs"—the bottom of the hospital's pecking order, whose main function was to do anything they were told. Residents asked them, "Did Mr. Jones get his chest X-ray?" Go fetch. "Did you fill out the form to get Mrs. Smith transferred to that nursing home? No?" Bad dog! Interns were the "we" residents referred to whenever they said, "*We* should do this."

Interns got some payback by supervising the guppies—the second-year students like Bob. Fortunately, the interns' lot was so miserable they actually appreciated their guppies' help, despite the students' near-total lack of useful skills. If a student was very cooperative and relieved them of some "scut"—like drawing blood or retrieving test results from the rat's nest of paper slips in the laboratory's shoe box—an intern might earmark a few minutes of his ninety-five-hour workweek to teach the student a thing or two about medicine, or life. It was a quid pro quo out of *Clockwork Orange*.

So the Team was a Band of Brothers and Sisters—trench buddies—and often it was "us" against "them." *Them*, in this case, was usually the system: hospital rules, hospital forms, and hospital bureaucrats, all of which seemed like land mines strategically buried in the path of getting anything done. Sometimes it was the nurses, though with them you learned quickly to bite your lip, since the nurses possessed the power to bail you out or make your life a living hell (the latter could come in the form of the 4:30 A.M. page: "Hello, Doctor. Just wanted you to know I'm about to draw Mr. Banzhaf's blood cultures"). Sometimes it was even the patients or their families. Now, don't get us wrong: These young doctors cared dearly about their patients and wanted only the best for them. But when you had a patient "on the launch pad"—ready for discharge—after a harrowing three-week stay, and *then* he develops a new complaint, being pissed *at him* was one of the many unattractive emotions that slithered to the surface of the sleep-deprived, anxious brew of our psyches.

So on this, the second day of his rotation, Bob entered the hospital—Philadelphia's Veterans' Hospital—concerned about taking good care of his patients, but even more concerned about meshing with the team. Like the kid transferring into a new school, fitting in was the most important goal. Everything else—learning, eating, bodily functions—was secondary. He resolved to be cheery, helpful, ingratiating, and benignly inquisitive. Anything but annoying.

The location of his rotation didn't help. The VA hospital (called the "Vah-Spa" by jaded doctors-in-the-know) was a drab old building that ran a poor second to the Hospital of the University of Pennsylvania (HUP). HUP was Penn's Mecca, its Holiest of Holies. The famous faculty stalked its halls like priests and peacocks. A letter of recommendation from one of them carried ten times the weight of one from the VA. HUP was the equivalent of Wall Street to a young banker; the Vah-Spa was the regional branch in Poughkeepsie.

Still, the VA had its advantages. The patients—all U.S. military veterans—were considered virtually indestructible. They seldom complained and didn't mind taking directions from fuzz-cheeked, almost-physicians. They had, after all, survived worse things than we could throw at them; and what soldier didn't know how to grin and bear it when a green-as-grass second lieutenant gave him orders? And Bob's first day had gone well enough. He'd located all the labs, stairwells, men's rooms, and the cafeteria. He'd learned the pecking order of his particular team and what nurses would and wouldn't do for you on the wards. He'd stayed out of trouble. Still, his biggest worry on this scorcher of a day, honest to God, was how stupid he'd look making rounds in a sweat-soaked shirt.

One of each student's jobs is to "pre-round" on his patients. Pre-rounding is a kind of reconnaissance mission, in which the intern or the student gives his assigned patients a quick once-over and tries to reconstruct what happened to them overnight. Then, at 8 A.M., the entire team (minus the attending) gathers together to begin "work rounds," during which the student or intern "presents" each patient to the resident, who checks their work and decides on the plan for the day. Later in the morning, they once again summarize all their findings and present their plans to their attending for his blessing, and possibly a little teaching. Together, Bob and his intern had eight patients to pre-round on. In keeping with their relative efficiency, Bob was assigned three to check; his intern would pre-round on the other five.

The pre-round routine was always the same. If patients were asleep, wake 'em up. Ask how they feel (sleepy didn't count as an answer), check their vital signs, and briefly listen to their hearts and lungs. Quickly scan the chart to see if there had been any "events" (changes in status or new medications during the night), then move on. Bob arrived at 6:30 A.M., which gave him ninety minutes to pre-round on three patients. Piece of cake.

Unfortunately, his first patient took a bit more time than he had budgeted. He was a ruddy, jovial guy from Northeast Philly who rose early and chatted endlessly about the weather, the Phillies, the lousy VA food, and his colorful military career. He would've undoubtedly started on his analysis of the Big War if Bob hadn't found a polite way to extricate himself. It was now 7:10—ten minutes behind schedule.

Bob hustled to the second patient's room. As we say, this was an older VA hospital, so its amenities would have made Florence Nightingale feel at home. This particular room was a mini-ward, with a single sink and four beds separated by flimsy curtains that provided only the illusion of privacy. All were filled, and each patient sat up as Bob came in. But his quarry was Mr. Adams, a seventy-one-year-old who was showing signs of congestive heart failure after a recent hip operation. The room's big window faced east, so the morning sun bore into it like a laser. The atmosphere was stuffy and oppressive.

Mr. Adams sat upright in his bed, sweating profusely and panting like an overheated pug. He looked terrible. Bob checked his lungs with his stethoscope, straining to hear the crackling sounds of pulmonary edema—a sign that his failing heart was getting worse. Nope—in fact they sounded pretty clear. He then checked the vital sign log sheet—a periodic record of a patient's heart rate, respiration, temperature, and so on. He found Mr. Adams's heart and respiratory rates had both increased, but he wasn't feverish. He did look awful—his forehead dripped with perspiration and his bed rattled with every heave of his chest—but he didn't seem to have heart failure or, without a fever, pneumonia. From his classes, Bob knew a lot about embryogenesis (how babies develop in the womb) and mitochondrial biochemistry (don't ask), but he really couldn't think of anything that would explain Mr. Adams's peculiar symptoms and signs. So—when in doubt, ask the patient.

"Well, Mr. Adams, looks like you're having a rough morning. What do *you* think is going on?"

"It's really hot in here, doc," Adams panted. And it was. That's what it must be, Bob thought; overheated like an old car.

Bob completed his checklist and told Adams that the rest of the team would be around to see him again at about nine. The patient smiled gamely and gave a feeble good-bye wave. Bob left the room with as much dignity as he could muster, trying not to feel like a complete impostor.

The good-bye wave turned out to be appropriate. At 8:40 A.M., Bob's team was assembled and rounding on its fifth patient when the loudspeakers blared, "Code Blue, Room 307. Code Blue, 307."

"Who's that?" the resident shouted, already sprinting down the stairs.

"Oh, shit—" the intern answered, two steps behind her. "Adams is in that room."

The team arrived to find Mr. Adams motionless on the sweaty sheets. While the resident went right to work on CPR, the intern drew the flimsy privacy curtain, separating Adams's terrified roommates from the Code Blue scene. It was an absurd gesture: The three patients could hear every sound and see the bulging outlines of the doctors and nurses through the curtains. The resident turned to Bob.

"Wachter, what did he look like when you saw him this morning?"

"He told me he was a tiny bit short of breath. But he looked OK," Bob lied. He couldn't help himself: The words just came out. Shame replaced the humid heat in his red cheeks.

Mr. Adams's autopsy showed he had suffered a massive pulmonary embolism—a big gooey blood clot had formed in his legs, broken off, and found its way to his lungs, in an instant knocking out half of his breathing capacity. Looking back, Bob realized the patient's "presentation" (the symptoms he reported and his findings on exam) was textbook—heavy perspiration, shortness of breath despite clear lungs, the time interval between major hip surgery and the onset of respiratory problems—all of it fit.

The only problem was that it was a textbook the second-year med students hadn't yet read, and Bob was too naive, scared, insecure, proud, and anxious to fit in to ask a real doctor to help out when it might have done some good.

In *Complications*, Harvard surgical resident Atul Gawande describes the terrible paradox of medical training:

> In medicine, we have long faced a conflict between
> the imperative to give patients the best possible care

and the need to provide novices with experience. Residencies attempt to mitigate potential harm through supervision and graduated responsibility... But there is still no getting around those first few unsteady times a young physician tries to put in a central line, remove a breast cancer, or sew together two segments of colon. No matter how many protections we put in place, on average, these cases go less well with the novice than with someone experienced.

This is the uncomfortable truth about teaching. By traditional ethics and public insistence (not to mention court rulings), a patient's right to the best care possible must trump the objective of training novices. We want perfection without practice. Yet everyone is harmed if no one is trained for the future. So learning is hidden behind drapes and anesthesia and the elisions of language.

We remember all too well our own days as students, interns, and residents. And how could we not? The adrenaline-pumping, high-stakes encounters with seriously ill patients is drama enough, but the overlay of uncertainty, anxiety, and embarrassment renders them literally unforgettable. Take, for example, our first attempts to place an IV into a live patient: "Ow! What the hell are you doing?" they exclaim, unlike the docile grapefruits we practiced on. We toss one citrus and grab another; but the live patient still confronts us, as we nervously search his sterilized, outstretched arm for a site for our second or third attempt.

As bad as these IV attempts were, at least they were a solitary slice of hell; the early procedures we did with the resident present were worse. For our first spinal tap, we stood behind the patient— who was uncomfortably contorted on the bed in the shape of a human question mark—our resident stood beside us, and we tried to sound confident despite the overwhelming feeling of nausea.

"OK, Mr. Driscoll, you're gonna feel a little bee sting, then some pressure—"

Meanwhile, our resident is gesturing frantically that our entry angle is all wrong, wordlessly signaling that our needle's path has as much chance of striking oil as spinal fluid. All this patter and pantomime is pulled off in an atmosphere of cheery professionalism, as we try our best to hide our sense of quiet desperation from the patient, who remains awkwardly coiled on his side. It's a show, put on by very amateur actors.

But, as bad as trainees feel, we now know that supervisors feel even worse. Novices can only do what they can do, and if they screw it up, well—they're novices, what do you expect? Residents and attendings, though, sweat both the novice *and* the procedure. We know we could do things better, faster, and safer ourselves; but that's not what teaching is about. Instead, we grit our teeth and follow our pre-procedure briefing with a few well-placed grunts and "uh-uhs" and the body English of parents watching their teenager back a car from the garage.

In 1970, Charles Bosk, the Penn sociologist who tagged along with surgical residents for eighteen months and shared his experiences in *Forgive and Remember*, wrote of the teaching supervisor:

> On the one hand, he needs to restrain himself from taking charge of situations too quickly, lest he damage a subordinate's confidence. On the other hand, he needs to know when to rescue a subordinate—and patient—lest a surgical accident shake the novice's belief in his abilities.

For those of us who supervise doctors-in-training, the critical issue is not whether we will "grab the steering wheel"—of course we will, if the danger is obvious and imminent. Rather, the dominant question is: How long do we wait before doing it? Most experienced professionals—certainly those with experience teaching—can see many slips and errors coming long before students have any inkling they're headed for trouble. Most of us modulate our coaching to the abilities and attitude of the student. A good, conscientious learner responds well to subtle suggestions until, eventually, such suggestions aren't needed. A massively talented but cocky apprentice, on the other hand, may need a few trips to the precipice—a good scare or two—before *he convinces himself* that more caution and humility is in order. This is nothing unique to medicine, but the consequences of misreading a student, or a situation, in our profession can be particularly devastating.

Medical faculty members and supervising physicians are terribly conflicted about all of this. To closely supervise a trainee, we must be in the trenches with them most of the time, including nights and weekends. That's not practical for any profession, at least over the long haul. When a teacher or supervisor says, "You can't pay me enough to do that," they usually mean you *won't* pay them for the hours and psychic involvement everyone knows the task demands.

Consider a patient admitted to the hospital with severe congestive heart failure at 10:00 A.M. In an academic hospital, the patient is usually admitted by the ER or by a community doctor to one of our medical teams. He is quickly assessed by the resident, assisted by the interns, who then calls the supervising physician (us) with a one-line synopsis of the case. (Fifteen years ago, even *that* call wouldn't happen; the attendings often didn't hear about a new patient—for whom they were legally responsible—until the next day's rounds). Our practice now is to run down to see the patient— putting everything else in our very busy, multitasking academic life on hold: answering e-mails, returning phone calls, preparing lectures, writing or editing research journal articles, preparing for committee meetings, working up next year's budget, or seeing other patients in the clinic—the list goes on and on.

Now we arrive at the patient's bedside. The resident describes the case in greater detail and we briefly examine the patient. The intern follows us intently. We make a few observations, do a little teaching ("Make sure you consider the possibility of pericardial tamponade in a cancer patient with elevated neck veins"), ask our trainees a couple of follow-up questions—and recommend initial treatment. Then *bang*—we step back on our academic treadmill, while the residents stick with the case: consulting specialists, ordering tests, reviewing the patient's previous chart (these can be voluminous with chronically ill patients), looking at X-rays. At some point, we submit our bill to the insurance company for clinical services—it's typically about seventy-five bucks for an hour's work. Even if we spent the next ten hours with the patient, we wouldn't receive another dime. And even if the patient benefited from that extra one-on-one attention from senior staff, our other duties would go unfulfilled—those e-mails and phone calls (many of which deal with other patients) would go unanswered; our well-prepared lecture would turn into a rambling, improvised monologue; those research proposals and journal articles would never get written—leaving our institution and our profession just a little bit poorer.

So we tell the residents to "carry on"—implement their treatment plan, perform the needed procedures, and "call us if you need help." Of course, they sometimes do; but mostly they don't. The next morning—after most of the clinical dust has settled—we all sit down for formal "attending rounds," at which time we review the patients in more detail and spend an hour or so teaching our trainees. We also make mid-course corrections in the treatment plan, which are sometimes needed.

This admonition to "call for help"—Bosk calls it the "no surprises" rule—has several unspoken meanings. Decoded, it means (at one level) "call if you need help; but if you call *too* often we're going to wonder about your confidence and competence." At another level, it also means, "If you screw up, be sure you call me *first* before I hear about it from someone else." In this tug-of-war, students and residents generally learn that it is safer, career-wise, to deliver bad news personally than to have it reported behind their backs. But there is a lot of guesswork that goes into this calibration.

As a result, many residents hesitate to call—either to ask for help in a genuine crisis or report a screwup they caused themselves. As one trainee said, "The way you learn as an intern is by being put on the spot and coming through it. You develop a self-awareness that you can handle a lot of situations. The problem is learning what situations you can't handle. There's a lot of pressure not to ask, a lot of fear of appearing foolish."

The attendings are torn about this, too. We can't pitch, catch, and play first base at the same time, no matter how badly we might want to; and accepting other obligations—in classroom teaching, research, or administration—means letting go of some of the things we used to do. An attending surgeon interviewed by Bosk summed it up this way:

> I know a lot of patients complain that they don't see us around; they think we're not concerned. What they don't understand is that just because we're not there doesn't mean we don't know what's going on. I talk to [the chief resident] every day... I have complete confidence in [him]. I've helped train him for the last five years. When the year started I really stood over his shoulder; but now I know that if he runs into anything that he can't handle, he'll call me... Look, everybody expects Mehta to conduct the orchestra; but they don't expect him to play every instrument himself.

The traditional model of medical education—dominated by unfettered resident autonomy—is, thankfully, giving way to something better. We now recognize that "learning from mistakes" is fundamentally unethical when it is built into the system: using patients as disposable training aids by student-doctors who are, by definition, unqualified, or marginally qualified, for a procedure is indefensible. It is also flawed thinking to assume trainees will even *know* when they need help, particularly if they are thrust into the performance arena with little or no practice and supervision.

This has led not only to some system reforms, but also to a crack in the dike of academic medical culture. The two of us now stay regularly at our hospital late into the evening while our residents admit new patients. That practice—two senior attendings simply *being there* as routine tasks unfold—would have been judged as pathologically obsessive only twenty years ago. We remember from those days one conscientious, forward-looking attending who did what we're doing now—and was derided by colleagues as "the world's oldest intern." If by that they meant he was a physician who never quit learning and demanded quality care for every patient, we agree, and would happily accept the epithet ourselves.

In the late 1990s, Bob was in the hospital at 11 P.M. as his team admitted a patient with multiple organ failure. As always, he gave his team first crack at a workup and diagnosis—the "good supervisor" playbook tells us to give trainees a chance to evaluate a patient before stepping in, like Moses, and laying down the law. The patient was terribly ill. Nothing in her body was working right. Blood oozed from every break in her skin and IV site, her lungs choked with edema fluid, and she was stuporous. The results of her blood tests looked as if they came from a random number generator. The situation was dire—and confusing.

"What do you think?" Bob asked a bit tersely—this was one of those situations where you didn't have time for a lot of Socratic questions and hand-holding. "Shall we call in some consultants? Maybe a hematologist? Somebody from infectious disease?"

"No," a second-year resident said resolutely. He had been out of medical school for all of thirteen months. "I think I've got a handle on this."

"Well, I've been at this for fifteen years," Bob said, marveling yet again at the unalloyed confidence of the novice, "and I don't have the foggiest idea what to do. Let's get some help."

And so they did. In cases like these, the medical lesson—the patient had a rare but treatable hematologic disease called thrombotic thrombocytopenic purpura—is probably less important than the life lesson: Know when you're out of your depth. And harder to inculcate.

Thankfully, the old culture of guess-and-stumble, and "If you can't be right, be certain" is changing. Both residents and faculty realize the need for better oversight of training, especially when it comes to hands-on healing. The obstacles now are mostly financial. Contrary to lay opinion, teaching time is *not* reimbursed, so material incentives that might put more attendings back on the floor are lacking. Altruism is great and it's why most of us joined the profession, but if we're going to break up physicians' families and send those practitioners to early graves, we should at least compensate them for their time.

Some old-school teachers raise other questions. They fear that too much clinical oversight will create a generation of timid, buck-passing doctors—the same way overcontrolling parents create kids who grow up to be insecure or bossy. Seeking the right balance between autonomy and interdependence is what education is all about. In medicine, the pendulum had swung too far toward the former and, in our high-tech, error-prone system, a swing back toward collegial caregiving—mutual support openly solicited and freely given—is a necessary and welcome correction.

There are many things that are very broken in American health care, but the training system works relatively well. Despite being buffeted by the winds of the marketplace, we've managed to retain our reverence for education and service, and we're beginning to find the sweet spot between autonomy and oversight. But we can do better. We continue to suffer from the lack of compensation and support for teachers, no real systematic approach to teaching trainees about systems thinking, and a paucity of methods for training the doctors and nurses of tomorrow to act like players on the same team, a point we'll return to later in the book.

* * *

Ask the average person why residents and interns make so many mistakes and he or she will likely reply, "Oh, it's those backbreaking schedules. The poor dears never get any sleep!"

Like so many myths and legends, there's more than a grain of truth to this one. The typical residents' schedule hasn't changed much since we were in their shoes. At its core is the ritual of being "on call," which means staying in the hospital overnight—sleeping only if you can—to care for sick patients. Bad as things are now, they have improved since the mid-1900s. Back then, many residents actually *lived* at the hospital (giving us the term "house officer," which we still use today to refer to interns and residents) for months at a time and never went home at all. If they were married, their spouses came to the hospital for a quick cafeteria meal and an even quicker embrace, much as they would with a prisoner. Even as recently as twenty years ago, many residents were on call every other night, which meant the young physician would go to work at 6 A.M., put in a thirty-six-hour shift—leaving the following afternoon—then go home to get some sleep, only to repeat the ordeal beginning at six the next morning. If you do the math, this equates to a 120-hour workweek—pretty impressive, since a full week only contains 168 hours.

Today, most call schedules keep residents at the hospital every third or fourth night, which cuts the commitment down to 80 to 100 hours; but some schedules are worse. Some surgical programs are so rigorous that the only way residents ever get an entire weekend off (known as the "Golden Weekend," it's often referred to in the same hushed, reverential tone as great sex and single malt scotch) is to trade time slots with another colleague and pay them back with a

"Power Weekend": arriving at the hospital at 6 A.M. on Friday and working straight through until Monday night—an eighty-four-hour shift with little or no sleep.

The origins of this sadistic rite of passage are obscure. Nobody (least of all medical schools) sat down and "designed" a resident training program in which sleep deprivation was a considered part of the curriculum. This is not true in other skill-based, high-risk occupations. Military personnel (especially in critical combat career fields) *are* intentionally subjected to extended periods of sleeplessness during advanced training. This is partly to build confidence—to let them know they can function under such trying conditions when they have to—but also to let them experience their own heavy-eyed symptoms of degraded performance so they'll know when to pull back or call for help. While many mature physicians and other caregivers *do* find themselves having to work under such duress later in their careers—after a natural disaster, say, or a major epidemic—the notion that one-hundred-hour workweeks were thoughtful preparation for a life in medicine implies far too much foresight on the part of the medical establishment. In truth, "resident abuse" arose mostly as a convenience to faculty and administrators who saw such semiqualified physicians as a source of cheap labor for hospital patients who needed twenty-four-hour care. They rationalized this by telling each other that they were instilling a patient-comes-first attitude in the trainees, and telling trainees that since *they* had to do it as interns and residents, why should the newbies get a free ride? ("And look how good we turned out!" was the unspoken message). Gradually, this simple expedient became a hallowed tradition.

Believe it or not, some physicians, even today, think trainees need these brutal hours to realize their full potential. Others think, with a straight face, that those anointed by God to be doctors are, as a breed, simply impervious to the consequences of fatigue. One such doctor posed several telling questions to the *Journal of the American Medical Association*:

How did earlier generations of physicians achieve such clinical excellence with even less hours of sleep than current residents receive? Are current medical trainees under the assumption that medicine should be a profession with normal working hours? If residents are afraid of being involved in a motor vehicle crash [when leaving the hospital after a marathon shift], why can't they sleep in the call room before driving home?

Let's answer this last question with a quick thought experiment. Suppose you are a typical resident who's been at work in the hospital—immersed up to your ears in the blood, stool, and sputum of desperately ill patients—with no sleep and barely a meal for thirty hours. Finally, the blurry hands of your trusty Timex tell you your shift is over. Now, which are you going to do: Go home, pop a beer, and veg-out for the first fifteen minutes of a *Seinfeld* rerun before collapsing on your own comfy bed, or flop on a lumpy hospital cot (PA system still blaring Code Blues and pages) for a restless nap before "risking" the fifteen-minute drive home?

Not all of the concerns raised about work-hour limitations are nonsense; a few thoughtful commentators have sounded alarms that, at least on the surface, have merit. Dr. Jeffrey Drazen, editor of the *New England Journal of Medicine*, wrote that long hours

> ... have come with a cost, but they have allowed trainees to learn how the disease process modifies patients' lives and how they cope with illness. Long hours have also taught a central professional lesson about personal responsibility to one's patients, above and beyond work schedules and personal plans. Whether this method arose by design or was the fortuitous byproduct of an arduous training program designed primarily for economic reasons

is not the point. Limits on hours on call will disrupt one of the ways we've taught young physicians these critical values... We risk exchanging our sleep-deprived healers for a cadre of wide-awake technicians.

These concerns are real, but they should be put in perspective. There is a tendency for professionals to recall their earlier training sacrifices fondly; we call this the "Days of the Giants" syndrome. It is particularly acute among older physicians who, not coincidentally, think other aspects of our culture are going to hell in a handbasket. Yet even those of us (present authors included) who believe no human being should be forced to make complex, weighty decisions on a thirty-two-hour-long "lactic acid high" must concede that potential problems lurk if we reduce trainee hours too much, or create a shift-work mentality.

One thing we know for sure: Fatigue does degrade performance. One study showed that twenty-four hours of sustained wakefulness results in performance equivalent to a blood alcohol level of 0.1 percent—legally drunk in every state. Although early researchers felt that this kind of impairment occurred only after very long shifts, we now know that chronic sleep deprivation, or *sleep debt*— burning the candle at both ends for too long—is just as harmful. In an experiment in which healthy volunteers performed math calculations, researchers found the subjects were just as impaired after sleeping five hours per night for a week as they were after one twenty-four-hour wakefulness marathon. They didn't check to see what happened when both these disruptions occurred in the *same* week, which is the norm for medical residents.

"Sleep inertia" is another factor whose significance researchers are only now beginning to understand. During the first ten or fifteen minutes after waking, our reflexes are slow and our judgment is faulty. We tend to substitute automatic behaviors for conscious choices, which makes slips even more probable. One sleep researcher told us of a resident who, awakened by her pager three times in one hour during a call night, brushed her teeth three times—one for each page—then went back to sleep each time before she finally realized the electronic *beep* probably wasn't a reminder to floss.

Although it defies common sense to believe that fuzzy brains and bad medical decisions are not related, hard proof of this intuitive link has been surprisingly hard to come by. One reason is that most sleep studies involve "healthy volunteers" who are subjected to tests (usually of some cognitive task) in a controlled environment. Medical residents live in a completely different world. First of all, they start off where most volunteer studies end: in a state of chronic sleep deprivation. Researchers who study them are usually comparing the effects of acute versus chronic sleeplessness, not episodes of sleeplessness punctuating a normal, rested condition. Second, residents don't wake up and do math problems: They make life-or-death decisions about sick patients. This often involves some kind of hands-on procedure, from placing a breathing tube to administering an assortment of life-sustaining drugs. Most of the time, the adrenaline is pumping and they are processing signals—often conflicting ones—from nurses, technicians, colleagues, the patient, and pieces of paper containing Latinate words and strange-looking numbers.

Most of the studies using surgical simulators or videotapes of surgeons during procedures *do* show that sleep-deprived residents have problems both with precision and efficiency. It takes them longer to do specific tasks and the fine motor skills they need to complete them are diminished. You can perform this experiment at home. Before you go to sleep tonight, set the alarm for 3 A.M. and leave a note to yourself that the first thing you're going to do upon waking is to thread a needle, or set the table for dinner— as fast as you can. Keep track of how many times (and how much time) it takes to get that thread to go through the needle's eye, or how many trips you make to the kitchen to get all the silverware and dishes. You'll quickly appreciate the problem.

Studies of nonsurgical trainees are less conclusive. One showed that interns who averaged less than two hours of sleep in the previous thirty-two made nearly twice as many errors reading EKGs, and had to give them more attention, especially when reading several in a row. On the other hand, different studies showed that tired radiology residents made no more mistakes reading X-rays than those who were well rested, and that sleepy ER residents performed physical exams and recorded patient histories with equal reliability in both tired and rested conditions.

So does that mean that ER doctors are in tip-top shape after a grueling, marathon shift? We doubt it. One study found that more than half of nearly one thousand ER residents reported at least one near-accident driving home, and 8 percent had actually been in crashes. Virtually all of these incidents followed a night shift and most residents were driving alone. Both of us recall dozing off at intersections while waiting for red lights to change following thirty-six-hour stints at the hospital. Fortunately, we just drew a few honks, and not an ambulance ride back to the ER, but these situations can't help but give one pause. After an Englishman was convicted of manslaughter after falling asleep at the wheel of his Land Rover and striking a train, killing ten people, two British orthopedic residents wondered about the legal liability for trainees and hospitals if surgeons performed procedures in a similar condition. "If the law judges us unsafe to drive in this state," they wrote, "what are the implications for operating?"

The most ambitious project to try to sort out the influence of sleep deprivation on residents' performance is a federally financed study by Charles Czeisler and his colleagues at Harvard's Brigham and Women's Hospital. Czeisler—a tall, distinguished Harvard professor with a lantern jaw and impressive résumé both as a physician and as a neurophysiologist—has studied sleep for thirty years. He was lead scientist on John Glenn's sleep experiments during Glenn's historic second flight into space in 1998. Normally, sleep research is considered a medical backwater, but the burgeoning medical resident work-hours controversy has suddenly put Czeisler's work in the limelight.

Czeisler divided interns in the Brigham ICU into two groups. In the first, the young doctors adhere to the classic on-call, up-all-night schedule. In the second, interns are relieved at night by other colleagues. Both sets of interns wear a handful of electrodes fastened to their head to measure brain activity and eye movement. Every hour, they spit into special beakers so that technicians can measure their levels of melatonin, a sleep hormone. Needless to say, these study subjects raise eyebrows among new staff and patients wandering the hospital halls. One resident, clueless about the study, told us, "I saw this one intern with these electrodes and wires on her head. I thought, Oh, that must be tough—to be an intern and have a seizure disorder. And then I saw another intern with the same headgear and I knew something was up." The results of the study, which will include both groups' rates of errors, episodes of nodding off, and car crashes, should be out in 2005.

If the problem of excessive work hours seems obvious, the solution isn't. After the Libby Zion case in 1984, in which a young woman died at the hands of fatigued and undersupervised New York Hospital house staff, the uproar (generated in part by Zion's father, a *New York Times* reporter) led the state to limit resident work hours. Several years later, a *JAMA* study showed that the number of complications in New York hospitals actually went *up*. Experts disagree as to why this happened. Some speculated that, while residents got more sleep, the handoffs between them became more frequent, creating more opportunities for fumbles. There was also some evidence that residents and their bosses weren't observing the new rules: "Routine rule violations," we now know, are a part of the medical landscape when safety rules butt heads with efficiency or culture. Finally, it dawned on observers that maybe those residents enjoying a little extra free time weren't using it for shuteye. Believe it or not, some actually used their newfound off-duty hours to moonlight at private hospitals to make a few extra bucks, like overworked police officers who double as security guards or bouncers. (Don't confuse residents with Rodeo Drive plastic surgeons: The average resident's debt load from medical school is $100,000, more than twice their annual salary.)

But even if New York failed to stumble onto the magic formula, the logical connection between fatigue and errors, and the periodic high-profile cases—like the anesthesiologist who fell asleep during a child's ear surgery, resulting in the boy's death—have made it critical to tackle the problem of sleep deprivation in residents. Regulators have begun to do just that.

In July 2003, the Accreditation Council for Graduate Medical Education (ACGME—the group that blesses the nation's 7,800 residency programs involving over 100,000 trainees) finally limited resident schedules to a more human maximum of eighty hours per week, with no shift lasting longer than thirty consecutive hours and at least one day off per week. The ACGME acknowledged the absence of data supporting "eighty" as a magic number, or even that observing it would automatically improve patient safety. But the act did signal their belief that the public felt long work hours were contributing to errors, and that voluntary action by the profession now might forestall more onerous and disruptive legislative intervention. Of their decision, the Council wrote: "The public could interpret lack of action as the medical profession's abrogating its responsibilities, disregarding public opinion, and ignoring the scientific evidence on sleep and performance."

We applaud the ACGME for taking this action, but the central question remains: Will these new work rules make patients safer? Believe it or not, we—like virtually every patient safety expert we know—think the new residency work limits will, unfortunately, probably *increase* the number of medical errors, at least in the short term. Here's why:

Suppose you are admitted to a hospital one evening at 6 P.M. A resident reviews your record, interviews you and the family member who brought you in, and briefs her attending. The whole thing takes about an hour. She also consults a specialist for input on your case, then returns to ask you a few more questions based on this new knowledge. She sends off a dozen lab tests and schedules three different X-rays to help sort out what may be wrong with you. She makes full use of all this input from her attending and several consultants and comes up with a plan to begin treatment and monitor your progress. She then follows your course, analyzing test results as they return and making mid-flight corrections to your treatment plan. Suddenly, she sees one lab test that doesn't jibe with the others, so she rethinks her diagnosis. You're not getting better—though you should be—so she's stymied. She calls for more tests and consults another specialist. Now she's been on your case (as well as several others) for about twelve hours. She's tired. But with your case in flux—at a point when a few more bits of information could tip the diagnosis in one of several ways—you want this doctor to see you to the goal line. Under the old system, she would, even if her eyeballs were a bit scratchy for want of sleep.

Now let's switch the scenario. Under the new, more humane scheduling system, this resident's shift ends halfway through her initial workup. She's talked to you, but not your family. She's put in a call to the first consultant but he hasn't yet called her back. She did talk briefly with a surgeon, but he asked more questions than she could answer. Some of your blood work is back, but a half-dozen other tests are pending. Now she signs out to her well-rested colleague. Are you safer?

The problem, of course, is that the replacement resident is juggling more balls than the Cirque du Soleil. He has some notes on a chart and some cryptic lab reports, but he can't know everything that was going on in his colleague's mind as she followed that intricate ballet between cognition and intuition known as Bayesian reasoning. He'll do the best he can, of course, and maybe he'll make sense of those later lab reports and have some clue about what the second specialist wants to talk about when he finally returns her earlier call—but you as a patient shouldn't have to depend on luck for these things to happen.

Although it is certainly demoralizing to see our post-call interns dozing off during our scintillating lectures, even the educational balance sheet could tip in either direction. Something special happens when a trainee follows a patient's illness from mysterious beginning to climax. It's not just a part of medicine, it's the *heart*—presiding over that wonderful passage from sickness to health that every doctor lives for. To head for the door at shift-change is like walking out in the middle of a good movie, or having one art student finish a painting begun by another. Of course, no one is going to argue that the same doctor needs to attend to you for all ninety-six hours of a four-day hospitalization, but that's not necessary. Most acute illnesses are reliably diagnosed by the first day after admission, and if you make the handoff before that important fact-finding and fact-interpretation cycle is finished—say, by cutting a work shift down to ten or twelve or even eighteen hours—you've virtually guaranteed that the patient will be handed off at the time of greatest flux and educational opportunity, short-changing both the patient and the trainee.

This is where many analogies between health care and other industries break down. Yes, it is true that commercial pilots can't fly for more than eight hours straight without relief. And truck drivers are supposed to leave the road after ten hours for a mandatory break. But between these shifts, their machines either sit idle or (as in the case of ships at sea) are operated by another crew. Operational or maintenance status is either relayed electronically or in a written logbook, so that discrepancies or instructions from the first shift are transmitted concisely to the second. New problems may arise in the second shift, but it's usually not because the first shift had to quit in the middle of a critical function. (You don't change airline pilots on final approach, but only after the airplane is cruising or at the terminal gate.) Fumbles may occur in all of these high-tech handoffs, but they're quite unusual. In medicine, on the other hand, they're dangerously routine.

In fact, we can't think of another industry in which the intake and processing of information is as complex and fluid as medicine. This means that the real question—the one patients should really care about—is not whether a fatigued doctor makes more mistakes, but whether the errors *caused* by fumbled handoffs and more subtle information seepage will exceed those caused by fatigue—a Hobson's choice if there ever was one. Our experience suggests that handoff fumbles will "win" this perverse contest, at least in the short term, and the real losers will be the patients.

This might sound like we're arguing against the ACGME work-hour limits, but we're actually not. Hundred hour workweeks *have* to be bad for young doctors, their loved ones, and ultimately their patients. We've seen colleagues—well-meaning, empathic people—explode at patients, curse out nurses, and even (once or twice) commit suicide, in situations in which fatigue played a role. So we support the new regulations, but strongly believe that they must be accompanied by thoughtful research to assess both the benefits and the dark sides of work-hour limits, and by aggressive programs to improve information transfer.

In any case, the new rules are now in place and we'll await the experiment's outcome. And one of the outcomes, you can be certain, is that some of the results will be fudged.

New York, as we said, has now had work-hours limits, enacted soon after the Libby Zion case, on the books for a decade. Unfortunately, since the limits came as unfunded mandates (just like the present ACGME changes), the primary method for bringing 100-hour-a-week residents down to 80 is to have their colleagues on lighter rotations (50 hours/week) come into the hospital and cover for them in their "free time." Many of the residents themselves don't find this trade-off attractive (they generally prefer to be "beaten up" for a month if they can catch their breath—and do their laundry—

the next). In 2002, for example, the New York State Department of Health cited 54 of the state's 82 teaching hospitals for violating the work-hours limits. Residents also worry that work-hour regulations will squeeze their educational time. Finally, the culture of residents makes them reluctant to sign-out a patient with serious, unresolved issues to a colleague. Part of this is professional pride: If you start something, you finish it and you don't abandon a patient who needs you and is beginning to trust you. Another is the unwritten law among residents: Thou shalt not dump a big load on thy brother.

And there is yet another risk—one that could actually undermine academic medicine in the United States. With our residents at home in bed, attending physicians like us will undoubtedly jump into the breach, especially if fumbles increase dramatically, which they very well might. Dr. Debra Weinstein, residency director at Massachusetts General Hospital, wrote, "Teaching hospitals can recruit and train faculty members...at salaries below the market rate because coverage by residents...insulates [them] from many responsibilities related to direct care and allows them to treat many more patients, often while pursuing research and teaching." Some patients may benefit from this extra attention by a senior physician, but the sick system that produced the problem to begin with won't get any better, and, ultimately, the best faculty will find other, easier things to do. Our system of training physicians and conducting biomedical research—the world's envy—will be the poorer for it. "Junior attendings are fearing for their lives," said one young Pittsburgh surgeon of the new regulations.

As of this writing, it's not clear if other states will follow New York's example of "routinely violating" the new work-hours rules. In 2002, Yale University's surgery program was placed on probation by the ACGME, a noisy shot-across-the-bow that put other prestigious and opinion-leading programs on notice. And in case any of us missed that one, the internal medicine residency at Johns Hopkins Hospital—perennially "America's #1 hospital" according to *U.S. News & World Report*—was stripped of its accreditation in

August 2003 for work-hour violations. The ACGME is playing hardball, probably for good reason. Without active enforcement, violations will multiply like bacteria in a Petri dish. We've heard of residency directors who all but plead with their trainees to lie to the accreditors about their work hours, using the argument that the loss of accreditation would devalue the resident's own pedigree. One residency program staged a skit in which an intern was asked by a mock accreditor (played by another intern), "So, how many hours did you work this week?"

The fatigued intern, playing himself, chanted, "Ninety-five hours, *sir!*"

The pretend program director then pulled him aside and asked, "Do you think you might have overestimated that by twenty?" He dangled a twenty-dollar bill in front of the intern's face.

"Sure," the intern said. "I worked seventy-five hours!"

We know of no cases of actual bribery, but money may be the least motivation for earnest young doctors trying desperately to succeed. Perhaps the twenty-dollar bill was a metaphor for something else—a good recommendation, assignment to challenging cases, a Golden Weekend or two—there are lots of ways to influence people.

"Nobody likes a whistleblower," confessed one resident.

All of this kicking and screaming is not just resisting change simply for inertia's sake. Something *will* be lost with the end of traditional scheduling rituals. Whether that loss will be compensated for by parallel gains in safety remains to be seen. At least for a short period—one year, three years, five years?—we'll see an increase in handoff fumbles, reduced educational time, and increased costs for all hospitals, many that can ill afford them. We may even see the physicians' culture change from a "do whatever it takes" mindset to an "it's not my problem, it didn't happen on my watch" mentality.

On the other hand, as society changes, its caretakers must change with it. We must take seriously the public's rational concerns about sleepy doctors. This is a problem that must be addressed, and now is as good a time as any.

Policymakers at the national and local levels have roles to play. Everything has a price, and the cost of more humane or publicly palatable medical training is funding to improve the system that makes it possible: to make handoffs safer, to relieve residents of their mountains of superfluous paperwork, to provide decent rest facilities in hospitals, and to compensate alternate providers (whether physicians or nonphysicians) who can cover for sleepy residents. We need to be more creative about limiting work hours without compromising patient safety—a time bomb that *will* go off if we start running residency programs like the Teamsters. We can learn lessons in how to do this from other industries, but those lessons won't change the basic nature, or challenges, of medical care.

Finally, even while adhering to the new regulations and sorting out the logistics and systems to make the new schedules safer, medical educators must work tirelessly to instill the ethic that medicine *is* a special calling, and when the rubber of the shift-change meets the road of a sick patient who *really* needs her doctor to stay another hour, the patient still wins.

CHAPTER 12: HUBRIS AND TEAMWORK

In the autumn of 1995, a radar operator aboard a U.S. aircraft carrier off Newfoundland signaled the bridge that their ship was on a collision course with a Canadian vessel. The captain got on the radio and the following exchange ensued:

U.S. CAPTAIN:

>"Please divert your course five degrees to the south to avoid collision."

CANADIAN RADIO OPERATOR:

>"Recommend you divert your course fifteen degrees north to avoid collision."

U.S. CAPTAIN:

>"This is the captain of a U.S. naval vessel. I say again, divert your course."

CANADIAN RADIO OPERATOR:

>"No, sir. I say again, you divert your course!"

U.S. CAPTAIN:

>"This is the aircraft carrier U.S.S. *Coral Sea*. We are a large warship of the United States Navy. Divert your course now!!!"

CANADIAN RADIO OPERATOR:

>"This is a lighthouse. Your call."

—The Lighthouse Parable

"Code Blue, Room 426! Code Blue, Room 426!"

Like the order to crash-dive a submarine, the PA blasted in every corner of the hospital. All it lacked was a klaxon and exploding depth charges. This was an emergency. This was no drill.

The Code team scrambled to the scene. Like cops at a robbery-in-progress, they got the facts while they deployed. A young swing-shift nurse, Jane Hyatt, had just found her patient gray-blue, not breathing, and without a pulse.

Code Blues used to be a medical secret—hence the word, "Code"—but the public is well familiar with them now thanks to a generation of TV hospital dramas. Shows like *ER* and *Chicago Hope* generally get the details right, especially the first few moments when nobody knows what's going on and has nothing to fall back on but established procedures. Like a choreographed battle scene, a half-dozen doctors, nurses, and respiratory therapists dash into the patient's room and prepare their gear. On TV, after a half-minute of great acting, orchestral precision, and some vigorous chest thumping that never musses the hero's hair, the patient miraculously recovers, smiles gratefully, and thanks the self-effacing doctors—unless, of course, he or she has been written out of the script, which happens only a third of the time. The truth, unfortunately, is much more grim. In real life, only one in eight patients who receive CPR for an in-hospital cardiac arrest survives to leave the hospital. Perhaps unsurprisingly, the general public's estimate of the chances of full recovery after CPR is precisely the same as the wildly inflated TV survival rate.

The other thing television gets wrong is the energetic but otherwise unruffled portrayal of the start of most TV codes. The truth is that chaos often reigns supreme. Some hospitals have no formal system for responding to Code Blues. The hospital operator just calls it on the PA and hopes that some CPR-trained doctors and nurses are nearby and respond—the hospital equivalent of a flight attendant asking passengers, "Is there a doctor on the plane?" Others have a slightly more organized approach, paging specially equipped caregivers who are scattered around the hospital and never really train together. In either case, the people running into the patient's room when a Code Blue is called are really a collection of trained passersby.

So in Room 426, the Code—as it *really* plays out—is under way. One doctor inserts a large catheter into the patient's arm so that an IV can be started. Syringes of powerful, lifesaving drugs— epinephrine, bicarbonate, amiodarone, atropine—are passed over the patient's chest like cheese puffs at a spirited dinner party. The team's doctors and nurses, most of whom have never worked with each other before, shout instructions, yell questions ("Who's got an eighteen catheter?" "Does anybody know this guy?"), and run in and out of the room on special errands. It is semiorganized bedlam.

In this case, the focus of all this attention is a man in his late seventies with a face of gray stubble. A respiratory therapist squeezes oxygen into his lungs with a big rubber balloon. The therapist pauses every fifteen or twenty seconds to suction sputum from the patient's throat. One doctor compresses the patient's chest—down and release, down and release—like some terrible metronome. Another doctor, feeling for a pulse in the patient's groin, where the big femoral artery passes close to the surface, yells "STOP!" He detects a pulse—a faint one, but it's there.

The chest compressions stop, but the Code work continues. A nurse goes to the floor's central nursing station to phone the ICU to reserve a bed. The Code team leader asks again if anybody knows why the patient went into cardiac arrest. This is crucial: Even though many Codes are treated identically at first, with standard CPR, some cases—such as a collapsed lung, pericardial tamponade (fluid accumulation in the sac around the heart), or a major blood chemistry problem, such as a potassium buildup—require special treatment.

"Come on—does *anybody* know this patient?" the team chief shouts again.

Nobody answers, including Nurse Hyatt, who has just started her shift. The Code enters its fifth minute. Bystanders have now gathered by the door. Some are staff—they trickle in to see if they can help. Others are just curious—including visitors from other rooms, like rubberneckers at a car wreck. The shouting begins again.

"OK," the team leader barks over the din, "everybody who doesn't need to be here—out!"

Aaron Riegel, a physician who just happened to be on the floor when the Code was called, dashes off to the nurse's station to find the patient's chart. Riegel is a decisive guy—a senior resident already accepted into an ICU fellowship—and thus no stranger to stress. He thrives on it and radiates confidence, which is good, although some of his colleagues think his confidence borders on cockiness. But whether you like his style or not, you can't help but notice him. He looks like a TV doctor, with a Hollywood haircut and well-toned physique. And he looks great in a set of scrubs, a pair of clogs, and the fleece vest he habitually wears to tote his doctor paraphernalia. This combination of professional zeal, *M*A*S*H*-like informality, and yuppie accessorizing shouted not just "good doc," but "super doc." His patients adore him.

Riegel returns to Room 426 a moment later, chart in hand. He skids to a stop, flips a couple of pages, then looks at the team in horror.

"Oh my God!" he gasps. "This guy is No Code."

Everyone stops what they're doing.

In some hospitals, the No Code (more formally called "Do Not Resuscitate," DNR) order is flagged with a big stop sign—literally, like you see at an intersection—taped to the front of the medical record. Riegel's hospital used an eye-catching, blood-red form—duly executed by the patient and required witnesses—stashed with the rest of the patient's chart. Despite the Code team's can-do, SWAT-like attitude, they're trained to stand down when a DNR is identified, no matter how much it aches. In fact, when the patient is a DNR, the Code is not to be called—no pages to the Code team, no PA announcements—at all. *This* was a giant screwup.

A second or two after the word sinks in, the team begins slowly and deliberately to undo everything they've done. They unplug the IV, pack up their paddles, tubes, syringes, and medicines, and file quietly from the room. Nobody likes to lose a Code, but that's part of the business. But when all that effort and adrenaline is wasted, unappreciated, unwanted—especially by the patient himself—well, it's tough. Really tough.

"I'm gonna fill out an incident report," one of the residents fumes to a colleague as she stalks down the corridor toward the elevator.

"Somebody really blew it. I don't want to do this again. Ever."

"Yeah," her colleague, not quite so distraught, replies. "I think I remember a case where somebody filed battery charges against a doctor who tried to revive a DNR. Or maybe it was assault."

The angry resident cuts him a sharp glance.

"I'm just saying," he shrugs, "you gotta be careful about these things."

Back in Room 426, a somber Nurse Hyatt begins cleaning up the patient's room. Just out of nursing school and as yet unaccustomed to the roller coaster of hospital life, she sometimes feels like a total fraud. And, as a twenty-two-year-old woman who wears her red hair in a ponytail, patients frequently mistake her for a candy-striper. But she had been a good student and wanted to be a good nurse. She paid attention to things. She knew about DNRs and was surprised nobody mentioned at shift change that the sick old man in 426 had been changed to No Code. She also didn't remember seeing the order in his chart. But Dr. Riegel had spoken with such authority—who was she to question him? And she hadn't seen the chart for the past hour—maybe one of the doctors had changed the patient's status that morning and had forgotten to tell the staff. After all, that's what the chart is for, to convey information, to bridge those kind of gaps.

She thinks briefly about looking into it, curious about who put the order in the file, and when—but what would be the point? So she decides to put the whole thing behind her and chalk it up to experience.

She glances at the elderly patient, who now looks even more tattered and beaten up. She tucks the sheet and blanket up under his chin, smoothes out the wrinkles, and feels his pulse. A few slow, irregular beats... and then his heart winks out like the embers on a doused campfire. Looking up, she notices Dr. Riegel has left the chart on the foot of the bed—just sitting, like grandma in the wheelchair beside the dance floor at the wedding, while everyone buzzes around it cleaning up the room. Another floor nurse comes in with a tray to carry off the empty syringes, used tubing, and bloody towels—the detritus of a lost battle—and picks up the chart. Idly, she flips it open.

"Hey, Jane," she says softly. "Do you know the patient's original diagnosis? I mean, before the Code?"

She picks out the red form—yes, it was there, just as it should be, and Jane relaxes a bit. Reading upside down, she even sees the patient's name stamped on the bottom right-hand corner of the page. The only problem is...

"Omigod!" Jane covers her mouth. "That's not this patient! Dr. Riegel pulled the wrong chart!"

The other nurse looks up, eyes like saucers. "What are you talking about?"

"This patient is full Code. Oh, God! Always has been—I'm sure of it. I'll go pull his chart. You stay here."

A few moments later, the PA blares again. "Code Blue, Room 426. Four-twenty-six, Code Blue." Heads cock in a hundred places around the hospital—there was no obvious explanation for a re-called Code.

Dutifully, the Code team rushes back and picks up where they left off—though it has been twenty minutes since the first call and the patient isn't responding. They compress and thump and inject and shock, but the tired old heart is finished. The team leader pronounces the patient's death and pulls the sheet up over his face. For the second time in half-an-hour, the team files dejectedly from the room.

Dr. Riegel is not among them. He had moved on to other duties and was not on the floor for the second Code. The nurses look at each other, bewildered, and go back to their jobs.

The first story here, as in so many medical mistakes, seems obvious. It's easy to blame Dr. Riegel for plucking the wrong chart from the crowded rack and for not checking the name against the patient's wristband. That a well-meaning provider made a careless blunder is beyond debate. But the case's second story illustrates numerous and significant blunt-end problems as well: a poorly trained Code Blue team, inadequate procedures for identifying patients during Codes, deficient systems for documenting advance directives in charts, and so on. After this case— it always seems to be *after*, never before—the hospital changed many of these procedures, and added a rule that at least two physicians and a nurse needed to confirm a patient's identity before a Code could be cancelled. Other ideas were floated and discarded for one reason or another. One, to create a "DNR wristband," was rejected as too stigmatizing for the patient ("I am *not* my DNR order," said one nurse tartly, ending the debate). Another was to put a special sign over the patient's bed, but inevitably someone would forget to take it down when the old patient left and a new patient crawled under the sheets.

None of these ideas, though, addressed the root cause of the blunder: Jane Hyatt's hesitancy to speak up when it mattered. That error had nothing to do with DNR forms or wristbands, but had everything to do with most hospitals' thin culture of teamwork. We see here, as we have in so many other cases, a nurse who felt something was wrong but failed to raise her concerns with the physicians. It would be easy to simply say she was a novice intimidated by the doctors' mystique (and by one charismatic, brash doctor in particular), but that would be missing the point. Was the hospital's culture one that encouraged or inhibited cross talk and challenges—among colleagues or between levels in the caregiver hierarchy? Answering this question is the only way to understand what really happened in Room 426 on that terrible evening. And to fix it.

To many patients as well as practitioners, doctors and nurses seem like the original "odd couple." Sometimes, they seem to inhabit different universes: Doctors are from Mars, Nurses are from Venus. Doctors are stoic, competent, and sometimes brilliant; nurses are caring, tireless, and sometimes heroic. And while we're dealing in stereotypes, let's not forget those doctors who are arrogant or absentminded and those nurses who are careless or rude. Sometimes we imagine a handsome doctor and beautiful nurse sneaking off for a quickie in the residents' call room, and that's been known to happen. At other times, we actually hear them arguing—in each other's faces and at each other's throats—about a patient's condition or treatment.

Although it's less dramatic than any of this Hollywood hyperbole, in truth, doctors and nurses get along fairly well. With the exception of some specialties (surgery, for example, still tends to be a "boy's club" with die-hard chauvinist traditions), modern-day differences are due more to professional hierarchy than sexual discrimination. This is especially true for the newer generation of caregivers, since the old "Doctor is God" archetype is fading from medical culture, pushed along, no doubt by the increasing feminization of the MD workforce (nearly half of today's medical students are women). "Plays well with others" is a new category on the scorecard for evaluating medical professionals, and it's long overdue.

Yet, for two groups that have historically—and necessarily—worked closely together, there is still remarkably little understanding and appreciation of each other's roles. Too often, doctors still see nurses as glorified clerks and housekeepers whose main role is to do what they're told—to clean bedpans, deliver pills, and focus on being kind, not smart. For their part, many nurses view physicians as arrogant clods who are genetically incapable of collaborating with "underlings," those who do the real work of actually *caring* for sick people.

A recent exchange overheard at our hospital perfectly illustrates this rift. One nurse had the chutzpah to actually question an "order" by a young resident, asking him to clear it first with his supervisor. "MD!" the young doctor barked. "Do you know what that means? It stands for *makes decisions*!"

"And RN," the nurse retorted, "stands for *rejects nonsense*!"

Such exchanges are not the hallmark of a healthy relationship. In one survey of more than seven hundred nurses, 96 percent said they had witnessed or experienced disruptive behavior by physicians.

Nearly half pointed to "fear of retribution" as the primary reason such acts were not reported to superiors. Thirty percent of the nurses also said they knew at least one nurse who had resigned as a result of boorish—or worse—physician behavior, while many others knew nurses who had changed shifts or wards to avoid contact with particular offensive doctors.

The importance of this tension grows as the U.S. nursing shortage gets worse. According to the American Hospital Association, demand for nurses now exceeds supply by 126,000; and one in seven hospitals report vacancy rates of over 20 percent on their nursing staffs. Since a third of all U.S. nurses are over age fifty, there will be more nurses leaving the profession than entering it by 2020, leaving a shortfall of nearly a million nurses to care for the aging Baby Boom generation.

This means that the nurses who remain will feel even more stressed, unappreciated, and underpaid. It's no surprise that burnout is their major occupational hazard. As early as 1960, a nursing historian wrote, "What is exceptional in nursing is the nature of the work: the continuous and intimate association with pain and not infrequent contact with death.... Not every man or woman would feel themselves able to undertake the duties of a nurse." Since then, the pace of hospital stays—the increased throughput and more extensive use of lab tests and procedures, not to mention the staggering increase in the number and types of medications—means that the nursing shortage will only increase the chance for slips and errors. A 2002 report concluded, "Most healthcare workers entered their professions to 'make a difference' through personal interaction with people in need. Today, many in direct patient care feel tired and burned-out from a stressful, often understaffed environment, with little or no time to experience the one-on-one caring that should be the heart of hospital employment."

Although nursing has traditionally been a profession of women (95 percent of nurses in the U.S. are female), young, career-minded women now have many other challenging (and less draining) professional opportunities. Even those already in nursing are leaving, many to take less stressful jobs in other venues, such as in health care administration, in call centers, even in law offices as malpractice consultants. A 1999 survey of Pennsylvania nurses found that 41 percent were dissatisfied with their work and that one in four planned to leave their jobs in the coming year.

Initially, studies defining minimum nurse-to-patient ratios were based on nurses' efforts to avoid burnout and flex their muscles at the collective bargaining table. However, recent data suggest that medical errors do in fact increase with higher ratios of patients to nurses. One study by University of Pennsylvania nursing professor Linda Aiken found that surgical patients had a 31 percent greater chance of dying in hospitals when the average nurse cared for more than seven patients. Aiken estimated that 20,000 deaths per year could be linked to inadequate nursing care—and remember, these are not just errors and slips by nurses, but mistakes committed by doctors and technicians that nurses simply didn't have time to catch. For every additional patient added to a nurse's average workload, patient mortality rose 7 percent, and nursing burnout and dissatisfaction increased 23 percent and 15 percent, respectively.

Lots of metaphorical "sponges" have been thrust into these gaping wounds to help stanch the bleeding of our nursing corps, but so far none has proved very effective. All over the country, administrators are raising salaries, offering signing bonuses, and abolishing mandatory overtime—but still the hemorrhage continues. Broadcasters air public service announcements touting the rewards of a nursing career, but it doesn't take too many conversations with real, live nurses for promising students to see that high-tech or nonmedical service jobs offer more money with less aggravation.

Although some of the answer to the nursing shortage will come through the traditional dance of competitive bargaining—better pay, benefits, and working conditions—new technology could play an important role as well. Even as it improves safety, technology can relieve some of the paperwork burden and allow nurses to spend more time with their patients. Next time you're in a hospital, watch a nurse take a patient's vital signs to see one tip of this particular iceberg. Most hospitals now use digital blood pressure cuffs, which give readings in numbers instead of lines on an analog dial, the old-fashioned way. But instead of feeding this luminescent number—composed of bits and bytes—into a digital computer, where it could be instantly available to everyone, the twenty-first-century nurse still writes the blood pressure reading down on paper (or the back of her hand, or the cuff of her scrub suit) and takes it back to the nursing station, where she manually copies it again onto a bedside flowsheet and a third time, most likely, into her notes on the patient's chart. (After looking at these records, interns, residents, and attendings may copy the numbers *again*, ever-multiplying the chance of a transposition or ID error.) This procedure is just plain nuts, yet it goes on hundreds of times during a typical shift and is one reason nurses—justifiably— think so much of their time, training, and talent is wasted.

The nursing shortage has begun to shake up hospital administrators, many of whom have been forced to close down whole wards due to lack of staff. For a time, some went so far as to charter whole jets to bring candidates in from Ireland and the Philippines. This tactic has abated in the past few years, both because of post-9/11 immigration complexities and the fact that it is now seen as politically incorrect (the moral equivalent of exporting tobacco) since the source countries face their own nursing shortages. Not only have the administrators been out shaking trees for more nurses, but they've also begun to try and create a more positive work environment. A hospital spending hundreds of thousands of dollars trying to recruit nurses is going to come down like a ton of bricks on a doctor who harasses the nurses or makes their lives miserable by being an arrogant cad. "Hon, can you get that chart for me"—accompanied by a wink and a pinch—now thankfully survives mostly as the stuff of physician-redneck legend, although regrettably, it is not yet wholly eradicated.

Yet all this attention to recruitment and retention can feel awfully corporate, as if we're just trying to fill our quota of bodies to keep the beds open. What it neglects is the key role that nurses play in making and keeping their patients, and the system, safe.

Suzanne Gordon, co-author of *From Silence to Voice: What Nurses Know and Must Communicate to the Public*, counsels nurses to promote themselves a bit more—to teach patients and professionals that their life's work is anything but trivial: "People don't understand that if a stroke patient isn't assessed correctly, if the food's going down the wrong tubes, they may die or be sent to the ICU. If someone isn't helped out of bed and walked, their blood won't circulate and they could end up with a pulmonary embolism and die. All of these so-called unimportant tasks are really about life and death."

Adds Barbara Blakeney, President of the American Nurses Association, "Nurses prevent bad things from happening. And it's much more difficult to measure what doesn't happen as opposed to what does."

Fostering teamwork and creating more satisfying nursing roles isn't as simple as pumping up nurses and cutting doctors down to size. Teamwork is not a zero-sum game, in which one team member gains status and recognition only by diminishing the perceived worth of the others. The tragedy in Room 426 shows that making care safer requires active effort to foster collaboration, mutual appreciation, and a willingness to speak out when doing so challenges the hierarchy. It shows that passing out job descriptions, schedules, equipment, and nametags doesn't make a team.

Unfortunately, this lack of teamwork isn't confined to doctors and nurses. Similar problems bedevil relationships among physicians themselves.

Much of medicine is hierarchical. Physicians generally see themselves as having authority over nurses—any nurses—even head nurses with advanced degrees and decades of hard-won experience. This, of course, bugs the hell out of highly qualified nurses, the same way order-spouting junior officers—"ninety-day wonders"—annoy veteran sergeants. Residents see themselves as lording it over interns, just as residents themselves defer to attendings. Things get fuzzy, though, when a resident or fellow in one department comes up against a "peer" in another and they disagree over a clinical matter or a piece of turf. The same is true for attendings and senior physicians from different specialties.

For instance, a surgeon and an anesthesiologist may differ over what is prudent or necessary for a patient during a particular operation. The anesthesiologist may see fluctuating vital signs and want to stabilize the patient. The surgeon may insist that completing the procedure quickly is the only way to save him. Both may be right. Both are liable for their actions. Both feel equally responsible. Who has final authority?

The play-by-play announcer couldn't tell you—it's not written down anywhere. But the color commentator would explain that the surgeon is like the field commander—up to his waist in blood and gore; while the anesthesiologist is like the chief of staff—in a better position to see the bigger picture. Without a clear chain of command, the physicians must work things out on the fly, and they usually do. In case of disputes, such differences are often settled by who has the stronger personality, the most seniority, the best track record, or has intimidated (or earned the respect of) the rest of the OR crew.

In one notorious example of how *not* to work things out, a surgeon and an anesthesiologist at the Medical Center of Central Massachusetts prepared to operate on an elderly woman. Both physicians were of roughly the same age and experience level. The OR team was prepped and ready to go. Then, for some unknown reason—as the surgeon was about to make the initial incision—the two began to argue. The argument turned into a brawl. The anesthesiologist swore at the surgeon and the surgeon threw a foot-long cotton swab back at the "gas-passer." They lunged at each other and grappled on the floor at the feet of their stunned associates. After a moment, they separated and went back to their respective corners. As if the whole thing never happened, they told the wide-eyed staff that the operation would continue, which it did, without further incident. After the patient was taken to recovery, the bizarre event was reported to the state medical board and both doctors were fined $10,000 and ordered to undergo psychotherapy. Perhaps the patient was told in the recovery room that she had survived a hard-fought operation.

Whether it is in the OR or at a Code Blue, medicine has not done a great job in delimiting roles and responsibilities, fostering teamwork, and reflecting on the interpersonal relationships that often define success and failure. Even after a Code Blue, there is never a formal debriefing, except in those situations where a case goes forward to an M&M conference. The team just breaks up and wanders off, to resume their regular duties. When the CPR is unsuccessful, which is most of the time, we may ask ourselves individually why we failed ("Should I have given another dose of epi?"), but our failure as a *team* is never considered.

In fact, neither of us can recall ever sitting down and discussing what was going through each team member's mind as a Code Blue unfolded, why providers reacted as they did, and if their attitudes or actions might have been part of the problem. This lack of introspection, or critical analysis, is built into the system. And so, if the second story really *was* a teamwork problem, it goes untold.

Aviation is often held up as a model of how professionals working in high-risk, high-demand, high-tech environments can collaborate successfully without letting hierarchy, tradition, or prejudices get in the way. While it's easy to overestimate aviation's accomplishments in this area (after all, planes still crash), a few lessons from the aerospace world unquestionably apply to medicine, particularly as they relate to the culture of teamwork and open communication.

While pilots are lauded for their receptiveness to collaboration, surgeons are seen as poster-boys for inflexibility. The unflattering comparison has some merit. One study compared the attitudes of flight crews regarding teamwork to those held by surgical teams.

The surgeons themselves thought the team functioned well (three-quarters rated teamwork as "high"). The other members of the "team" begged to differ: only 39 percent of anesthesiologists, 28 percent of surgical nurses, 25 percent of anesthesia nurses, and 10 percent of anesthesia residents agreed that the level of teamwork was good. Nearly half the surgeons felt that junior team members shouldn't question the decisions of the senior physician. In contrast, 94 percent of airline cockpit crews rejected this sort of hierarchy—possibly because when the captain makes a mistake, everyone else goes down as well.

Of course, some would argue that the last thing you want with your chest cracked and your pulsing heart cupped in the hands of a surgeon is an indecisive, nurturing consensus builder, rallying the troops for a nice round of Kumbaya. But even those who favor George Patton–style surgical leadership recognize that there are situations—for instance, when the lead surgeon is fatigued, misinformed, or simply wrong—in which one would want a culture of collaboration, not a chorus of "yes men."

Unfortunately, the doctors who discourage such cross talk are the kind who need it most. In the survey just described, 70 percent of attending surgeons agreed that, "even when fatigued, I perform effectively during critical times." Among pilots, only a quarter self-assessed as such. In other words, while most pilots aren't afraid to ask for help when they're feeling below par—due to fatigue, doubt, or any other reason—tired or confused doctors think nothing of pressing ahead, and refuse even to acknowledge that this intransigence just might cause their patients harm.

This kind of macho denial and swagger was once part of pilot culture, too—but in an age when few passengers depended on them. In its early years, flight was often a solo enterprise. Best typified by barnstormers and airmail pilots in their leather helmets and silk scarves, they simply had no copilots or ground-based infrastructure to help them out. The aircraft were unreliable, too, so most pilots were also their own mechanics—a situation akin to a cardiologist taking time between patients to install a new circuit board on his computerized EKG.

As planes got bigger and more reliable, the airlines began to grow and crewed aircraft became the rule. Still, the old barnstormer tradition was slow to die. As late as the 1950s, at least one major airline still had an explicit policy warning First Officers against pointing out mistakes made by the captain. Even when such policies were replaced by commonsense regulations, some senior captains—the "chief surgeons" of their day, trained and acculturated during aviation's so-called Golden Age—held onto the old routine. They might still be holding on today, except for one problem: It sometimes proved to be deadly.

On March 27, 1977, KLM Flight 4805 departed Amsterdam's Schiphol Airport with 235 passengers and a crew of fourteen. At the helm was KLM's chief 747 instructor pilot, Captain Jacob van Zantent. Van Zantent had trained nearly all other KLM pilots to fly the 747. So great was his reputation that he was featured in KLM ads, including one in the in-flight magazine in the seat pockets aboard Flight 4805. The flight was scheduled to stop at Los Palmas airport in the Canary Islands, but was diverted to Los Rodeos airport when a terrorist bomb exploded in the Los Palmas terminal. Such curveballs often set the stage for accidents in both the sky and the OR: You start off planning to do one thing, then wind up having to do another, putting a premium on clear communications and good teamwork.

Flight 4805 eventually landed safely in Tenerife, on the other side of the Canary Islands. Once set to depart for the original destination, van Zantent was under some pressure to make his scheduled takeoff window. After some accidents attributed to fatigue, KLM had recently instituted strict regulations limiting continuous work hours for aircrews, and the company's most senior captain undoubtedly figured he had to set a good example (another case of the unforeseen consequences of safety regulations). Taxiing out for takeoff, his cockpit received two near-simultaneous transmissions. One was from the control tower: "Stand by for takeoff...I will call you." The other was from another jumbo jet, Pan Am Flight 1736, that had just landed somewhere ahead of them in the fog: "We are still taxiing down the runway."

For reasons we'll never know, van Zantent ordered his plane onto the runway. Even if he intended to hold in position, which he did for a short time, this was a serious breach of procedure. When the tower wants you on the runway, but to wait there for a separate takeoff clearance, they tell you to "position and hold." Van Zantent made this decision himself—perhaps misunderstanding the "stand by for takeoff" from air traffic control as permission to go onto the runway but not yet begin his takeoff. This alarmed his copilot, who reacted at once.

"Wait a minute," he said. "We don't have ATC clearance!"

"No, I know that," the captain replied confidently. "Go ahead."

As the KLM "heavy" prepared for takeoff, the Tenerife Tower asked the Pan Am pilot to report when he had turned off the runway—again, fog obscured the view in all directions and, in those days, airports had no ground-control radar to spot planes moving on the surface.

"OK," the Pam Am skipper replied. "We'll report when we're clear."

The official report of the Spanish Secretary of Civil Aviation recounts what happened next:

> On hearing this, the KLM flight engineer asked:
> "Is he not clear then?" The [KLM] captain didn't
> understand him and [the engineer] repeated, "Is he
> not clear, that Pan American?" The captain replied
> with an emphatic, "Yes" *and, perhaps, influenced by
> his great prestige, making it difficult to imagine an error
> of this magnitude on the part of such an expert pilot,*
> both the co-pilot and the flight engineer made no

further objections. [emphasis added]

Captain van Zantent advanced the throttles and KLM 4805 began its takeoff roll. A few seconds later, the Pan Am pilot saw the KLM's landing lights burst through the fog.

"There he is! Look at him! Goddamn... that son-of-a-bitch is coming!"

Van Zantent managed to get his plane airborne, but could not clear the huge 747 in front of him. The underside of his plane smashed through the fuselage of the Pan Am airliner, resulting in a tremendous explosion, strewing wreckage all over the runway. The crash killed 583 people on both planes: the worst aviation collision in history.

Today, the culture is different. Even highly trained, aggressive fighter pilots "fly by the book" with no discernible loss in combat effectiveness.

The contrast between aviation's long climb from silk-scarf barnstormers to disciplined, integrated flight teams and health care's struggle to create a similarly collaborative system is striking. Even among private pilots, "flying doctors" (both physicians and dentists) have among the worst safety records of any occupation group. There are several theories to explain this observation. One is that doctors are inherently overconfident, another is that they too often fly when they are tired or distracted, and a third is that doctors are used to leaving certain details to others—risks you just can't take when you're the only pilot on board. We suspect that many flying-doctor accidents occur simply because the physicians fail to use all the resources a team-oriented aviation system provides.

Consider the contribution teamwork—or lack of it—makes in a typical medication mistake. A resident thinks the dose of medication ordered by her attending is incorrect, but assumes the highly experienced attending knows what he is doing. The attending hasn't ordered this medication in a long time, and assumes the young resident—who carries around that fancy PDA—is up to speed on the latest meds and knows all the doses. Besides, wouldn't a conscientious colleague correct him if he was wrong? The nurse and pharmacist assume that if two doctors were in on the order, there can't be a mistake, so they process and administer an obviously faulty prescription. The result is a needless medication error that could've been prevented if *any* member of the attending's "cockpit crew" spoke up when something looked funny.

But the answer isn't simply to bring the high-and-mighty down a peg or two. Teamwork is a two-way street—everybody on the crew needs to feel that they "have permission" to speak up when they have concerns. Crashes like Tenerife convinced everyone in aviation that better teamwork could be lifesaving, and resulted in crew training that not only forces senior captains to be part of the team, but encourages other flight officers to assert themselves when safety is at stake. This training technique is referred to as Crew Resource Management, or CRM, and it is just now being tried in medicine.

CRM recognizes that while machines can break, they don't make mistakes; people do. Factors contributing to these errors include fatigue, perceptual errors (such as misreading an instrument or mistaking an oral instruction), and the occasional clash between personal styles and the cultures of different specialties in a high-tech, high-stress environment. Some CRM programs teach participants how to "trap" errors, as well as how to resolve them quickly once a situational "ambush" occurs. Participants learn the warning signs of unconscious conflict, and how to prevent or handle such conflicts when they do occur. Aviation expert John Nance explains:

> How do we prevent a misunderstood instruction from leading to a crash? By expecting such an error, and by training other pilots to listen in order to catch and correct mistakes... Now, instead of an environment in which the captain is God and is

addressed only when he or she approves, captains are required to listen carefully to their fellow crewmembers, and the other pilots are virtually required to speak up if they think the captain is making a mistake.

For example, the first rule in any flying emergency is to "maintain aircraft control"—it won't do you any good to consult the rest of the crew and solve a complex electrical problem if the airplane spirals down while you're doing it. So aircrews at all stations know the captain will likely have his or her hands full just controlling the plane and have a reduced ability to tell everyone else what to do. In these cases, manufacturers and test pilots contribute greatly to air safety by trying to foresee possible malfunctions and develop specific procedures for dealing with them. Even when immediate action is needed and nobody has time to whip out the flight manual, aircrews are trained to have emergency procedures—including coordinated responses—memorized; then refer to the written checklist when things have settled down. After a crew has trained together like this for a while, they become sensitive to each others' personal styles, strengths, and shortcomings. More importantly, they know what should happen when things are going right, what it looks like when things go wrong, and what *the team* should do about it.

A good example of the importance of team training and resiliency is seen in organizational expert Karl Weick's analysis of an August 1949 fire in Mann Gulch, Montana, that took the lives of thirteen young firefighters. Here, the smokejumpers miscalculated the path of the fire and panicked as they tried to outrun the oncoming blaze, which was moving at 600 feet per minute up a hill with a 76-degree slope. Taught to hang onto their heavy packs filled with valuable instruments and equipment, all of them perished—except one. Group leader Wag Dodge dropped his tools, set an "escape fire"—which burned away brush and grass in a big circle ahead of the main blaze—and then laid down at its center and covered himself as the firestorm blew through. Dodge tried desperately to get his men to lie down with him, but it takes a lot of guts to face a roaring freight train by lying in the center of the tracks, so they continued their fatal retreat.

Weick describes the Mann Gulch debacle as a failure of "sensemaking"—the inability to sort out the best course of action because of miscommunication, indiscipline, lack of mutual trust, and ultimately, panic. His recipe for the collapse of sensemaking sounds suspiciously like the screenplay for many health care errors made under emergency conditions: "Thrust people into unfamiliar roles; leave some key roles unfilled; make the task more ambiguous; discredit the role system; and make all of these changes in a context in which small things can combine into something monstrous."

Weick describes other ways to make task-oriented teams more responsive and resilient. One, which he calls "respectful interaction," applies especially to medical team building. "If a role system collapses among people for whom trust, honesty, and self-respect are underdeveloped," Weick explains, "then they are on their own. And fear often swamps their resourcefulness. If, however, a role system collapses among people where trust, honesty, and self-respect are more fully developed, then new options... are created." Here we see that teamwork training does more than enhance performance in routine procedures and predictable emergencies; it allows teams to function and prevail even when the inconceivable happens, as witnessed by the miraculous rescue of Apollo 13 due to extraordinary teamwork among, and between, ground-based and space-bound crews.

Team training like this has barely begun in health care. Although better teamwork on all floors of a hospital will help, it's most useful in situations where time and psychological pressures are critical, as in the OR, ER, ICU and CCU, and within the Code Blue teams.

Consider our approach to heart attack victims in the ER. Evidence clearly shows that the time from arrival at the ER to insertion of the catheter for an angioplasty (the so-called door-to-balloon time) is tightly correlated with a patient's outcome. Patients with two-hour door-to-balloon times have a 50 percent higher death rate than those whose times are below one hour. Yet few hospitals hit the one-hour benchmark, and ER physicians and cardiologists usually blame each other for the poor performance. Rare is the hospital that views the *entire process* as a team effort; if they did, they'd almost certainly begin team training involving the two departments. Few do.

Compare this to a NASCAR pit crew, a team that can change out a long list of parts on a racecar—and refuel it—in twenty seconds. How do they achieve this extraordinary "pit-to-track" time? According to master mechanic Alistair Gibson:

> We do loads of practice back at the factory. We've got a simulation wheel that comes in with a catapult and stops. At the races we practice on Thursday and again on Sunday morning. If Thursday didn't go well, we'll slot in another... we're always looking for ways of making it quicker, safer and more simple.... We are ready for anything. Late calls, clutch-less stops, wing adjustments, rear jacking bracket failure, gun man run over, fuel man run over, we have quite a few eventualities.

In both medicine and aviation, CRM training involving a simulated crisis always incorporates a debriefing session that begins with a videotape review of the entire episode. As it plays, the instructor points out what's happening, since that's not always apparent to team members preoccupied with their own tasks. In medical CRM drills using realistic mannequins, these scenarios—coupled with the debriefing—can be surprisingly dramatic and illuminating. Kaveh remembers one very sophisticated Code Blue simulation more vividly than any of his actual resuscitations, which tend to pass in a blur. During the simulation, the intern handling the defibrillator couldn't figure out how to make the damned thing work, which led to several sweaty minutes as everyone tried his hand at it, jiggling and whacking the machine as if it were a temperamental toaster. Watching that on the videotape not only taught the intern how to deal with such technical issues, it showed all team members how best to react—and not react—when a procedure hits a snag.

Jody Hoffer Gittell, a management expert at Brandeis University, argues that while checklist routines and advanced planning may serve other industries well, health care's triple whammy of limited time, parallel tasking, and decision making under uncertainty create a unique demand for "relational coordination." While most service industries tend to focus on individual encounters between providers and consumers, she points out that medicine stands apart because of its need for regular improvisation and interactions that involve a complex combination of specialized knowledge, technical skills, psychology, and rapid use of both sketchy data and instant feedback.

To test her hypothesis of medical exceptionalism, Gittell studied patients undergoing joint replacement surgery at nine hospitals. She found that patients' quality of care, pain control, and postoperative functioning were all far better when there was improved relational coordination—better communication, shared problem-solving, common goals, and mutual respect—among caregivers.

In an effort to decrease the chances of wrong-site surgery, many hospitals (including our own) have recently begun to mandate a "time out" prior to the first incision. This is similar to a team huddle before the snap in football. All the providers—doctors, nurses, OR techs—gather around and agree on what the operation is supposed to be; something like Jack Nicklaus visualizing that perfect swing, or Yo-Yo Ma playing those complicated opening notes in his head. The immediate goal is to ensure that the right surgery is being done on the right patient, but it clearly goes deeper than that. One UCSF cardiac surgery nurse described the process this way:

Yes, it is useful for us to go through the checklist and for everyone to agree on what the procedure is. But it is more than that. For the first time in my career, all of us gather around, and the surgeon says, "This is Mr. James and we'll be doing a two-vessel cardiac bypass on him." And we briefly chat about it. In the past, we would start the operation and many of us wouldn't even know what the procedure was going to be. It really feels like we're part of a team.

Clearly, we must do much more to create a collaborative culture in health care—one in which all providers at all levels feel free to report and learn from their mistakes, act in concert, and voice their concerns while there is still time to do something about them. This new culture will require substantial new training, in-service coaching, and patience. Physicians in particular have to see themselves in a new light: not as "captain of the ship" but as an integral part of a multidisciplinary team in which no role, or voice, can safely be ignored.

CHAPTER 13:
THE OTHER END OF THE STETHOSCOPE

Each patient carries his own doctor inside him. They come to us not knowing that truth. We are at our best when we give the doctor who resides within each patient a chance to go to work.

— Albert Schweitzer (1875–1965)

June Washington is everyone's "favorite aunt." She is gregarious and unfailingly friendly, inquisitive without being nosy. Her laugh spreads through a room like ripples on a sunny pond. She is a true delight.

A lifelong asthma sufferer, she's managed to raise six children, organize her PTA chapter, and crusade for safety as a member of Mothers Against Drunk Driving. But now, in her seventies, the asthma is taking its toll. She gets winded walking up and down the hill near her home carrying a bag of groceries. She sees a lung specialist, Dr. Michael Stevenson, every month or so for what she calls, "my tune-up." It's a good match between caregiver and patient.

Dr. Stevenson is a throwback to a bygone era. Favoring bow ties and tweed jackets when he's not in a crisp, knee-length white coat, he is passionate about his patients and clinically aggressive when it comes to keeping them well. "Costs are somebody else's problem," he likes to say, and his patients love him for his unwavering focus. His gruff manner, they argue, is part of his charm—another way he gets them to "take their medicine." He has read the literature encouraging physicians to discuss advance directives with their patients before the need arises, but has never agreed with the practice. "If they were dying and I brought it up, it would just push them over the edge. And if they're healthy, why ruin their day?"

So when June Washington had a severe, acute asthma attack and called an ambulance (you could hear her labored wheezing throughout the ER), her preferences about life-sustaining treatment were not written down. The fact is, she had never talked about the subject of an advance directive with anyone.

She was admitted to the hospital by Dr. Stephanie Chan, an attractive, lively intern who was Phi Beta Kappa at Princeton and near the top of her med school class at Yale. Chan is that rare intern who looks cheery and rested after an arduous night on call. Mrs. Washington took an instant liking to her when they met in the ER, and the feeling was mutual.

Dr. Chan had been trained to elicit resuscitation preferences from all her newly admitted patients. When she saw that Washington had no advance directive on her chart, she dutifully sat by the bed and began her carefully worded speech. They had only a couple of minutes before a gurney would transport Mrs. Washington to the step-down unit: a facility not quite as elaborate as an ICU yet capable of giving seriously ill patients closer observation than a regular ward.

"I have this conversation with all my hospital patients," Chan began, putting a reassuring hand on Washington's arm, hoping to make her feel she hadn't been singled out for some dire reason the doctors weren't telling her about. "If you ever get to the point that you can't breathe on your own—that you need a breathing machine to keep you alive—we need to know if you want us to do that."

Chan saw Mrs. Washington's eyes slowly sadden. The brave smile wavered. From her look, Chan could see her patient suddenly focusing on the ominous rattle inside her lungs, on the horrible hunger for air inside her chest. Death, always a potential visitor, was suddenly on her porch, and Dr. Chan had just rung the doorbell. Chan's question brought forth a torrent of emotions— mostly worries— about being "hooked up to machines," being "a vegetable" for the rest of her life. Sure, friends would visit in the beginning, but after a while.... She recalled her friend Lucy's death, like that for months. Couldn't eat. Alone and pathetic. A horrible way to go. Absolutely no dignity. No, she couldn't bear an existence like that.

"I wouldn't want that," Mrs. Washington said haltingly, breathlessly, but in a surprisingly calm and resolute voice. "No way, honey."

Chan nodded empathetically, gave her arm a little squeeze, and left the room. She stopped and checked the "DNR" box on her checklist for Mrs. Washington.

The rest of the night was busy. Chan spoke to her supervising resident, Dr. Ron Lebow, briefly between patients. At one point they discussed Mrs. Washington, and the resident agreed with the intern's findings about the patient's condition and her plan of action.

"Sounds good," he said. "Continuous albuterol by nebulizer, IV solumedrol, and some antibiotics. Anything else?'

"Oh, yes," Chan said. "She wants to be a DNR."

"OK," Lebow wrote "DNR" next to an open checkbox on his own index card, then put the card in the breast pocket of his jacket. Silently, he resolved to confirm the patient's DNR status himself. Chan was very bright and thorough, but with only two months on the job, she was still a little green. It was now past midnight—Lebow knew his attending physician needed to co-sign the DNR form within twenty-four hours, so after confirming the DNR with the patient himself, he would write the order on the chart and discuss it with the attending when he came on duty in the morning. It never occurred to him to call Dr. Stevenson, listed in the chart as the patient's lung specialist. Chan already confirmed that an ER clerk had called Stevenson's answering service and given notice that June Washington had been admitted. Dr. Stevenson had called back to say he would come to see her in the morning, so he was already in the loop. The patient seemed stable. There was no reason to call him again.

At about 1:30 A.M., Mrs. Washington got out of her hospital bed to go to the bathroom, and suddenly collapsed. A nurse in the step-down unit heard her fall and called for Lebow, who just happened to be standing outside the room reviewing Washington's chart before meeting her. The nurse and the doctor rushed in together. Mrs.

Washington wasn't breathing, and had no pulse.

Surprisingly, this was a rather unusual situation—and it put Lebow in a stunning predicament. It was a "witnessed arrest"—one of the few times when CPR has at least a fighting chance to succeed. On the other hand, his intern had just told him that the patient didn't want to be revived. He hesitated a second—an eternity in such situations—then immediately called the Code. "After all," he thought, "we might quickly bring her back—and I never did get a confirmation of her preferences."

His instincts were good. The Code went like clockwork and CPR saved Washington's life. After about ten minutes of chest thumping and three different heart-starting medications, she began breathing. They returned her to her bed and as the nurses plugged her back into the various tubes and monitors, Lebow—sweaty and weak-kneed—sat down to collect his thoughts. He wrote up the incident in Washington's chart and placed a call to Dr. Stevenson to tell him his patient had Coded, but had been brought back to life.

"By the way," he concluded, "she told my intern earlier she wanted to be a DNR. I hope we did the right thing."

"What the hell are you talking about!" gruff old Stevenson roared. "June Washington loves life. She gets along just fine—completely functional. I can't imagine her declining resuscitation. Thank God you ignored it!"

As it turns out, Stevenson was right. Later that day, Mrs. Washington—still aching where the vigorous chest compressions made hairline cracks in her breastbone (already fragile from years of cortisone treatment for her asthma)—had recovered enough to talk.

"When that sweet young Dr. Chan spoke to me about DNR," she said to the attending, "I assumed she was asking me what I'd want the doctors to do if I was a *vegetable*. I never wanted to be stuck on a breathing machine like that. But of course I wanted you to bring me back if you thought I could come back and be like I was before."

Involving patients in their own medical decisions seems like such an obvious proposition that it's hard to believe that it can cause harm. But caregivers have no monopoly on miscommunication. Particularly as we traffic in complex or emotion-laden messages, we invite the possibility that either the caregiver or the patient will misinterpret something, employ selective listening, or just plain ignore or deny the facts. So the case of June Washington shines a light on how patients can help prevent—and how they sometimes unwittingly promote—medical errors.

The so-called patient autonomy movement—emphasizing the rights of patients to full disclosure about their conditions and participation in treatment decisions—really began outside of health care. Prior to the 1950s, doctors were trained to be paternalistic, and patients were conditioned to be subservient. All the accoutrements of a medical encounter—from a chart that's available to everyone but the patient, to the flimsy hospital gown designed to keep the patient's body accessible and immobile—intentionally or inadvertently reflects this imbalance of power. Even so simple a device as a stethoscope symbolically separates the all-knowing, technology user (the doctor) from the weak and ignorant patient by bits of cold metal and a long rubber tube. According to the old adage, a lawyer who pleads his own case has a fool for a client, and that went double for patients who tried to play physician.

Then came the 1960s and '70s. Ralph Nader's *Unsafe at Any Speed*, Rachel Carson's *Silent Spring*, Vietnam, Woodstock, Watergate, and *Our Bodies, Ourselves* made social policy and professional ethics everyone's business. For many, "Question Authority" was more than a bumper sticker, it was a way of life. Patients not only insisted on participating in decisions about their own health, many took time to learn about their options and the underlying issues.

Fast-forward to the early twenty-first century. The "empowered patient" is no longer the exception, he or she is an expectation of the system. Hospitals and private practices are awash in consent and disclosure forms, and informational booklets and phone numbers for resource and support groups. Patients frequently show up for a consultation or a procedure armed with the latest information about their condition—some of it abject nonsense, of course, lifted off guerrilla Web sites or from sources with hidden agendas, like pharmaceutical companies ("Doctor, how come you haven't given me the 'purple pill'") or advocacy groups "raising awareness" about their special diseases.

Accommodating this new clamor for information and participation did not come easily to doctors. It's pretty tough to cover all the bases with a flu patient in a twelve-minute office visit; much less go through the pros and cons of MRIs for bad headaches, angiograms for chest pain, and (perhaps hardest of all) CPR. So, doctors mostly avoid these subjects unless they're specifically asked about them. The exceptions—areas in which standard practice has become detailed engagement with patients over their own preferences—are those unusual decisions that physicians see as true toss-ups, such as hormone-replacement therapy for symptomatic perimenopausal women or prostate cancer options for men with elevated PSAs— both of which remain controversial topics at this writing.

The fact remains, though, that despite all the forms and forums and mandates, doctors still don't include patients sufficiently in care-related decisions. One study analyzed over one thousand audiotaped doctor-patient discussions about diagnostic tests or treatments, and found that less than one percent of moderately or highly complex decisions could be considered "truly informed" from the patient's perspective. Another showed that the average doctor waited only twenty-two seconds before interrupting a patient's own recitation of his clinical complaint. Some of this impatience undoubtedly occurs because doctors spend all day listening to similar stories and twenty-two seconds, in some cases, is enough to turn the fragments of a layman's story into a well-understood clinical mosaic. So, like spouses completing each others' anecdotes, we jump in, risking the possibility that this particular patient's finale will turn out a little different ("Oh, I almost forgot to mention, I've also been coughing up blood..."). Interestingly, left uninterrupted, 80 percent of patients will finish their story in just under two minutes, so the doctor had better put that stolen minute-and-a-half to pretty good use!

Discussions about resuscitations present special challenges to those on both sides of the stethoscope. It's hard enough to talk about such things with patients who already know they are at death's door—even those who have been on life support for an extended period and are "sick and tired of being sick and tired"—let alone those who are feeling fine and just want to get to their grandchild's soccer game. For patients in between—those with a serious chronic or acute illness who may be overwhelmed, confused, or a little unfocused because of their diseases or medications—such "discussions" can quickly turn into soliloquies by the doctor or long stares out into space. Besides, is it even realistic to expect patients who have never experienced an end-of-life scenario to understand the nuances of treatment, the contingencies of a prognosis, or the possible consequences of decisions involving dozens of life-taking illnesses? Finally, what makes us think doctors are better than anyone else at negotiating these treacherous waters when they have had virtually no training to do so?

It may not surprise you to learn that physicians often do a pretty poor job eliciting these preferences with patients. Duke researcher Dr. James Tulsky taped thirty-one residents as they discussed resuscitation options with hospitalized patients. The residents knew they were being taped (having brought the recorder into the room themselves), so we can assume they were more motivated than usual to get the discussion right. Nonetheless, the resulting conversations about end-of-life preferences were highly flawed. While all of the young doctors mentioned the possibility of mechanical ventilation, only half mentioned CPR and just one-third the ICU. None gave his or her patient a realistic estimate of the chances of surviving a Code Blue. The doctors also talked much more than they listened: The physician's monologue took up most of each ten-minute discussion. They closed their "pitches" with a solicitation for the patient's overall values and goals in only 10 percent of the cases.

In a subsequent survey, Tulsky found that these residents, whose average age was twenty-nine, were confident in their abilities to hold these delicate conversations (90 percent said they did a "good job") but one-third admitted they had never been observed or critiqued when discussing resuscitation with a patient. As a whole, the house staff seemed inadequately trained, overconfident, and far too fond of hearing their own voices instead of the patient's; their talkativeness undoubtedly reflects their discomfort with the situation, like an awkward first date. The results also raise another obvious question: Can *any* healthy twenty-nine-year-old really understand how a critically ill seventy-five-year-old feels about life and death without taking the time to ask them, then really listen? Too often, the "discussion" became a forum for residents to promote their own preferences. Ninety-two percent admitted, "if I were in this patient's condition, I would want a DNR order."

But Tulsky resisted the urge to fully ascribe this behavior to youthful inexperience. He next turned his microphone to a group of older physicians in five primary care practices in North Carolina and Pittsburgh. Unfortunately, they did no better. In the outpatient setting, DNR conversations lasted an average of 5.6 minutes, with the doctor speaking two-thirds of the time. For the most part, the scenarios painted for patients were grim, to say the least. One example: "If you were very sick with a terminal illness... if you had something that could never be cured and there was no cure available for you and you started to get really, really sick..." *OK*, thinks the patient, *I can see where this is going....*

On the other hand, a few doctors went to the other extreme. The pictures they painted were at least a shade *too* rosy: "Sometimes what ends up happening is that you have problems with your breathing and you need to be on a respirator breathing for you for a short period of time." These doctors failed to point out that two-thirds of patients revived by CPR need to be on a mechanical breathing machine, and that they can't talk while on a ventilator. The doctors didn't even describe what a ventilator (which patients often confuse with the little nasal oxygen tubes) looked like or was supposed to do.

Not surprisingly, both of these simplistic methods generally led patients to the responses the doctor probably wanted, subliminally at least. One patient said, "Oh well, if my heart stopped and I wasn't out of it, then I guess I would want it... But if I didn't know what I was doing, like a vegetable, then I would not want to live"—just as June Washington affirmed, once she'd actually been through the experience.

Clearly, if we doctors are going to have meaningful and reliable discussions with patients about resuscitation, we've got a lot to learn. As Tulsky concluded, "A poorly worded conversation risks many harms, including violation of patient autonomy, psychological distress, loss of trust in the health care provider, and, most seriously, unwanted attempts at resuscitation that result in prolonged and severe neurological impairment." To this we would add one more obvious error: *failure* to resuscitate because of a misunderstanding of the patient's preferences. This is the one that would have killed June Washington, but for one on-the-ball resident.

Stripped to its essence, the DNR problem is one slice of a bigger challenge: how to turn the informed consent process into a reliable instrument for patients to express their true preferences, while at the same time ensuring that the process lives up to its potential to block some medical errors. June Washington provided "informed consent" for her DNR order, just as Joan Morris provided "informed consent" for her cardiac EPS procedure in the "wrong patient" case. Clearly, without better systems and training, informed consent can simply be another gaping hole in the metaphorical Swiss cheese.

We recall a simple case that really drove home the hazards of relying on patients to protect themselves. An intern was directed to remove surgical staples from a Mr. Garcia. The intern entered the ward and, wary of making a mistake, asked the patient point-blank, "Are you Mr. Garcia?" The man smiled and nodded, so the doctor proceeded to remove the sutures from a wound that, as it turned out, should have been left untouched. He later learned that the patient was very hard of hearing and made a habit of smiling and nodding politely whenever anybody asked him anything.

This is the simple stuff—making sure we get these kinds of identification procedures right is a straightforward matter of teaching our doctors and nurses how to ask open-ended questions ("please tell me your name") and not put words in patients' mouths. Eliciting patient preferences, and making sure patients have the information they need to care for themselves safely, are much bigger kettles of fish. Even when well-educated patients, speaking the same language as the physician, discuss highly charged—or even routine—medical issues, communications gaps can appear. And whenever there is a difference in understanding about facts or intentions, all of the assumptions behind "informed consent" and patient autonomy go out the window, which is left open for more mistakes.

Health literacy is a comparatively new concept that has begun to teach us that patients need better grounding in health care basics before they can reliably understand the often compressed and arcane messages they get from harried and hurried health professionals. Some studies show poor health literacy in up to half of adult patients, and a few have linked it to poorer outcomes in diseases like diabetes. Low health literacy—and doctors' failures to appreciate it—is particularly risky in outpatient settings and at the time of hospital discharge, when we count on patients' abilities to carry out some often extraordinarily complex instructions entirely on their own.

Take the case of Mitch Winston. A sixty-six-year-old gentleman, Winston came to a local ER with shortness of breath and was quickly found to be in atrial fibrillation—a potentially dangerous, fast and irregular heart rhythm in which the top of the heart quivers like a bowl of Jell-O. The physicians planned to sedate Mr. Winston, then shock his heart back into a normal rhythm with the defibrillator. A big danger of this plan is that any blood clots created by the quivering heart can be jarred loose by defibrillation, setting the stage for a stroke. To decrease this risk, physicians usually ask patients to take Coumadin, a powerful blood thinner, orally, for about a month prior to scheduled administration of the jolt.

Winston was sent home with verbal and written instructions to take a three milligram Coumadin tablet alternating with a four milligram tablet every other day—a reasonable starting dose. Unfortunately, an ER is a noisy place and this one was slightly quieter than a subway station. To make matters worse, the doctor instructing Winston was interrupted twice: once by the pharmacy, paging him about another patient's prescription, and a second time to tend to an emergency patient who had just arrived with a stab wound.

"Sorry," the doctor said when he finally returned to Winston, "where was I?"

The physician picked up where he thought he left off, and gave Winston three separate appointment slips: one for a specialized anticoagulation clinic, another for the hospital's cardiology clinic, and a third for his regular doctor. The patient listened attentively while all this was explained to him, nodded agreeably at all the right times, and left the ER with his various instructions tucked into his wallet.

The first sign of communication breakdown occurred when Winston failed to check in for his first follow-up appointment at the anticoagulation clinic, which had been scheduled three days after his ER visit. Ten days after that, he was brought back to the ER by ambulance after passing out. This time, he was passing large, tar-like black stools and vomiting what looked to be old coffee grounds—classic signs of gastric bleeding. His lab studies showed he had lost about half his volume of blood this way, and that what serum remained was about three-times "thinner" than intended, rendering his blood incapable of clotting even after a trivial internal or external bruise.

"Have you been taking Coumadin?" the ER doctor asked him.

"Yes, I've been taking these pills every day," Winston replied, showing the doctor that he had been taking *both* Coumadin pills every day instead of the 3 mg pill one day and the 4 mg pill the next.

Flabbergasted, the doctor corrected him immediately, reread the instructions on the medication, and asked how he could've misinterpreted them. Sheepishly, Winston confessed that he hadn't really understood the original oral instructions ("Everything was happening so fast, and everybody was so busy") and that he couldn't read the discharge sheets or the medication label because, well, he couldn't read. The appointment slips were still folded neatly in his wallet, just where he had put them two weeks earlier.

At least Winston had a fighting chance to get things right. He spoke English and, if he hadn't been quite so intimidated, could have called his regular doctor, or the hospital, or a pharmacist, and gotten his questions answered. When a patient doesn't speak English, or is a non-native English speaker with a limited vocabulary and different cultural habits—as is increasingly the case in America—the doctor might as well be talking to an empty chair. Few clinics can afford to have multilingual interpreters on call and, in a hospital setting, the average patient is seen dozens of times each day by many different caregivers, all of whom exchange at least a few words, if for no other reason than to explain to the patient that they are there to draw blood, update the chart, take the patient's order for dinner, or whatever.

So we muddle through as we always do in such situations, whether as tourists in a foreign land or doctors in a big hospital. We point to the patient's stomach and yell "PAIN?" (All societies seem to think that VOLUME is the universal translator.) Sometimes family members are present, so we conduct our interview through them—although their interpretations are not always reliable. It's also awkward for all concerned to ask a twelve-year-old child to translate his middle-aged aunt's description of her bowel and bladder problems. Sometimes a member of the patient's ethnic group is on staff (give me a clerk, an orderly, a security guard—anybody!) and we make ourselves understood that way, never mind how badly that breaches the patient's right to medical privacy. One study at an outpatient clinic in Boston found thirty-one translation errors per outpatient visit; two-thirds having potentially adverse clinical consequences. The errors were even more dangerous when ad hoc volunteers (relatives, bystanders, etc.) were used instead of professional interpreters. In one case, the amateur interpreter told a mother to place the oral antibiotic amoxicillin into her child's ears instead of her mouth.

Even in those cases when a professional interpreter is available, as sometimes happens at big San Francisco hospitals where a substantial number of patients speak Chinese, Spanish, or Tagalog (the Filipino language), something inevitably gets lost in translation. We both recall times where patients gave us long, impassioned answers to our questions—accompanied by significant body language and facial gestures, followed by dramatic silences, then another burst of information. Anxiously, we'd turn to the official translator who, half the time, would simply say, "He says he feels fine."

As you've seen, problems with communication between caregivers and patients do cause some errors, but there is a larger issue when it comes to the role of the "customer"—can patients ever protect *themselves* from medical mistakes? Some patients certainly believe so. Almost the mirror image of Mitch Winston, they approach every medical encounter grimly determined to double-check and second-guess everything their caregivers do. If a medical error is going to happen during their hospital stay, it's *not* going to happen to them!

These folks now come prepared with reams of Internet printouts on their illnesses, brochures from alternative health care providers (many of which are critical of Western medicine on principle), and stacks of self-help books, mostly written by nonphysicians, with titles like *Take This Book to the Hospital with You* and *How to Get Out of the Hospital Alive*. Even the Joint Commission on Accreditation of Healthcare Organizations, JCAHO—the staid hospital regulator that shares nothing with the Chicago Seven other than a hometown—has launched a campaign urging patients to "Speak Up!" Its president, Dr. Dennis O'Leary, says, "In the traditional medical model, the doctor has the parental view and the patient is childlike. But today, as a doctor in this highly complex, litigious and risky environment, I appreciate a patient helping me out because I'm less likely to make a mistake."

In the "Speak Up" campaign, JCAHO tells patients, "Don't assume anything," and "Educate yourself about your diagnosis and tests." They recommend that you "ask a family member or friend to be your advocate," "know your medications," and "participate in decisions about your treatment." Many consumer advocates go further, warning patients to question nearly everything—from your need for hospitalization to begin with to whether a particular blood test is truly necessary. Armed with evidence that providers fail to wash their hands before touching patients about half the time (in one study, doctors were the worst offenders, washing only 15 percent of the time), these people receive caregivers into their semiprivate suites like guard dogs at a junkyard, barking reminders to wash up before the doc can cross the room to the sink.

Some of this advice makes sense. If nothing else, knowing more about your condition, the reliability of various diagnostic tests, and the efficacy of procedures improves your health literacy and makes you a more informed consumer of medical services.

And you will catch an error from time to time. So go ahead and invite a family member or friend to be at your bedside, or accompany you to an outpatient visit, whenever you can. Make sure the nurse asks your name (or, even better, checks your wristband) before giving you medicine or taking you to a test. Ask your physicians and nurses to explain what they're going to do to you, and why, and remind anyone about to invade your body or give you a shot or a pill what medications you're getting and the reason you're getting them. And if they answer with something that sounds fishy, by all means: Speak up!

However, there are major limits on what you as a patient can do to protect yourself. No matter how much you might wish otherwise, the doctors, nurses, and administrators *will* stay in control of the hospital; and a lot of what seem like errors or oversights are simply the mysterious ways in which your healers work. For example, if you have a medical hand-washing fetish—fine. Just keep in mind that technology changes, and many hospitals, including our own, now use a special, alcohol-based blue goop that is much more effective at killing germs than conventional soap and water. Just as important, it encourages caregiver use because it only takes a couple of seconds to apply and evaporates rapidly—no towels required. To further confuse you, most hospitals place these gel dispensers *outside* patient rooms. The point is: Not all safety precautions are apparent, and some have actually been very well thought out and are followed regularly, whether the patient sees them or not.

If you do choose to act as your own safety advocate, we can share with you some pointers we've learned, and observed, over years of experience:

• Don't be a "Who is your supervisor?" or "I'll call my lawyer" kind of patient. This is unlikely to improve your level of care and it only encourages providers to ignore you. (Think about it: who wants to go into a room, even for routine matters, when they know they'll be abused?) If you demand a certain "minimum" level of service, that's probably what you'll get.

• Do be as friendly and open with your caregivers as your condition permits. The worst any true professional will do is perform to expected standards. If your caregivers bond with you personally, even a little, they're more likely to go that extra mile—the cheapest medical insurance you can buy.

• Use the limited time you have with your caregivers—both doctors and nurses—well. Don't waste it with a lot of extraneous conversation, observations, and complaints about things they can do nothing about, such as parking, the noisy ward down the hall, or the cost of prescription drugs. Most hospital staff are overworked. Chitchat is fine if they have time, but you'll do everyone a favor if you deal with business first—tell them if you're in pain, or are having an odd reaction to a procedure or medication—then let them get on with their many duties.

• Do persist in getting any substantive questions answered. Be firm and inquisitive, but patient and sympathetic. If a caregiver can't answer your question and says, "I'll get back to you," make sure she does so by reminding her in a courteous but timely way. In an extreme case (your need is urgent, but not an emergency), use the phone in your room to contact someone else—a relative or friend who can follow up for you, or even your primary physician or local pharmacy—if you're having trouble getting what you need.

Of course, if things go south in a hurry—and you've seen that they can—then by all means do whatever it takes to protect yourself. A few years ago, a woman in her forties took a bad spill on an icy street in Manhattan's Chinatown. A local shopkeeper called 911 and, after a short ambulance ride, the woman found herself parked on a gurney in Roosevelt Hospital's ER, where she began to age gracefully, like a forgotten piece of furniture. After several hours of neglect, she borrowed a visitor's cell phone and called the police. "Help!" the woman told them, "There's a woman being held hostage at Roosevelt Hospital!" When the cops showed up a few minutes later, she quickly received more attention than she knew what to do with. Sometimes, speaking up *is* just what the doctor ordered.

Philosophically, we believe that the burden of ensuring patient safety should not be on sick patients, but rather on health professionals, health care systems, and policymakers. Patients have enough to worry about without feeling responsible for their own safety. We recognize that you might see this as recommending that you "know your place," and you would be well within your rights to accuse us of paternalism—or even a bit of hypocrisy in a semiconfessional book that, if nothing else, has made the point that our present system cannot simply be trusted to keep you safe.

But we *must* make it so. And in Part III of this book, we'll begin to consider how.

PART III: CONSEQUENCES

CHAPTER 14: SPILLING THE BEANS

Everyone will be famous for fifteen minutes.

— Andy Warhol (1928–1987)

Died of complications after gallbladder surgery

As medical stars go, Dr. James Jaggers was one of the brightest. A pediatric heart surgeon, his professional life had been a string of small miracles.

One of his two specialties was the Ross Procedure, a rare open-heart surgery in which two of the four heart valves—in a child, each as fragile as tissue paper and no larger than a dime—are replaced. At the conclusion of this nearly impossible procedure, a tiny coronary artery is reattached to the beating heart—the equivalent of sewing a tube the size of a pencil lead onto a pile of quivering pudding. The tiniest slip will end the child's life.

Performing this procedure takes a special breed, and Dr. Jaggers had the Right Stuff as surely as any Mercury astronaut. With his surgical acumen, roguish good looks, and winning personality, his patients and their families, quite naturally, placed him on a pedestal, and the shadow it cast was long indeed. As one former patient recalls: "When Dr. Jaggers was done talking to me a warm feeling overcame me and I knew I was in good hands. I could relate to what he was saying...."

As if his regular services weren't enough, Jaggers periodically volunteered to help poor children in developing countries. His latest trip: In late 2002, he led a delegation of volunteer physicians to Nicaragua.

Jaggers's second specialty was pediatric heart transplants. Only a few hundred of these marvels take place each year. Everything about them is astounding—and the nine-hour operation in which the tiny, diseased heart is removed and replaced with a donor organ (which must be removed from the deceased and installed within six hours) is just one part of the process. High drama surrounds even the selection of candidates, and thousands die annually simply because a suitable organ can't be found or transported in time. The financial stakes are high, too. The cost of a transplant starts at a half-million dollars—and that assumes everything goes perfectly.

Transplants of any kind depend on the astonishing advances we have made in immunology. In earlier decades, the importance of matching blood groups (A, B, AB, and O types) between donor and recipient was well understood, as was the significance of the Rh factor (the "positive" or "negative" that further modifies each type). We also understood a bit about the complement system, which amplifies the immune system's attack on foreign invaders: bacteria, splinters, literally anything entering the body. More recently, the greatest advances in transplantation have come not so much from better surgical technique (although hooking up the plumbing is far from trivial), but from divining how to keep the body's own defenses from destroying the new organ intended to save it. Suppressing the immune system, even in the service of a good cause, opens the door to other problems, from opportunistic infections to fatal cancers. Decreasing these complications—while protecting the transplanted organs from attack—is key. And we've largely succeeded: The three-year survival rate for most transplants is now up to 75 percent, and several Nobel Prizes have been awarded to the researchers whose discoveries made this possible.

One of the Meccas for transplant technology is Duke University—the "Harvard of the South"—in Durham, North Carolina. Duke's medical center is a study in contrasts: a modern edifice of chrome and marble rising from an almost medieval-looking campus of ivy-covered stone buildings bedecked with turrets and gargoyles; a world-class medical crossroads that began as a truck stop on the road to Florida. Although many Americans know Duke best as a basketball powerhouse, its massive medical center has an equally awesome reputation among physicians, medical schools, and hospital administrators.

Duke's motto—"Brilliant Medicine, Thoughtful Care"—is nowhere more evident than in its transplant programs. Duke performed the nation's first successful outpatient bone marrow transplant and one of the nation's first kidney transplants. Today, Duke runs the largest lung transplant program, and one of the largest heart transplant programs, in the nation. Not surprisingly, the facility became America's clinical Cover Girl in 1998 when *Time* magazine published a special issue on high-tech medicine, featuring "A Day in the Life" of Duke Medical Center.

Consequently, Dr. Jaggers (who received his training in fine, but not world-class facilities—the University of Nebraska, Oregon Health Sciences University, and the University of Colorado) was surely thrilled when he was invited to join Duke's faculty as head of its pediatric heart surgery department in 1996. A virtuoso with medical instruments; he would now perform on the stage of medicine's equivalent of Carnegie Hall.

It should have come as no surprise, then, that Dr. James Jaggers and his program would become media stars; internationally recognized examples of the breathtaking potential of modern medicine.

But the script turned out to be by Alfred Hitchcock, not Frank Capra.

Jesica Santillan was the kind of patient James Jaggers was put on Earth to save. The pretty seventeen-year-old girl from Jalisco, Mexico was born with restrictive cardiomyopathy, a disorder of the heart that limits its ability to accept blood from the lungs and pump it effectively to the rest of the body—like a party balloon that won't fully inflate because the rubber is too stiff. Even worse, the back-pressure this exerted on her delicate lungs was ruining those organs, too. As she got older, her condition grew worse, until her parents—a truck driver and laundress—sought treatment for her in the United States, the place where so many impossible dreams had a way of coming true.

They raised the $5,000 necessary to smuggle Jesica across the border in the back of a truck, after which she joined relatives living in a windowless trailer in Louisburg, North Carolina. That's where her poignant story caught the eye of a wealthy local businessman, Mack Mahoney, who founded a charity— "Jesica's Hope Chest"—to raise $500,000 for her heart-lung transplant. As luck would have it, one of the nation's premier pediatric transplant facilities lay a stone's throw away, led now by a master surgeon with a soft spot in his heart for children from developing countries. On April 5, 2002, Dr. Jaggers first met and examined Jesica, and he put her on Duke's heart-lung transplant waiting list. Her chances seemed remote—just six pediatric heart-lung transplants were performed in *all* of America in 2002—but remember, Jaggers trafficked in miracles. Both he and Jesica began the wait for a suitable donor.

Quickly, Jesica became a star in her own right. A local newspaper wrote a touching profile of her a month before her transplant. Because her parents worked, and she needed constant care because of her weakened condition, she spent most of her time at the Mahoneys' Louisburg home. When Christmas 2002 rolled around, Jesica appointed herself "chief tree decorator" for her generous hosts. This was Movie-of-the-Week stuff; all that remained was for the inspiring final act to be written.

For Jaggers, Jesica's was an extraordinarily high-profile case, and both the surgeon and his staff undoubtedly felt crushing pressure to find a suitable donor. Some of this pressure was humanitarian— Jaggers and his team passionately believed in the good they were doing. But part of it was pragmatic. Success in a high-profile case like Jesica's brings favorable headlines for the surgeon and the facility, and converts instantly to more patients, more income, and more grants—the lifeblood of any big medical center.

So Jaggers must have been elated (as much as any humanitarian can be elated when new life is possible only after someone else— worst of all, a child—has died) after receiving a middle-of-the-

LEADERS / THINKERS

DR. DONALD BERWICK A pediatrician and president of the Boston-based Institute for Healthcare Improvement, Berwick helped catalyze the writing of the IOM report on medical errors.

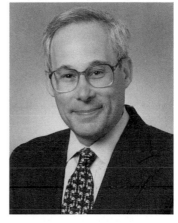

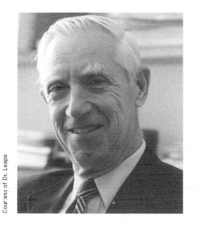

DR. LUCIAN LEAPE The Harvard pediatric surgeon was the first prominent physician to turn his focus to medical mistakes.

DR. ATUL GAWANDE While still a surgical resident, Gawande introduced many readers to the human dimensions of medical errors with his columns in *The New Yorker* and then his book, *Complications*.

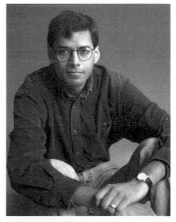

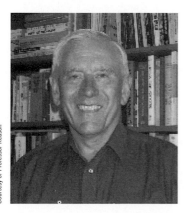

PROFESSOR JAMES REASON

A psychology professor in Manchester, England, Reason's "theory of error" has been used in virtually all high-risk fields, but, until recently, was ignored in medicine.

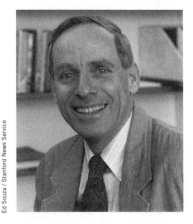

PROFESSOR AMOS TVERSKY The late Stanford psychologist helped pioneer the study of decision-making under uncertainty, promoting a deeper understanding of cognitive and judgment errors.

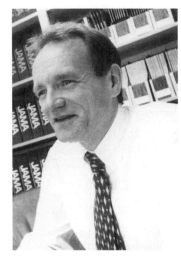

DR. TROY BRENNAN The Harvard physician-lawyer led the Harvard Medical Practice Study, from which the IOM's famous death estimates ("a jumbo jet a day") were drawn, and has been the nation's leading thinker on medical malpractice and patient safety.

VICTIMS

JESICA SANTILLAN The young girl who died in 2003 at Duke Medical Center after she received a heart-lung transplant of the wrong blood type.

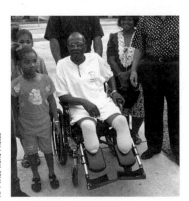

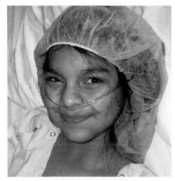

WILLIE KING The 51-year-old diabetic man from Tampa, Florida became a nationally known icon for wrong-sited surgery when his incorrect leg was amputated.

SCENES AND SET-UPS FOR ERRORS

A typical "team" in an academic teaching hospital includes a supervising physician (the "attending," second from left), a resident (two or more years out of medical school), two interns (one year out of medical school), and several medical students.

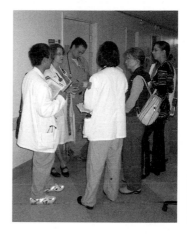

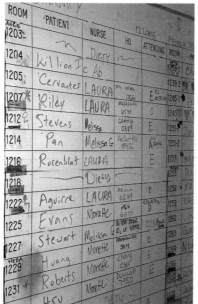

A nursing station whiteboard, with hastily scrawled patient names, along with each patient's nurse, house officer (HO), and team (letters A thru E). Think there's a chance of a mix-up? (Patient names are fictitious.)

A typical nursing station on a hospital ward, including a ward clerk, nurses, and a physician. Notice the rack of patient charts at left.

Insulin or heparin? In a busy, chaotic ICU, would it surprise you that a nurse might grab one when she intended the other?

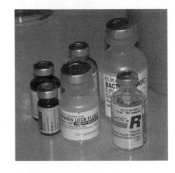

An electrophysiology (EPS) laboratory, with a draped patient and the EPS nurse and fellow at her bedside. The attending physician sits at a console in the next room, following the case through the glass and on the computer screen.

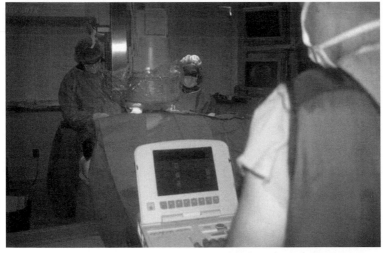

A not-too-unusual sea of IV drips in a modern ICU.

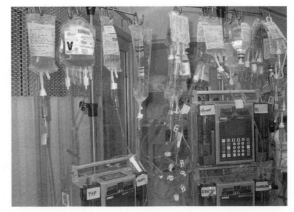

FIXES

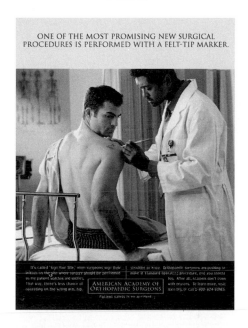

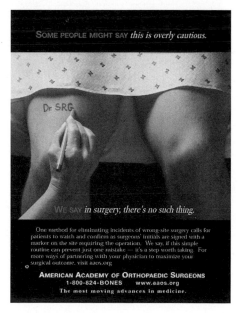

Posters promoting the American Academy of Orthopedic Surgeons' campaign to get its members to initial their surgical sites prior to operating, in an effort to prevent wrong-sited surgery.

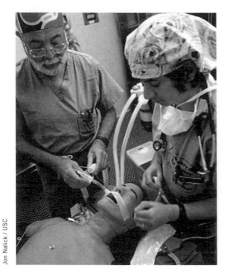

Training doctors in the age of technology: Increasingly sophisticated and realistic simulators allow doctors to learn new techniques and practice teamwork without the risk of harming patients.

A medical bar-coding system in action, as a nurse scans a patient's bracelet. An alarm goes off if the bar code doesn't match, for example, a medication label or a surgical schedule.

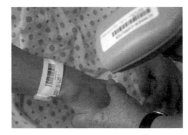

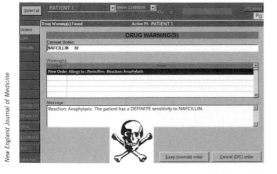

No more doctors' handwriting: A computerized physician order entry (CPOE) system eliminates medication errors due to bad penmanship, and sets the stage for doctors to receive sophisticated electronic decision support.

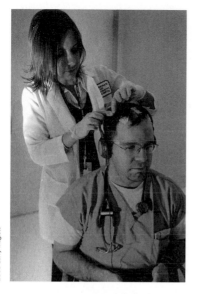

An ongoing study at Brigham and Women's Hospital measures the impact of sleep deprivation on physician performance and error rate. In addition to monitoring brain waves, the doctors produce an hourly saliva sample to measure levels of the sleep hormone melatonin.

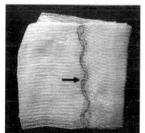

A

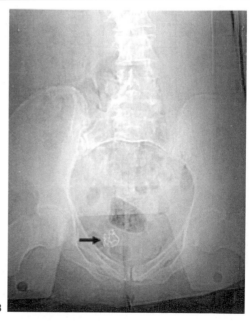

B

American Journal of Roentgenology

A four-by-four-inch surgical sponge with an interwoven radiopaque thread (arrow) (panel A). Panel B shows an intra-operative X-ray, performed because of an incorrect sponge count, demonstrating the marker (arrow) in the pelvis. The sponge was identified and removed.

U.S. House rejects homophobia
*Hefley amendment to overturn
executive order goes down to defeat.*
                                    page 19

Banner days
*More on the just-completed
Gay Games from Amsterdam.*
                    page 22 – 23

Perversely pretty
*Photographer Pierre
Molinier in Santa Monica.*
        see Arts section

BAYAREAREPORTER

Vol. 28 • No. 33 • 13 August 1998

Serving the Gay & Lesbian Community for more than 27 years

No obits

by Timothy Rodrigues

Readers of the *Bay Area Reporter* who regularly scan the obituary page for familiar faces – friends, ex-lovers, former tricks, that guy you used to see at the gym who has not been around for a while – will have to forgo that ritual this week. No obituaries were filed with the paper for this issue, a first since the AIDS epidemic exploded in San Francisco's gay community.

That doesn't mean that there were no AIDS deaths in the past week; next week's issue may have more obits than usual. Nevertheless, after more than 17 years of struggle and death, and some weeks with as many as 31 obituaries printed in the *B.A.R.*, it seems a new reality may be taking hold, and the community may be on the verge of a new era of the epidemic. Perhaps.

"It is certainly refreshing, and I think we deserve a break

health for the Department of Public Health (DPH), told the *B.A.R.* "We all deserve a little bit of respite," he continued.

Derek Gordon, director of communications for the San Francisco AIDS Foundation (SFAF), who has been living with HIV for many years, talked about scanning the obituary page, looking to see who had died, and feeling "it was just a matter of time before I would see my own face.

"I remember my grandfather said he knew he was getting near death because he used to scan the obits," he told the *B.A.R.* "I used to think how tragic because I was doing the same thing at 30."

Gordon cautioned that the epidemic is not over, but acknowledged that the decrease in the number of obituaries reflects a parallel trend in his personal experience. He said he no longer feels the same sense of "doom and despair," and added, "I don't have any [recent] obits to personally tell."

Dick Pabich, AIDS policy advisor to Mayor Willie Brown, and someone who has lived with AIDS for many years, has had the opposite personal experience. He has recently had

had to deal with for some time.

"I have frankly had a concern that we are seeing a shift in the opposite direction," he said, mentioning an increase in the number of people he knows who have died, gotten infected by HIV, or been diagnosed.

While acknowledging that the lack of obituaries is symbolically very important, Pabich warned that it is important not to overstate the situation and said there should be no lessening of efforts to fight the epidemic.

If current estimates are correct, 10 people may have been infected by HIV in the last week, and it is estimated that 15,000 people living in San Francisco are HIV-positive.

Although scientists, reporters, and government officials have commented that AIDS deaths have been declining since the introduction of new anti-HIV drug regimens, several of those interviewed mentioned that many people cannot obtain, choose not to take, or do not benefit from currently available treatment options. Also, the incidence of HIV/AIDS is in-

The war can eventually be won: The August 13, 1998, front page of the *Bay Area Reporter*, the newsweekly for San Francisco's gay community. The paper had, for a decade, devoted up to a quarter of its space to AIDS obituaries.

night call from the New England Organ Bank (NEOB) on February 6, 2003. The call informed him that a dying donor with organs perfectly suited to young Jesica had been found. This by itself was a minor miracle. Death takes people in many nasty ways, and donor organs must not only be undamaged by trauma, they must be free of the disease that killed the previous owner. And for pediatric transplants, the organs must also be of a size that fits the recipient, which is often the most challenging match of all.

The youth in question, a seven-year-old boy at Boston's Children's Hospital, was the perfect donor: His heart and lungs were pristine. Upon his death, the NEOB had immediately informed the United Network for Organ Sharing (UNOS), which acts as a clearinghouse for patients on transplant waiting lists across the U.S. As the clock began ticking on the highly perishable donor organs (the heart cells start dying about six hours after being removed from the donor), the UNOS computers switched into overdrive. UNOS looked first in New England—good organs don't matter if you can't get them to the patient in time. When no local matches came up, the net widened and reached Duke Medical Center. UNOS's first call, routed through a transplant intermediary—the nonprofit Carolina Donor Services, CDS—went to Dr. Carmelo Milano, Duke's adult heart transplant surgeon, who had two patients with Type A blood (the donor's blood type) on his waiting list. But they weren't good candidates: The replacement heart and lungs were just too small for an adult's torso.

The UNOS computer next identified a child at Duke—not Jesica—who seemed to fit the criteria, so CDS got Dr. Jaggers, head of pediatric heart surgery, on the line. Awakened from a sound slumber, Jaggers discussed a few technical matters, including the organs' size, and told CDS that the computer-chosen patient was not appropriate for the operation (that child was too sick for the surgery), but that he had another patient, seventeen-year-old Jesica (who was not yet registered in the UNOS system), who *was* a perfect fit. CDS's usual procedure at this point was to confirm the blood-type match between donor and recipient, but for reasons unknown, they did not do so in this case.

As soon as Jaggers got off the phone, he dispatched a colleague, Dr. Shu Lin, to fly to the donor's hospital in Boston and "harvest" the organs. Lin, an eighth-year transplant surgery resident, expertly removed the organs from the just-deceased young boy. The heart and lungs were "triple bagged" and placed in an icy bath. Incongruously, the lifesaving vessel for this half-million-dollar venture was, as always, a sterilized Igloo cooler that can be purchased at Toys "R" Us for less than twenty dollars. At the time, Lin was told the donor's blood type—Type A—on at least three occasions, but he did not know Jesica's blood type. He had a single job to do, and reconfirming the match was not part of it. Like everyone else, he assumed that a match had already been made by his colleagues back home. Between his arrival at Boston Children's Hospital and his return to Duke on a chartered plane (which waited with engines thrumming at Logan Airport), he and Jaggers spoke three separate times. The question of the blood types never came up.

While the harvesting surgery proceeded 530 miles to the north, Jaggers's ten-member surgical team swung into action. They scrubbed together and entered Duke's OR number 7, one by one, walking backward with hands aloft to avoid any accidental contact with contaminated surfaces. Jesica (whose family had been called with the good news only hours earlier) was now prepped and anesthetized. With a deft hand, Jaggers made the incision in Jesica's bony chest (her illness had reduced her weight to a mere eighty pounds), "cracked" her sternum, and began removing the diseased organs that had ruined her childhood. In the transplant business, this is the equivalent of football's two-minute drill. It is essential to remove the diseased organs just moments before the replacements arrive, so as to avoid further deterioration of the new set, allowing the "installation" to take place as soon as possible. In Jesica's case, Duke's official chronology of the surgery showed that the new organs reached the OR at about the same time as the old ones were being lifted out of Jesica's thoracic cavity.

Lin arrived in OR number 7 a few minutes before 5 P.M., and handed off his precious cargo. The Igloo cooler was placed on the floor, out of the way—its work was done. Large letters on its side read, "Blood Type A." But all eyes were on Jesica, and on Jaggers.

As we might expect from a surgeon of Jaggers's caliber, the operation went flawlessly—at least for the first five hours. At about 10 P.M., an alert technician in Duke's immunology lab made a startling discovery: The new organs' blood type (Type A) didn't match Jesica's (Type O). This realization must have been so incomprehensible to the lab staff that they undoubtedly considered it an error. Since the blood type matching was simply their first test—completely *pro forma*—before they undertook a battery of more sophisticated immunologic assays, nobody expected any disconcerting results—let alone a heart-stopping blunder. So they ran the test again. The results were the same.

Encountering a Type O patient is usually good news for blood banks: Their blood can be used by any other person needing a transfusion—they are *universal donors*. Type O blood lacks the antigens that trigger rejection—attack by the recipient's own antibodies. Jesica's problem was that this immunologic welcome-wagon doesn't work in reverse. Type Os can only receive blood or organs from other Type Os; anything else is like forcing a square peg into a round hole.

The lab notified the Operating Room immediately. Jaggers was staggered by the news—he must have felt like the captain of the *Titanic* after the first jolt of the iceberg slammed the starboard hull—and knew instantly what would happen. Without breaking the rhythm of his surgery, he ordered his team to close up, as they began administering large doses of anti-rejection drugs in an all-but-futile effort to stop the inevitable. What had begun as a heroic attempt to grant young Jessica a few more years—if not decades—of life had suddenly become a battle to keep her alive for a few more days, in the vain hope that a matching organ donor would be found and the disaster miraculously reversed.

"It's that deep sort of sinking feeling," Jaggers reported later, "a completely helpless feeling that there's absolutely nothing you can do about it."

After a tense hour or so in the ICU, during which the organs appeared to be working, the fatal attack from Jesica's newly aroused immune system finally began. Sadly, despite the high-tech heart-lung machine that kept Jesica alive throughout the operation, despite Duke's corps of Nobel Prize-winning scientists, despite a brilliant and dedicated surgeon whose OR team actually *functioned* like a team, the entire system lacked a method for ensuring that the simplest of all matches—known to doctors from the earliest days of transfusions—had been accomplished, checked, and double-checked.

Lloyd Jordan, Carolina Donor Services executive director, recalling his earlier coordination with the organ bank, later told *60 Minutes*, "We could have requested her blood type, and I wish we had." Jaggers himself recalled discussing the donor's size and cause of death with CDS, but "did not recall ABO [blood] typing being discussed... I assumed that after providing Jesica's name to the organ procurement organization and after the organs were released to me for Jesica, that the organs were compatible."

"That," Duke CEO Dr. William Fulkerson later said with Herculean understatement, "was an inaccurate assumption."

As of this writing, no one has established precisely how this mix-up occurred. Perhaps Dr. Jaggers misunderstood the CDS rep on the phone. Maybe the blood type *was* mentioned but Jaggers had a temporary lapse of memory (it was, after all, the middle of the night) and it simply slipped his mind that Jesica's Type O was the universal donor, not the universal recipient (that's Type AB). Most likely, in the high excitement of the moment—the triumph of finding a set of pediatric organs the right size for his celebrated and sympathetic patient—Jaggers just plain forgot to ask about such a prosaic detail, assuming that people lower on the system's totem pole had already checked.

If, as Einstein said, God resides in the details, so apparently does the devil. Like so many medical errors, this one occurred because people were so focused on the big picture that they completely overlooked the small stuff. A few weeks after the Duke case made news, Bob was addressing an audience of three hundred of America's top patient safety experts at a federally sponsored conference. He asked, "How many of you have seen an error at your institution involving the failure to accurately transmit a crucial piece of information at the time of a handoff?" Every single hand went up.

At its core, the Duke error was among medicine's most basic mistakes—what patient-safety guru Don Berwick means when he refers to "the banality of the screwup." In fact, the case perfectly fits James Reason's Swiss cheese model, in which multiple small errors align to reveal a single, massive hole in the system. By this point in the book, you already have a deep understanding of how a simple slip can snowball into a breathtaking tragedy.

But Jesica's case offers a number of additional lessons as we turn our attention to the *consequences* of medical errors. Among them: How do doctors deal with their mistakes; how and when (or even *if*) caregivers should tell patients and families about these mistakes; whether to tell the media; and whether regulatory agencies should be involved—and, if so, whether it should be in an informational or punitive capacity. In Jesica's case, these issues arose at once and with hurricane force; but in everyday practice they occur constantly, in far less public but equally dramatic and wrenching ways, in hospitals throughout America.

In Jesica's case, the first call administrators made was probably to the hospital's Risk Management department. The risk manager is usually a lawyer—paid by the hospital—whose role is to step in when a particularly horrific error has occurred. The title "risk manager" is a delicious euphemism, redolent with double entendre. Although many risk managers emphasize that their function eventually results in safer treatments (and many have, in fact, become more proactive in mistake prevention since the 1999 IOM report was published), the "risk" they seek to manage is mostly the hospital's risk of being sued. When called about a particular case, the risk manager's main tasks are to settle everyone down, assess the hospital's liability, and help control the damage.

After the initial heads-up, risk managers begin gathering all of the available facts—attempting to find out who did what, and when; who knew what, and when; and if things are really as bad as everyone thinks. This is not an objective investigation, the results of which are intended for the medical archives. It is legal case-building, and the information it generates is legally privileged; the hospital may or may not use it to increase its leverage in future settlement negotiations or litigation. Of course, the risk manager, like the other members of the medical staff, hopes that it never comes to that, but if it does the hospital needs to be prepared.

Part of this "crisis management" is to counsel the doctors and nurses and other staff members to keep their mouths shut—at least initially. Confession may be good for the soul, but it's ruinous in court. This advice, of course, is not unique to medicine—it's what lawyers tell any client faced with a potential lawsuit involving legal and financial liability. In a way, it's like reading the "Miranda rights" to parties who themselves may feel stunned or sorry about an unfortunate event, even when they are not directly responsible for it. For caregivers trained to be tactful and empathic—and to explain complex events to patients and their families—holding their tongues after an error is both counterintuitive and morally gut-wrenching.

Moreover, modern risk managers now realize that Watergate-style stonewalling (standard practice in the past) just doesn't cut it with patients or the press. As with other corporate disasters—such

as accidents at nuclear power plants, airline crashes, or oil spills—
"controlled disclosure" works better than stony silence. So current
practice calls for the hospital to acknowledge the tragedy and
sometimes even admit that "mistakes were made" (without getting
too specific), which does seem to go a long way toward tempering
initial reactions.

In the Duke case, you can bet that senior hospital administrators
were paged "stat" within minutes of the risk manager learning of the
error. A series of frenzied meetings undoubtedly followed, during
which hard facts were merged with mitigating circumstances and
plausible, buck-passing explanations. By the next morning, the PR
damage-control consultants were probably called in—the same
type of pros who handled the Tylenol poisoning and Firestone tire
blowout cases—and were given the hospital's story about what went
down. This is not as Machiavellian as it sounds. Duke Medical Center
is a billion-dollar-a-year business that trades on a hard-earned
reputation for quality care. Jesica's tragic story was a crackling
brush fire that—without proper handling—could quickly turn into
a conflagration that could burn down the whole institution.

Most errors, of course, are handled far from the media spotlight.
In less telegenic cases, the risk manager's role is simply to advise
providers as to the best way to manage the situation (and then, after
the legal dust has settled, to work with the staff and administration
to be sure a similar error doesn't happen again). When the plan is full
disclosure, the risk manager offers to sit at the doctor's side during
the family meeting—partly to show that the hospital really cares by
sending an administrative representative, but also to clear her throat
every time the doctor gets too weepy or confessional. Physicians often
feel this "service" feels too "lawyerish" and prefer to meet with families
alone. After they're done, the risk manager handles "phase two" and
consolingly offers what amounts to a settlement package: waiving the
hospital bill, for example (Duke waived Jessica's bill, which came to
$899,382), or moving the patient to the head of the line for a repeat
procedure, or offering to pick up the costs of ongoing care.

The compulsion to make things right—for both Jesica's and Duke's sakes—led to a final chapter that medical ethicists will be debating for decades. Since transplanted organs are an extraordinarily limited resource, there is a double tragedy in transplant cases where good organs are "wasted" due to error—not just the harm to the first victim, but to the *potential* recipients who were denied their chances at new lives. In the Duke case, this happened not just once, but twice. To atone for the first organ mix-up, Jesica was put at the head of the line for the next set of organs that came down the pipeline, and she received a second heart-lung transplant on February 20, 2003. This time, Jesica was so weak and her body so ravaged that the odds against her survival were astronomical. Even a brilliant doctor like Jaggers couldn't save her (yes, he was allowed to perform the second transplant, under the watchful eye of his boss, Dr. Duane Davis). She died shortly after the second surgery.

Although it is emotionally appealing to argue that "the system" owed Jesica a second chance, it is nearly impossible to make the moral case that this ultra-high-odds surgery was more justified than using these scarce organs in another patient with a far better prognosis.

As you can see, the ethical and emotional dimensions of medical errors—while outwardly similar to mistakes in other fields—are ultimately unique, and compound the psychological complexity of disclosure. As British psychologist Charles Vincent observed:

> First, patients are unintentionally harmed by the people in whom they have placed considerable trust, so their reaction may be especially powerful and complex. Second, they are cared for by members of the same profession, and in some cases the same clinicians, as those who were involved in the injury itself...

Because of this, continues Vincent,

The lack of an explanation, and of an apology if appropriate, may be experienced by the patient as extremely punitive and distressing and may be a powerful stimulus to complaint or litigation.

Although full disclosure is unquestionably the right thing to do ethically, what about its financial implications? Does a confession make a lawsuit *more* likely, as some risk managers fear, or *less* likely, as psychologist Vincent suggests?

Oddly, there is surprisingly little evidence on this point. One study, cited frequently by researchers exploring this issue, describes how a VA hospital in Lexington, Kentucky adopted a policy of full disclosure and was sued relatively few times over the following year. Although this appeals to the humanitarian instinct in all of us, the study was flawed in several ways. First, nobody measured how much "full disclosure" actually occurred *before* the new policy was in place. It's possible that the policy simply codified what was already common practice. Second, as most lawyers know, it's damn hard to sue federal facilities like the VA.

Notwithstanding these defects, proponents of full disclosure often cite the VA study as proof of their position: that honesty is always the best policy. While that's an easy position for researchers to take, the caregivers themselves—the ones who actually committed, or are accused of committing, the errors—often have a different opinion, since they face personal liabilities that the armchair advisers don't. One St. Louis physician gave voice to this skepticism: "Everything you read and everything that you're told says that you are supposed to tell what errors you make as soon as you can. Let [patients] know what your thinking is, what you are going to do about it. And your chances of having an adverse litigation are less if you take that approach. Now, the question is, how many of us believe that?"

Apparently, not a lot of doctors. Although patients understandably want their doctors and hospitals to come clean about mistakes, full disclosure remains the exception. One survey of medical residents found that 76 percent had not disclosed a serious error to a patient. In a national survey, only 30 percent of patients who felt they were victims of a medical error said that their doctor or nurse had told them about it. In a series of focus groups, patients unanimously wanted to be told about errors in their care, including the causes, consequences, and plans to prevent similar errors in the future. They also wanted an apology. One patient described how he would want a major error—a hypothetical insulin overdose caused by a prescribing error—disclosed: "[I'd want the doctor to say to me] 'You have my deepest sympathy... We're doing everything within our powers to correct this error and we can assure you that this problem will not happen again.... I'm available to sit down and discuss with you in detail what happened, and again, I'm sorry.'"

In the same set of focus groups, physicians expressed a powerful urge to apologize to patients about their errors, but felt the threat of malpractice suits prevented them from doing so. "You would love to be just straightforward," said one physician about a hypothetical mistake in which he overdosed a patient on potassium because he failed to check a crucial laboratory test. "Gosh, I wish I had checked that potassium yesterday. I was busy, I made a mistake... I will learn from my mistake and I will do better next time, because this is how we learn as people.'" Then he confessed, "But if you say that to a patient... we have this whole thing, the wait to cash in..." through a malpractice suit.

So the jury is still out regarding full disclosure—if not on a moral level, then as a practical fact of life. The two of us have seen lawsuits that grew out of a family's anger after stumbling onto an error they hadn't been told about; raising the possibility that patients (and juries) view cover-ups as worse than the crimes. But we've also seen lawsuits triggered by a heartfelt apology and full explanation—essentially handing the plaintiff's lawyer a case based on the physician's clinical goof and ethical scruples. You can be sure that the doctor receiving the subpoena in such a case will be less apt to confess after his next error—let the ethicists be damned.

In the Duke case, Jaggers disclosed the error to Jesica's family right away. "Jim Jaggers came right out and said there's been a terrible mistake," said a fellow Duke surgeon with obvious admiration. "He had the guts and the courage to go out and tell the truth." But Duke's openness did nothing to quell the family's anger and that of her patron, Mack Mahoney. "To me... they murdered her," was Mahoney's emotional response.

And it was Mahoney's fury that ignited the subsequent furor in the press. Duke, quite naturally, was not particularly inclined to alert the media about the mistake. Four days after the first transplant, Duke spokesman Richard Puff didn't mention the mix-up to a local reporter following Jesica's story. "Her doctors continue to monitor her progress in getting past the initial organ rejection," Puff told the reporter. "Initial rejection is somewhat typical for most transplant patients."

When the networks picked up the story and began a full-court press, *mea culpa* became Duke's only viable strategy. The medical center's CEO, Dr. William Fulkerson, issued a "mistakes were made" kind of statement, admitting Duke's wrongdoing while highlighting the flawed transplant matching system that was largely responsible for the terrible foul-up. "In our efforts to identify organs for this desperately ill patient, regrettably, a mistake occurred," Fulkerson said. "Human error occurred at several points in the organ placement process that had no structured redundancy."

Far from being a unique circumstance, the errors served to expose the system's underlying vulnerabilities. It turns out that similar transplant errors had occurred at least twice before, in 1991 and 1994, but had escaped public notice. (Ironically, both happened at Oregon Health Sciences University, where Jaggers received his surgical training.) Soon after Jesica's story hit the wires, every transplant hospital in the nation, including our own, created double- and triple-layer redundancies in their blood-type checking procedures. *There but for the grace of God...* was the prevailing sentiment of all those physicians and administrators who knew that such an error was not exactly unthinkable at their own institutions. "It is something I have nightmares about," said Dr. Michael Acker, chief of heart transplantation at the Hospital of the University of Pennsylvania. "This is an example of what can happen when you let your guard down and there are holes in the system."

As we watched reports of the Duke case stream across the CNN screen like an electronic boomerang, we got to wondering: What makes some medical errors newsworthy, and others not? It's not a simple matter of frequency. We've already seen how America's most oft-committed errors—medication mistakes—pass virtually unnoticed thousands of times each day. It's not even a matter of fatalities—several error-related deaths occur in every American hospital each month. What, then, turns bad news into big news?

This is not a minor question, since fear of media exposure runs neck-and-neck with fear of lawsuits in reasons for "failure to disclose" by caregivers and hospitals. To help answer this dilemma, we chronicled some of the most mediagenic medical mistakes over the last twenty years (presented here in chronological order):

*1984*An eighteen-year-old woman, Libby Zion (daughter of a prominent *New York Times* reporter), was a patient at Cornell's New York Hospital. She received the pain medication Demerol, which caused a fatal interaction with her antidepressant. The alleged root cause: Residents who were fatigued and inadequately supervised.

*1987*Pop artist Andy Warhol died at New York Hospital after semiroutine gallbladder surgery. The death was ascribed to inadequate postoperative monitoring and a fatal buildup of fluid in Warhol's body.

*1994*Health care reporter Betsy Lehman of the *Boston Globe* died after receiving a chemotherapy overdose during experimental treatment at Harvard's Dana-Farber Cancer Hospital.

The root causes were a young physician's unfamiliarity with the experimental protocols, and an inadequate system to guard against chemotherapy mistakes (Chapter 4).

1995 A fifty-one-year-old diabetic, Willie King, had the wrong leg amputated at a Tampa, Florida community hospital. The mistake was attributed to paperwork errors and an inattentive surgeon (Chapter 7).

1995 Rajeswari Ayyappan, the fifty-nine-year-old mother of an Indian film star, had tumor surgery on the wrong side of her brain at Memorial Sloan-Kettering Cancer Center in New York. A mix-up between Ayyappan and another patient was blamed (Chapter 7).

1998 Comedian Dana Carvey received a coronary bypass of the wrong vessel at Marin General Hospital in California. Carvey underwent a second bypass successfully at a different hospital in Los Angeles. The first surgeon blamed Carvey's unusual heart anatomy for the error.

1999 and *2001* In a pair of similar cases, two relatively healthy young volunteers died while participating in research studies: eighteen-year-old Jesse Gelsinger at the University of Pennsylvania (in a gene therapy experiment) and twenty-four-year-old Ellen Roche at Johns Hopkins Hospital (in an asthma experiment). Both deaths were attributed to adverse reactions to the experimental medications.

2002 Mike Hurewitz, a fifty-seven-year-old healthy former *New York Post* reporter, died after donating 60 percent of his liver to his brother, a physician, at New York's Mount Sinai Hospital. Inadequate resident supervision was blamed.

2002 Linda McDougal, a forty-six-year-old woman from northwestern Wisconsin, had a healthy breast removed unnecessarily at United Hospital in St. Paul, Minnesota. A pathologist mixed up her biopsy slides with the cancerous specimens of another patient.

2003 Jesica Santillan died at Duke University Medical Center after receiving transplant organs of the wrong blood type.

Lack of redundant systems for checking the match between donors and recipients was blamed.

What do these notorious top ten have in common? Half of them (Carvey, Zion, Ayyappan, Warhol, and Lehman) involved high-profile victims. Three of them (Lehman, Hurewitz, and Zion) made instant headlines because of the victims' connections to major newspapers. Several befell hapless Good Samaritans who had nothing wrong with them—the research volunteers at Penn and Hopkins, and the healthy man donating part of his liver to his brother: all dying, in a way, of altruism—a classic "human interest" lead.

What virtually *all* these stories had in common, though, was that the errors took place at teaching hospitals, particularly in the East. Seven of the ten are major academic centers on the Amtrak corridor. This may leave a subliminal impression that East Coast teaching hospitals are fundamentally unsafe, but that would be neither fair nor accurate. There is no evidence that teaching hospitals are less safe than community hospitals, and quality comparisons to date tend to favor the former over the latter. This is particularly noteworthy, given the extraordinary complexity of the many cases referred to academic medical centers—it's one of the reasons patients go there. This spotlight on academia has also led to disproportionate media attention on trainees as *the* major source of errors. Yes, residents need more supervision and more sleep, but it seems unlikely that a patient being cared for by house staff at Harvard or Johns Hopkins at 2 A.M. is in more peril than a similar patient under the care of a night nurse in a community hospital, and whose "attending" (the private doctor) is snug in his bed at home.

These academic institutions and professionals share another important trait—their core values center around learning. Our instinct (our workplace, UCSF Medical Center, is part of this same genus) is to present cases to each other, to learn from our successes and our mistakes, and to try to push the frontiers of medical care and training. Remember the "team" of attendings, residents, interns, and students you learned about earlier: Any mistake in an academic hospital is likely to have scores of observers, and sometimes dozens of participants. This makes academic medical centers pretty bad at one thing: hiding their dirty laundry.

But that's OK. In the end, a case like Jesica's, and its media coverage, helps make health care safer, through both the lessons it teaches and the resources it generates. But we won't get this type of exposure and the good it brings unless practitioners feel safe to share—even confess—their mistakes. Unlike some other industries, overcoming the code of silence in medicine takes a bit of doing. Downed airliners and leaky supertankers are pretty hard to hide; but most medical mistakes happen one at a time, often in the dead of night, and to people who are already very sick.

Thus opportunism, rather than any formal journalistic or public policy, seems to govern which mistakes come to public attention, and which do not. Prominent victims make good copy because the public feels, "if it can happen to them, it can happen to me." Prominent institutions make good targets, too, because Americans have an instinctive mistrust of big organizations—especially those that come across as arrogant and smug. And like so many items on the "infotainment" billboard, stories about medical errors tend to run in packs. After the public's interest is piqued by a particularly egregious case, editors keep their antennae out for similar instances, which—if they look hard enough—they're bound to find. It's not that the stories they come upon when they look under rocks are false; only that they present a chronic problem as being acute—a sudden crisis instead of an ongoing system failure. This is eye-catching but misleading, creating an Orange Alert of angst instead of reasonable concern about a complex but widespread problem, accompanied by a commitment to do the hard and sustained work of fixing things.

While one can raise legitimate concerns about the media's tendency to oversimplify medical errors—to portray them as individual screwups rather than system failures—and to arbitrarily focus on the academic powerhouses of the East Coast, the media's focus is an absolutely essential ingredient for creating the resources and attention that we need to make progress. Stalin was right when he said, "a single death is a tragedy, a million deaths is a statistic." The media's power to tell a dramatic, personal story (like Jesica's) then let the public expand that in their imaginations—to put themselves or their relatives in a similar situation—is where the real power for error reform will originate.

As the editors of *The New York Times* discovered in the spring of 2003 when a young reporter's fraud led the cameras and microphones to reverse direction, being the object of the media's attention after an error is not much fun. Yet even doctors and administrators who try mightily to avoid airing their dirty linen in prime time admit that press coverage has unquestionably helped patient safety. Michael Millenson, professor of health policy at Northwestern and Pulitzer Prize-nominated journalist, passionately argues: "It was the mirror held up to the profession by news media coverage that finally penetrated the self-protective shell of rationalizations, subverted the old paradigm, and prompted the current effort to develop a systems-oriented patient safety approach... In the case of medical errors, public scandal and the concomitant fear of public shaming finally broke through professional complacency."

Like Millenson, we too believe that media attention—even overkill—has had a big role in making health care safer. Whether the IOM report gained its luster from high-profile error cases or error cases suddenly became news because of the report doesn't really matter. While individual doctors and nurses may feel unfairly singled out for errors that can happen to anyone (the injustice is particularly acute when the true culprit is the system, as it usually is), the fact is: Somebody has to take a hit for the team if our safety score is going to improve.

So we are left with conflicting emotions over the Duke case, its disclosure, and the subsequent media coverage: tremendous sadness over Jesica's death; sorrow over the wasted organs of her young donors; general praise for the media for taking up the cause and pushing forward the safety agenda; and sympathy for Dr. James Jaggers, who will be remembered not for his selflessness, his skills, and his dedication, but for a late-night blunder that wasn't caught by a defective system—a blunder that served notice that he was human, nothing more, but quite assuredly nothing less.

CHAPTER 15: WHETHER REPORTS?

A doctor can bury his mistakes, but an architect can only advise his clients to plant vines.

— Frank Lloyd Wright (1867–1959)

When a case like Jesica's enters the media's crosshairs, questions about whether errors should be reported—to peers, to regulators, and to patients—seem almost academic. Who needs error reporting when there's *60 Minutes*?

But such cases are exceptional, in both meanings of the word. For the 99.999 percent of the errors that Mike Wallace won't hear about, what do we do? Should these errors be reported—and if so, to whom, how, and to what end? Despite their gravity, we have tended to approach these questions in a slapdash way, and the capacity of reporting systems to waste time, money, and goodwill is nearly limitless. There are lots of reasons for our chaotic and ineffective approach to reporting, but the main one is the huge gulf between passions and data.

And passions *do* run high. After the IOM report placed medical errors at the center of America's anxieties, there was a reflexive demand for more reporting of errors—and not just in the supportive company of colleagues. The fact that errors might be discussed behind the closed doors of an M&M conference seemed inconsequential, just one more circle of wagons by a profession hell-bent on protecting its dark secrets. In today's world, the pressure to report mistakes—by everyone, to someone (details to be sorted out later)—seems irresistible.

There are a number of basic truths that frame any consideration of reporting systems for medical mistakes. They include:

- Errors occur in hospital rooms and ORs, one at a time, to patients that are quite ill to begin with, rendering real the opportunity to hide them from view. This hurdle must be overcome for any reporting system to be effective.

- Some of the most instructive errors are "near-misses"—like two planes that nearly collide—and these can only reach the light of day when voluntarily reported by caregivers.

- The need to learn from errors permeates the system: Individual doctors and nurses, the floors or clinics they work in, their hospitals, their professional licensing boards, hospital regulators, the state, the feds, the media—all can claim a legitimate interest in learning about medical mistakes. Add to that the individual patient who suffered from the error, and maybe the patient's lawyer.

- This staggering mix of "stakeholders" creates huge logistical and political complexities when it comes to fashioning reporting systems. Each group has different ideas of what to do with reports, and each might need to receive very different snapshots of the exact same incident. It's a Rashomon-like mess.

- The public has a legitimate interest in learning about really bad errors—particularly when they form a pattern or are evidence of a truly dangerous provider or system of care.

- Caregivers appear to be quite willing to report errors for the purpose of learning—provided that they feel protected from being unfairly pilloried *and* that the system actually does something useful with their reports.

- The system can only do something useful with error reports if a whole lot of people and computers are assigned to sift through them and develop useful solutions from them. This is not free.

As you've no doubt noticed, there is simply no way to solve this multivariable equation successfully—many of the "truths" conflict directly with others. And yet, the stakes are too high—and the potential to learn from errors too great—for us to throw up our hands in frustrated resignation. The answer to the question, "Whether reports?" *must* be yes. But doing it poorly just makes things worse.

Let's take a brief tour of reporting systems, looking first at how doctors talk to each other about errors, focusing particularly on the remarkable ritual designed specifically for this purpose. From there, the questions get knottier, as we consider what happens when we expand the reporting universe beyond the closed doors of the conference room (reports to hospitals and outside agencies like regulators), and narrow it to the toughest and most important audience: the patient him or herself.

Nobody likes being sued or seeing his mug shot under one of those clever headlines—Doc Forgets to Give Medicine, But Remembers His Bill—but physicians have another reason for keeping quiet when the conversation turns to errors: Our training culture has never deemed them worthy of much discussion.

Unlike Harvard Business School case studies, which focus on both disasters (Enron, WorldCom) and successes (Microsoft, JetBlue), teaching hospital discussions tend to emphasize "Great Cases" and the Holmesian deductive powers of extraordinary clinicians. A favorite pastime is to present puzzling cases to famous clinicians at medical conferences—urine that turns dark in the sunlight, wheezing and a rash that comes on after a hot shower—and watch the diagnostic wheels turn. When these discussions appear in the literature (the most famous collection is the "Case Records of the Massachusetts General Hospital," published in the *New England Journal of Medicine*), we can't help but be impressed, often awed, by the displays of virtuosity.

However, learning to diagnose these obscure cases has as much in common with the daily practice of medicine as Olympic sprinting has with walking to the corner market. It's largely a parlor trick. Look ma, I solved The Riddle.

Little wonder that medical students and residents come to think of themselves as wizards-in-training, the anointed few. Like anorexic teenagers bred on a steady diet of supermodel photo spreads, the obsession with "The Great Case" has created unrealistic expectations about physician infallibility. David Hilfiker, a family physician, spoke movingly after reflecting on his own error in treating a woman he believed—mistakenly—was not pregnant, which led him to inadvertently terminate her pregnancy:

> Precisely because of its technological wonders and near-miraculous drugs, modern medicine has created for the physician an expectation of perfection. The technology seems so exact that error becomes almost unthinkable. We are not prepared for our mistakes, and we don't know how to cope with them when they occur.
>
> Doctors are not alone in harboring expectations of perfection. Patients, too, expect doctors to be perfect... The perfection is a grand illusion, of course, a game of mirrors that everyone plays.

Being perfect is tough. It means you can't spoil your image by discussing the boneheaded blunders, let alone the honest mistakes, you made during your brilliant career. The closest we physicians come to tearing down this wall is at the Morbidity and Mortality (M&M) conferences held in many hospitals.

The M&M conference is a remarkable institution, a generations-old ritual designed to provide a forum for physicians to confess their mistakes and help their colleagues avoid making similar ones. To facilitate this, the courts have agreed that discussions at M&M conferences are confidential and can't be used in litigation. Honesty, openness, and mutual support used to be the only ground rules—but like so many things in medicine, these too have changed over the years. Now M&M conferences often take one of two paths—both of which are flawed when it comes to preventing future errors.

The first path (which is especially common in our own field, internal medicine) generally begins with a war story, then drifts away from the real issue—the mistake that led to an adverse event, including a patient's death—and emphasizes instead the puzzling or peculiar aspects of the symptoms, the patient, or the treatment. In other words, it turns into another "Great Case" conference, and everybody has a hell of a time. Dr. Edgar Pierluissi, a young safety researcher, observed 332 hour-long M&M conferences in surgery and internal medicine at UCSF and Stanford, and found that only one in four sessions actually tackled errors head-on; and when they did, the discussion was perfunctory and generally blamed other departments.

Pierluissi did find that surgeons were more willing than internists to discuss errors, especially errors they committed themselves. Part of this may have to do with the nature of surgery—when you screw up under the glare of the OR lights, there's no place to hide. It also demonstrates that successful surgeons have healthy egos and thick hides. Whatever the explanation, surgeons seem to be less likely to avert their eyes from their own eclipses, which is good. However, surgical M&Ms more often end up on a second, equally problematic path: a ritualistic, penitential tongue-lashing of the offending doctors by their peers.

Harvard's Atul Gawande captured the essence of this public pillorying as a resident surgeon in the late 1990s. After committing a near-fatal mistake while attempting to intubate a comatose patient, he was called to task at his department's M&M conference. He later said, "I felt a sense of shame like a burning ulcer. This was not guilt: Guilt is what you feel when you have done something wrong. What I felt was shame: I was what was wrong."

This tendency to punish the person instead of the behavior is, thankfully, beginning to fade. But, in the "good old days," it was quite something to behold. Charles Bosk, the Penn sociologist who spent eighteen months shadowing a group of surgeons and trainees in the 1970s, attended dozens of M&Ms at the unnamed but prominent teaching hospital that became his second home. In the vivid language of the day, he described one surgical M&M conference this way:

After the case of Mr. Will was presented, [Dr.] Arthur [the surgical attending] sprang from his chair and said that he had a few words to say... "I think that this case represents all the things that are wrong with the hierarchy of a teaching hospital. Here we have one of society's unfortunates. Mr. Will came to us with no kith or kin...

"The first in the comedy of errors made on this man was made by the medical service. The decision by them not to dilate his abdomen was tantamount to gross neglect... I'm now going to turn to the errors we made in treating this man. First, I made a fundamental error this early in the training year in allowing the chief resident to operate solo in this emergency... The [other] guilty party is the chief resident involved. By not calling for help when he ran into trouble, the resident took undue risk with the patient's life... Now, Mr. Will is an old, unattractive, abandoned, cirrhotic black man whom we almost abandoned to surgical pathology. Our surgical responsibility rests even with our unattractive as well as our more attractive patients. In this case we have clearly committed surgical immorality."

This kind of pit-bull attack undoubtedly hurt the feelings of some people who may have thought they were doing the right thing. Will such a tongue-lashing make them more careful or just more defensive? Hard to know—it probably varies with the personalities involved and the particulars of the situations. Perhaps this tongue-lashing by Dr. Arthur was helpful, even necessary, for the people involved—but if it becomes standard fare at every conference, doctors will either start avoiding them or come prepared for gladiator battle—neither of which creates a healthy "culture of safety."

Having said that, we must acknowledge that some doctors find M&M "blamestorming" therapeutic, even cathartic. One physician, after finding himself on both the giving and receiving ends of a vitriolic critique, said, "You are supposed to give full disclosure [in the conference]. Don't hold anything back. And it is almost a religious experience. You get up, you confess your sins. They assign a punishment to you. You sit back down and you are forgiven for your sins."

If this psychology sounds faintly religious, it is. The problem is, confession to a priest is private, not public—or even semipublic, like an M&M conference. The opportunity for shaming (and all its unproductive accoutrements: Defensiveness, cover-ups, finger-pointing) are more likely to occur in the Town Square atmosphere.

But the public display has certain advantages as well. Bosk sees Dr. Arthur's *mea culpa* as one more example of putting the heroic myth into action—showing grace under pressure. For the surgeon-penitent, Bosk writes,

> putting on the hair shirt only emphasizes [his] charity, humanity, and the scope of his wisdom. It allows him to round out his professional self by adding to it the secondary qualities associated with the healer in our culture: humility, gentleness, wisdom, and a certain wry acceptance of the universe that allows him to accept the limits of human activity. It allows him to express guilt without being consumed by it.

The take-home lesson here is that, in medicine at least, "professional cover-ups" are frowned upon—as long as we're among friends. Inside the fort, there is considerable pressure to 'fess up, especially in teaching hospitals. For a field blasted so often for hiding our errors, the openness—and the intellectual honesty—on display at many M&Ms, particularly surgical M&Ms, is really quite impressive.

Bosk relates one telling conversation in which a senior resident was asked whether the wound infection of a patient named Carlos was on that week's M&M agenda. The student asking the question was well aware that this resident was partly responsible for the infection in question, and, coincidentally, was also in charge of planning the conference's agenda. He had the power to bury the embarrassing case simply by not bringing it up at M&M.

"You know that there's no one looking over your shoulder to check out what should be at the M&M," said the student.

The resident answered sharply. "That would be no good," he said. "A physician that doesn't own up to his own mistakes is no better than the shit that's draining out of Carlos's wound."

So, imperfect as they are, M&M conferences offer at least a starting point for improving patient safety. They prove that, given safe harbor, doctors *are* willing to take responsibility for their mistakes, share them, and learn from the experience. Unfortunately, as long as the focus remains on individual actions—whether for clinical, political, or egotistical reasons—the systemic problems that promote errors, or at least fail to stop them, will remain unfixed.

Can M&M conferences be improved? Some hospitals are experimenting with inviting nonphysicians to the conferences: administrators, nurses, pharmacists, technicians, and others connected with a particular case. While that obviously broadens the group's problem-solving resources and promotes the consideration of other troubles in the system, some doctors don't like this approach. They'd rather focus on the "clinical issues" than be distracted by all that systems talk. ("And who are all these other people, anyway?" one doctor might whisper to a colleague between bites of pizza. "The guy in the suit, is he a lawyer?")

Other hospitals are thinking about having trained facilitators run their M&Ms. This technique has been used for decades in other industries, where ego-driven peer managers tend to turn every conflict into a power struggle, and the pecking order, as opposed to fixing real problems, becomes the agenda. Facilitators understand healthy group dynamics and can steer groups away from blocking behaviors toward those that might actually improve the quality of care.

It's still too early to tell which of these methods—or perhaps something entirely different—will be the key to harnessing the full potential of the M&M as a problem solving, error-preventing forum. For now, it's good to know that the forum exists, just waiting for fresh approaches.

The same can be said—with a bit less optimism—about another staple of error reporting and prevention: the written error report.

Error reports—whether on paper or the Web, and whether routed to the hospital's risk manager or the state legislature—traditionally come in three flavors: anonymous, confidential, and open.

Anonymous reports—in which no identifying information is requested or offered—have the advantage of protecting the innocent, but they also protect the guilty. Since there is no accountability for the reports, the data are often unrepresentative: They can turn into complaint boxes for those with axes to grind. The biggest, problem, though, is simply the lack of follow-up: You can't contact the author to verify the facts or gather more information.

In a *confidential report*, the provider's name is known, but shielded from the legal system or regulators. Confidential systems cut down on spurious or vindictive reports. They also capture better data than anonymous systems, because investigators can contact authors for additional information—asking those systems-oriented questions that are frequently omitted from initial reports by sharp-end workers. The key to confidential systems working well is, of course, confidentiality. Users must trust the system. One experimental primary care reporting system at the University of Colorado, which allowed providers to choose either anonymous or confidential options, found that about 75 percent chose confidential reporting, suggesting that it is possible to achieve the required degree of trust.

The third option, *open reports*—where all people and places are publicly identified—has a poor track record in medicine. The potential for unwanted publicity and punishment vastly limits the number and types of errors reported (even when reporting is "mandatory"). Since it is so easy to cover up most health care errors, investigators seeking to learn the truth about errors generally find open systems to be unproductive.

What separates these three methods is the consequences, or lack of consequences, for the reporting party. It takes a great humanitarian to put his or her neck on the legal and media chopping block for the sake of improving the system. And even when individuals are willing to sacrifice themselves—out of guilt or altruism—there may be others on the team who participated in the error, or by omission facilitated it. It's one thing to torpedo your own career to expiate a bad mistake; it's another to ruin the lives of colleagues and coworkers who might not have favored reporting, or wreck the reputation of an institution that is otherwise performing well.

As a result of these competing philosophies and the dozens of interested parties, the field of error reporting has become a Tower of Babel. The present attitude seems to be to "let a thousand reporting systems bloom"—and we'll eventually sort out which ones are working. Perhaps. But for now, the patchwork of anonymous, confidential, and open systems—run by local hospitals, accreditors, states, the federal government, and others—is a mess, not only unhelpful but wasting millions of dollars that could otherwise be improving safety if put to better use.

Let's start our survey of error reporting systems with those run by local hospitals, since these—with some recent modernizations— are actually beginning to do some good. Most hospitals have long had a system—the submissions go under the intentionally bland and blameless moniker of "incident reports"—in which sharp-end workers can fill out a piece of paper describing an "incident" (everything from doing a procedure on the wrong patient, to a

near-miss, to an interpersonal fracas), stick it in a box, and then…
who knows? Reports (usually confidential, sometimes anonymous)
are tallied, and the bureaucratic machine spits out, at appropriate
intervals, analyses that say things like, "over the last quarter, we
had 243 incident reports. Thirty-seven percent were medication
errors, 18 percent were handoff errors, 7 percent were patient falls,"
and so on. As if we didn't know we had medication errors before
the quarterly report? So now what? Traditional incident reporting
systems lack a way to get the information to the blunt-end workers
who could fix the system (many don't even appreciate that there is
a system that needs fixing). Remedial action, when and if it comes,
often takes the form of platitudes and exhortations to "be more
careful." The end result is usually a big waste of time and trees that
caregivers—particularly doctors—learned to ignore, mostly for
good reason.

A 2003 survey of medical residents at a Connecticut community
hospital shows a typical response to such systems. While nurses were
found to use the system from time to time, only half the residents
even knew it existed and an even smaller fraction of physicians (three
out of the twenty-four who participated) had ever filed a report. In
addition to ignorance about the system, residents were strongly
ambivalent about it. They felt the hospital had a "nonsupportive"
attitude about reporting errors and an even worse track record for
dealing with them.

In the last few years, we've started to make some progress in
improving local incident reporting systems. Many hospitals' systems
are now Web-based, which makes it much easier to report errors
and near-misses, much easier to get the information to the right
people, and much easier to track the responses of managers. At
UCSF, for example, errors from the internal medicine ward reported
into the computerized system trigger an automatic e-mail to Bob
(who directs the ward), as well as to the floor's head nurse, chief
pharmacist, and the hospital's head of quality improvement. Each of
these people is expected to post responses, then—particularly if the

reports begin to form a worrisome pattern—put their heads together to fix the problem. It is a much better system, particularly when coupled with active steps to create a culture in which people realize that their reports are valued and acted upon.

But collecting, analyzing, and responding to reports is laborious; it's hard to do as a part-time job. Real progress will involve resources—people with the time, energy, and training to analyze the information and act on it. Right now, few new dollars have been committed, anywhere, to supporting the people who can make changes in response to the incident reports. If we persist in trying to do important and difficult work for next to nothing, we'll get what we pay for.

Even if we narrow our hopes from fixing errors to simply using incident reporting systems (either hospital or governmental systems) to do what they *can* do well—tally the number of errors—we still have a big problem. Just consider this seemingly straightforward question: Does a decrease in the number of error reports indicate that safety is getting better? Logically, you'd suppose so, but let's conduct a quick thought experiment:

Suppose you are a nurse or doctor who has witnessed or committed an error. You still have other sick patients to care for, so part of you feels justified in simply ignoring the slip (or out-and-out mistake) and just getting on with your job. When you do take time to think about reporting the error, the first thing that crosses your mind is not safety, but *malpractice*. You've also seen what the media can do with a really juicy medical mistake, so you fret that you, your department, and your institution may be crucified in the interest of selling a few more newspapers. You know that hospital incident reports are legally privileged, but third-party reporting systems (like reports to the state or medical specialty societies) have no such protection (several bills are pending in Congress to shelter "Patient Safety Organizations" from legal liability for the information they collect and disseminate, but so far none has passed).

But you're a charitable soul, and you really believe you've uncovered a systemic pothole that could swallow future patients. So you move toward the stack of incident reporting forms. But now you recall that nothing seems to happen at your hospital in response to incident reports—they seem to remain, untouched, on somebody's desk or in a hard drive. And you also wonder if you should report it through the hospital system, or the one run by your specialty society, or to a state agency (or, if it relates to a medication, to the pharmaceutical company or the FDA).

At the end of the day, after weighing all the pros and cons of reporting, you decide, quite understandably, to just go see your next patient.

Since this scenario can play out dozens of times a day in any institution, it is easy to see how a hospital that toasts its patient safety victory in response to a marked downturn in the number of error reports might just be deluding itself.

As you've seen, implementing a really effective hospital incident reporting system is pretty tricky. But once we take reporting systems beyond hospital walls, the opportunity to wreak havoc really accelerates.

As of the publication of this book, more than fifteen states have mandatory error reporting systems. For example, the New York State Patient Occurrence Report and Tracking System (NYPORTS) expects to log in 30,000 reports in 2003—and this is just for one state! It is not clear, even to hospital quality experts, what the analysts intend to do with all of this data. A similar system in Massachusetts gets 6,000 reports each year, although this system focuses mainly on falls by elderly patients in nursing homes. Virtually none of these reports are followed up by state regulators, and only half of the 600 reports from acute-care hospitals—where the clinical stakes are higher—are investigated. This pattern is played out all over the country, where millions of scarce health care dollars are spent on reporting systems without a dime being earmarked for analysis, feedback, and enforcement. But the people demand reporting, so the charade continues.

In its nascent attempts to find a reporting paradigm that works, medicine may again be able to take some cues from commercial aviation.

On December 1, 1974, TWA Flight 514—a Boeing 727—crashed into a hill on final approach to Washington's Dulles Airport, killing ninety-two passengers and crew. The investigation revealed that the crew had ignored high-terrain markers and was unclear about its instructions from air traffic control. Compounding these problems, the minimum altitudes on the Dulles approach routes were poorly defined—a fact previously reported by pilots and well known to the FAA. Despite these reports, nothing had been done to resolve or eliminate the problem.

A year later, the FAA launched the Aviation Safety Reporting System (ASRS) in an effort to "increase the flow of information" regarding "actual or potential discrepancies and deficiencies" in the aviation system. Because the FAA realized airline personnel might be hesitant to report directly to Big Brother, they contracted with a knowledgeable and respected—but legally and administratively separate—agency (in this case, NASA) to run the system and disseminate its lessons. This shrewd move assured users that the system would generate reliable data confidentially.

The ASRS rules are simple and straightforward. If any flight crew member (or even a ground crew member, like a mechanic) witnesses a near-miss (unfortunately, real aviation accidents don't need a reporting system), he or she *must* report it to ASRS within ten days. The report is made on a form that requires individuals to identify themselves, but only for purposes of follow-up fact finding (a *confidential* system). Once that additional information is collected, all individual identifiers are destroyed. In twenty-seven years of operation, there has not been a single breach of confidentiality, and trust in the system is exceptionally high. As an added incentive, if it later comes to light that a near-miss occurred and a member of the air- or ground crew was aware of it but did not report it to the ASRS, they can be disciplined retroactively. Thus aircrews know that their reports on file can later become their Get Out of Jail Free cards.

Just as important, ASRS has a feedback loop that would be the envy of any medical error reporting system. Cases are analyzed not only for their specific circumstances, but for patterns. These are published in the FAA's widely read newsletter, *Callback*. When an exceptionally hazardous pattern emerges, the FAA's Advisory Circular system (or, in the case of specific aircraft, an Airworthiness Directive) kicks in, based on ASRS data. These regulatory documents have the force of law and go directly to the facilities and equipment operators involved.

There is virtually no debate in aviation about the value of the ASRS. The system now receives over 30,000 reports per year, resulting in hundreds of upgrades to equipment and improved procedures—it is the linchpin in modern aviation's impressive record of safety promotion. It is no accident—literally—that aviation fatalities have decreased tenfold over the past twenty years.

The ASRS has five traits—ease of reporting, confidentiality, third-party administration, timely analysis and feedback, and regulatory action—that have led to its successes. We strongly believe that a health care reporting system that replicates these traits can also be successful, even in as decentralized and chaotic an enterprise as modern medicine.

Several interesting experiments are already demonstrating the potential value of this approach. The two of us edit a Web-based journal, *AHRQ Web M&M* ("webmm.ahrq.gov"), funded by the United States Agency for Healthcare Research and Quality (AHRQ), which receives hundreds of anonymous error reports per year and posts the most instructive ones, accompanied by analyses by recognized authorities. The site attracts nearly one thousand users each day—mostly providers seeking and sharing answers to dozens of quality questions. Dr. Peter Pronovost, a Johns Hopkins anesthesiologist and safety expert, has developed an ICU reporting system, also with support from AHRQ. Now up and running in twenty-four ICUs around the country, the system received more than 1,500 error reports during its first year and is feeding those reports back to participating institutions. Each participating ICU assembles a four-member team—a doctor, nurse, administrator, and risk manager—to review the reports and develop error reduction strategies. In both of these systems, we see the kernel of an ASRS-style system that might—just *might*—truly make patients safer.

Finally, assuming all of these other reporting hurdles have been overcome, quality crusaders are left with the problem of enforcement.

In aviation, everyone—pilots and airlines, manufacturers and ground-based organizations—operates under the thumb of the FAA. But in a profession that goes back to Hippocrates and the ancient Greeks—before the days of regulators—we medical providers tend to view self-regulation as a God-given right.

In 1998, Joint Commission on Accreditation of Healthcare Organizations (JCAHO), the hospital regulatory agency, began issuing "Sentinel Event Alerts," somewhat analogous to the FAA's Advisory Circulars and Airworthiness Directives. These alerts are issued in response to a clear and present danger—some safety issue that the agency feels hospitals and caregivers must deal with right away. But by early 2003, JCAHO had issued so many alerts—twenty-four, with new ones coming out every other month—that hospitals felt overwhelmed. They had neither the staff nor the financial resources to tackle every problem the regulators threw at them, so JCAHO was pressured into declaring a moratorium on new alerts until the old ones had been cleaned up. The same phenomenon happened when local administrators and safety committees bombarded staff with e-mails about local errors. Too many alarm bells, even if they're justified, only make people deaf—a Pavlovian response that indeed changes behavior, but not in the right direction. Once again, we see that improving safety takes resources—resources for the hospital to tackle the alerts; resources for individual caregivers or managers to develop and implement solutions—and finding these resources remains a huge challenge.

And, until sharp-end caregivers are fully on-board—and feel protected from undue blame, embarrassment, and lawsuits—no reporting system will ever realize its potential, no matter how well organized and funded. In 2002, a series of focus groups brought several St. Louis physicians and patients together to discuss medical errors. The physicians sat outside a circle of patients, who discussed their attitudes toward errors while the doctors listened quietly. Then the circles were reversed. The patients were shocked to learn how devastated many physicians felt as a consequence of their own mistakes. Symptoms of remorse ranged from general feelings of anxiety to chronic difficulty sleeping. One physician said, "This is one of the few businesses... where you have to hit a home run every time... and I find that the older I get, the longer I have been at this, the more I worry to the point that this is probably what is going to drive me out of it."

Dr. Albert Wu of Johns Hopkins calls these remorseful providers "second victims." He writes:

> Virtually every practitioner knows the sickening feeling of making a bad mistake. You feel singled out and exposed—seized by the instinct to see if anyone has noticed. You agonize about what to do, whether to tell anyone, what to say. Later, the event replays itself over and over in your mind. You question your competence but fear being discovered. You know you should confess, but dread the prospect of potential punishment and of the patient's anger.

Any reporting system that fails to account for the genuine guilt that providers feel when they have caused an error will be a practical—and a moral—failure.

In the end, we believe hospitals and outpatient clinics should file mandatory reports, but only on major errors that cause death or permanent disability. These reports should go directly to state or federal regulators or a national accreditor like JCAHO, to ensure that corrective action, once formulated, is effective, standardized, and enforced. But we feel strongly that, unless there is a pattern of errors by a particular caregiver or institution, or a mistake is so egregious as to create an immediate danger to public health, offenders should not be identified. In the vast majority of cases, public disclosure does nothing except further punish already remorseful doctors and nurses, reduce public confidence in a system that still does more things right than wrong, waste money that could be used for health care on defensive PR campaigns or litigation, and—most importantly—poison the environment of participation that is *essential* to keeping new information flowing into the system.

Within individual hospitals and medical groups, information about errors should be collected and disseminated through newsletters, conferences, and formal incident reports, but the focus should be on *system* safety, not individual or institutional blame. M&M-style conferences and investigative hospital meetings should remain protected from legal discovery, and new legislation created to expand these protections to other forms of reporting, such as online Internet forums. These systems should be modeled—in intent and impact, if not in detail—on the Aviation Safety Reporting System. The VA, in fact, is working with NASA to do just this for its vast network of hospitals, clinics, and nursing homes.

It is encouraging that the will and the technology to promote reporting are starting to materialize, but as we've seen, gathering data is only half the answer. Reported errors must be analyzed intelligently, with patterns recognized and practical solutions formulated. This can only be accomplished through a system that is widely accepted and adequately funded, and has regulatory teeth. The traditions long-established for M&M conferences make a good launching pad for bringing physicians into such a system, but others on the caregiving team must be included, too.

At a personal level, all patients on the receiving end of a significant sharp-end error deserve to be told about it. Medicine is, and always will be, an intensely personal service—anytime life and death issues are involved, professional ethics demand nothing less than candor. Having said that, we acknowledge that there are lots of ways to handle disclosure that don't unnecessarily alarm patients or expose the caregiver to unwarranted or excessive liability. More research into this woefully underexplored area is essential. We suspect that strategies involving straightforward apologies, prompt and fair settlement offers, family involvement, and highly visible institutional commitments to preventing similar errors in the future will go a long way toward defusing many potential problems.

In those comparatively rare cases where bad apples are found— lazy or intoxicated practitioners, or repeat offenders who simply refuse to use good judgment and follow the rules—we must deal with them aggressively. Such people have no more business in the OR, hospital ward, or the clinic than they would in a cockpit or behind the controls of a nuclear power plant. We will return to this point later.

Above all, we must never forget that caregivers are the key to making any reporting system work. We will depend on them to correct errors just as we depend on them for our diagnoses, treatments, and cures. The fact is, most providers who make mistakes are honest, hardworking, and skilled professionals trying to do their very best. When they make a serious mistake, they are either the first or second person to feel its pain. Like the patient, they are likely to carry its scars for the rest of their lives.

CHAPTER 16: MALPRACTICE

Rewards and punishments are the lowest form of education.

— Chuang-Tzu (369–286 BCE)

There wasn't much doubt that Cynthia Taylor, a vivacious middle-aged woman used to keeping up with her toddler grandson, had pneumonia. She had been ill for several days and her initial flu-like symptoms—chills, nausea, and vomiting—had settled in her lungs with a thud. What began as a tickle in the back of her throat blossomed into a cough that brought up thick green phlegm. Late on the fourth night of her illness, Cynthia bundled up and drove to the local hospital's E R.

The triage nurse, noting Cynthia's sweat-matted hair, labored breathing, and high fever, sent her right in to see Dr. Rubenstein, the ER physician, who ordered an immediate chest X-ray. The image revealed a large patch of white pus where healthy lungs usually showed black air. Through the stethoscope, each "deep breath, please" sounded like two strips of Velcro being yanked apart.

Yep, pneumonia, Rubenstein concluded, and a bad case at that. He ordered an immediate IV containing fluids and antibiotics. Taylor was admitted to a general ward, where she was "tucked in" by the nurses. The plan was to check on her every few hours, a standard plan that ordinarily works fine.

The 4 A.M. and 6 A.M. checks went OK. Taylor was sleeping, albeit restlessly. But appearances deceive: Deep inside her, the bacteria were working overtime, multiplying—one becoming two, then four, then eight, and ultimately thousands, even millions of teeming pathogens. The microbes, a breed called *pneumococcus* that commonly causes pneumonia, eventually overran both her powerful IV antibiotics and the defenses within Taylor's lungs. At that point, they spilled into her bloodstream, triggering an avalanche of symptoms that were in full bloom when Mrs. Taylor's morning nurse, Jody Benjamin, arrived at her room at 7:45 A.M. The night nurse's sign-out had said, "resting comfortably," so she was shocked to find her patient desperately ill. Taylor's blood oxygen level had plummeted, leaving her sweaty face a pale gray. Her breathing was shallow, rapid, and spasmodic.

The nurse immediately paged Dr. Andrea Harris, the physician who had just received sign-out from Dr. Rubenstein a few minutes earlier in the doctors' cafeteria.

"Taylor," Rubenstein had said wearily, adjusting his glasses as he stared at his clipboard over the Formica tabletop. "Fiftyish lady with pneumonia. Started ceftriaxone and doxycycline. She's a bit hypoxic, so she's on three liters of oxygen. Should be OK." He then went on to the next patient after a brief sip of his coffee.

But that was then. Within moments of answering the page, Dr. Harris knew the patient was anything but OK. Her oxygen level was so low and her breathing so shallow and rapid that it was almost inevitable that she would need mechanical ventilation—probably within the hour. The nurse covered Taylor's mouth and nose with an oxygen mask and, after a tense five minutes or so, the patient began to "pink up": Her oxygen saturation rose from the mid-70-percent range to 92 percent, a marginal but no longer critical level.

Despite the response, standard procedure for a patient this sick was to insert a breathing tube into her windpipe to ensure that her other organs would continue to get the life-sustaining oxygen they needed. That was a given, but Dr. Harris still had a quick—and difficult—decision to make. She could intubate the patient now—on the ward—or send her down to the ICU, where the experienced staff could perform the intubation more safely. Part of this trade-off was Harris's awareness of her own limitations. She had only done about eight intubations in her career, most of those under the guidance of an anesthesiologist in an unhurried, semielective setting. The nurses in the ward weren't any better—all fairly young and inexperienced, and not used to doing procedures on patients this sick. A third option was to call an ICU team to the ward, but that could take as long as transferring the patient downstairs.

The more she thought about it, getting the patient to the ICU seemed like the best choice. There, the intensivist physician and specialized nurses would have all the training and equipment to handle not only the emergency intubation, but any complications that might come up. It would only take a couple of minutes to get there, and the patient—though terribly ill—seemed to have stabilized for the moment.

Harris made her choice. She called the Unit and told them to stand by with their equipment—like fire trucks lining the runway for a smoking airplane. Reflecting later on her decision to move Taylor to the ICU: "In my mind it was a matter of what would be safest."

Dr. Harris, a floor nurse, and a respiratory therapist wheeled Taylor's bed to the service elevator—which mercifully was running just fine—and arrived at the ICU a few minutes later. It had been less than forty minutes since Dr. Harris had first laid eyes on Cynthia Taylor—and the first twenty-five had been taken up with the time it took her to assess the patient and the situation.

Unfortunately, as they say in the military, the plan usually goes out the window after the first shot is fired. In the ten minutes or so between notifying the ICU and actually getting there, Taylor's condition drastically worsened. The ICU team went right to work: The intensivist attempted to intubate the patient by gently depressing her tongue with a fiberoptic metal speculum while an ICU nurse began to administer sedation. But the airway was clogged and her trachea hard to locate. During the procedure, the ICU nurse monitoring her vitals reported that Taylor had lost her pulse. The team instantly began CPR. Frantically now, one doctor shocked the patient while another prepared for a second attempt at intubation. The first shock was unsuccessful in reviving the heart. So was the second. On the third, Taylor's heart restarted and they completed the intubation.

Though the patient lived, the loss of oxygen in an already oxygen-starved brain left Taylor with permanent brain damage. After another month in the hospital, she was released to her family—unable to recognize anyone, including her playful grandson.

Dr. Harris apologized profusely for the terrible outcome—though more out of empathy than guilt. In her mind, she had followed the book and made the right decisions at the right time. To have attempted an intubation herself on the regular ward, with none of the specialized expertise and equipment for what, in retrospect, turned out to be a hellishly complicated procedure, would've been pure folly. She felt terrible, but, like most doctors following a horrible "adverse event," she soldiered on.

Nearly two years later, Dr. Harris received notice that she had been named as a defendant in a malpractice case filed on Cynthia Taylor's behalf. It alleged she was negligent in delaying the intubation and not at least attempting it on the floor. She told us that the moment she received the news is seared forever in her memory—just like those terrible moments spent trying to save the patient whose family was now seeking to punish her.

"I was sitting in the ICU," she said, "and my partner calls me up and says, 'You're being sued... and that's why I'm leaving medicine.'"

Say "medical mistake" to a physician and the word you get back is *malpractice*. This conditioned response is the product of decades of experience. In our market-driven, litigious society, the malpractice system scars the health care landscape like the charred remnants of a lava flow. If we're going to shine the light of day on medical errors, we've got to understand the single most powerful force that keeps them in the shadows.

The need to compensate people for their injuries has long been recognized in most systems of law, and Western systems have a tradition of doing so by apportioning fault (*culpa*). This tradition is particularly muscular in the U.S., since the American ethos is so infused with notions of individual responsibility. *Tort law*, the general legal discipline of which malpractice law is a subset (it also governs product liability and personal injury) takes these two principles—compensating the injured in an effort to "make them whole" and making the party "at fault" responsible for this restitution—and weaves them into a single system. The system's yin and yang of linking compensation of the injured to the fault of the injurer (hoping at the same time to deter future unsafe acts and do all of this fairly) is brilliant in its simplicity and works reasonably well when applied to many human endeavors.

Unfortunately, medicine is not one of them.

We've already seen that most errors in medicine arise from circumstances in which the sharp-end provider is not strictly "at fault." Here we define fault as an act that could have been prevented, but wasn't; or an act that should have taken place, but didn't. Most errors involve slips—glitches in automatic behaviors that can strike even the most conscientious practitioner in any field. As slips, by definition, are unintentional, they are something like a force of nature: They cannot be deterred by threat of lawsuits.

Keep in mind, we do *not* refer to the acts of providers who fail to adhere to expected standards and whose slips, therefore, are not unintentional errors, but the predictable damage wrought by unqualified, unmotivated, or reckless workers. An analogy might be the difference between a driver who accidentally hits a child who darts into traffic chasing a ball, and a drunk driver who hits a child on the sidewalk after losing control of his speeding car. Both accidents result in death, and the first driver feels horrible because one should always keep a special eye out for kids on busy streets. But the second driver is clearly more culpable. If the malpractice system confined its wrath to medicine's version of the drunk, speeding driver, we'd be in far better shape.

And we do have them. Take, for example, Dr. Channagiri

Manjanatha, the Saskatchewan anesthetist convicted of criminal negligence for leaving the OR to make a phone call, leading to the death of a seventeen-year-old patient. Or the case of Dr. David Arndt, the Boston surgeon who left his patient anesthetized on the table with a gaping incision in his back to go cash a check at his local bank. And even these cases pale in comparison to those of psychopathic serial killer Dr. Michael Swango, whose crimes were chronicled to harrowing effect in James Stewart's popular *Blind Eye*; as well as Dr. Harold Shipman, a British general practitioner who killed more than two hundred elderly patients by injecting them with morphine during house calls. These horrific cases all occupy the darkest end of a very long spectrum. But between the extremes of innocent slips and breathtaking criminality, every society must draw lines as it tries to meet the goals of compensating the injured, deterring the dangerous, and doling out justice. In America, the line we have drawn tends to find fault when there is none, and to blame people instead of systems. This is not good for doctors, certainly. But more importantly, it is not good for patients.

A single slip or error, even if it results in a serious adverse event, does not make a doctor negligent any more than an out-of-bounds drive makes Tiger Woods a bad golfer. Yet our legal system forces judges and juries to look at each malpractice claim in isolation, as if years (or even decades) of error-free service meant nothing, or didn't exist.

Consider a doctor who performs a risky and difficult surgical procedure. Assume she has carefully and successfully completed the operation one thousand times in five years of practice, but slips during the one-thousand-first operation. The patient, being damaged, files suit, claiming that the doctor failed to perform to the somewhat nebulous "standard of care" expected for that particular procedure. It is no defense to demonstrate that the surgeon normally *did* avoid the error—a thousand times, as a matter of fact—or that some errors are a statistical inevitability if you do the procedure often enough. The tort system is amnestic as to these past successes—and thus fundamentally unfair to those whose jobs cause them to frequently engage in risky activities. As Alan Merry, a New Zealand anesthesiologist, and Alexander McCall Smith, Professor of Medical Law at the University of Edinburgh, observed, "All too often the yardstick is taken to be the person who is capable of meeting a high standard of competence, awareness, care, etc., *all the time*. Such a person is unlikely to be human."

Not all errors are slips. Some relate to judgment calls— decisions under uncertainty, the ones Amos Tversky warned us about—where the physician must choose between two or more alternatives, each of which has plusses and minuses. That's the conundrum Dr. Harris found herself in, and tragically, the outcome was disastrous (of course, neither we nor a jury can possibly know what would have happened had she chosen one of the alternative strategies). Physicians are called upon to make judgment calls like this all of the time. Since the tort system reviews these calls after the fact, we have a powerful instinct to assign blame. "The tendency in such circumstances is to praise a decision if it proves successful and to call it 'an error of judgment' if not," write Merry and Smith. "Success is its own justification; failure needs a great deal of explanation."

How can patients and their lawyers (let alone judges and juries) avoid the distorting effects of hindsight and deal more fairly with caregivers doing their best under difficult conditions? James Reason recommends the Johnston Substitution Test, which does not compare one act to an arbitrary standard of excellence, but asks only if a similarly qualified caregiver in the same situation would have behaved any differently. If the answer is, "probably not," then, as the test's inventor Neil Johnston puts it, "Apportioning blame has no material role to play, other than to obscure systemic deficiencies and to blame one of the victims."

Using the Johnston test, was Dr. Harris negligent? We don't think so. She reacted in a timely way to a crisis that was thrust upon her, and made a difficult judgment call which she believed to be best for the patient. The outcome was tragic, but there is no guarantee it would have been any better if Harris had tried the intubation herself on the ward, and a great deal to suggest that it could have been worse. Had that been the case, she would have been crucified by the plaintiff's attorney, and probably with more justification.

Liability seems more justified when rules or guidelines have been violated, since these usually *do* involve conscious choices by caregivers. Some organizations believe strongly in this principle, fearing that if they leave too much discretion to the rank-and-file, chaos will follow. A classic example of a type of organization that assumes that all rule violations are blameworthy is government, which tends to call its rules "laws."

But—in health care at least—even rule violations may not automatically merit blame. As we've seen, bureaucratic institutions like hospitals tend to spawn so many rules that the rules themselves often become contradictory, or, at times, even dangerous. Take, for example, a Joint Commission (JCAHO) policy that strongly discourages physicians from phoning new orders into a medical ward ("verbal orders") for fear they will be misunderstood. This makes common sense, but there are two problems. First, the only study to ever test this hypothesis found precisely the opposite effect: that there were *fewer* errors from verbal orders than written ones, possibly because both parties recognized the potential for miscommunication and were more careful. Second, a doctor who scrupulously follows this policy—never using verbal orders—may periodically inflict needless pain or put some patients at risk—as they wait for him to leave the OR or come across the street from the clinic to write an order in the chart. So even competent, law-abiding physicians—the ones who come to full stops at intersections, even when no one's watching—may violate this rule from time to time in the name of Hippocrates. (A reliable computerized order entry system, available on every ward, will ultimately resolve this conundrum.)

Similarly, a compulsive JCAHO stickler may lock up every medication vial (it's the rule, after all) and thereby place patients in danger when a drug is needed fast. Frontline caregivers joke that there are two days where it is best to avoid admission to a teaching hospital: One is July 1 (when new interns report for work, having just unwrapped their med school graduation gifts), and the other is the day before a JCAHO accreditation inspection—when everyone scrambles to "fix" the normal system. God forbid a Code Blue happens while the accreditors are on site—the medications the poor patient needs are likely locked in the Crash Cart, where regulations say they are supposed to be kept but, for practical reasons, never are.

It is not that we favor health care anarchy—routine rule violations should cause us to rethink the rule in question, not hand medals to scofflaws. And clearly, some rules must never be broken ("Sign your site," for example). Our point here is simply that the malpractice system will seize upon evidence that a rule was broken when there is a bad outcome, ignoring the fact that some rules are broken by nearly everyone in the name of efficiency—or sometimes quality.

If justice demands that the guilty be punished, it also demands that the innocent be exonerated. In this respect, the U.S. malpractice system fails badly. In its present form, every physician knows that his or her career can be ruined with a single slip. This ever-present pressure comes to the fore when we must act in an emergency, or make judgment calls based on scanty evidence. Just when our complete concentration should be focused on the patient, we reserve a little bit for self-preservation. How did we get into this mess? How can we get out of it?

The gradual evolution of malpractice law into a weapon against sharp-end providers has occurred gradually and been driven by forces that extend well outside the bounds of medicine. In a nutshell, our society—you know, the one that sues fast-food chains because they failed to warn people that the cheeseburgers might be fattening—has become an orgy of blame.

There are several reasons why. America prizes individual responsibility and the exercise of free will, and we are profoundly unsettled by vague blunt-end explanations. Even worse, the idea that a horrible outcome could have been an "accident" or "fate" strikes us as unscientific and conspiratorial—we seek an explanation as a moth seeks a light. As physicians, we see a parallel tendency when we care for patients who literally beg us to give them some reason other than "shit happens" when they develop a life-threatening disease for which we have no explanation. Since the days of Greek mythology, the human need to explain scary events has been our way of domesticating the harrowing uncertainties of life.

Moreover, the last forty years in America have seen a continuing erosion of professional privilege and a questioning of all things "expert." In malpractice suits, this has tipped the balance between plaintiff and defendant even further, but it was already an unfair match: Faced with the heart-wrenching story of an injured patient or grieving family, who can possibly swallow an explanation that "things like this just happen" and that no one is to blame, especially when the potential source of compensation is "a rich doctor," or, even easier to hate, her insurance company?

The role of the expert witness further tips the already lopsided scales of malpractice justice. Experts are usually chosen because they are well known in their fields, often widely published academicians. (In the interest of full disclosure, Bob has served as an expert witness, on both the plaintiff and defense sides, in about a dozen cases.) Almost by definition, they are particularly well informed about the small slivers of the medical world that are the sources of their reputations and the subjects of the lawsuits. Although the expert is asked to take on the mindset of "the reasonable practitioner" (in other words, someone operating under the same resource and time constraints as the doctor being sued, who has to keep up with not just the specialized literature of the expert but all the areas that might present themselves, who can't attend the latest cutting-edge conference on every patient's problem she might see, and who lacked the special wisdom of hindsight at the moment of truth), it is clear that this is an exceptionally difficult task, especially as the case becomes confrontational and experts assume more polarized positions. One Canadian judge articulated the standard: The reasonable person [which is the expected performance standard for the practitioner] "is not an extraordinary or unusual creature; he is not superhuman; he is not required to display the highest skill of which anyone is capable; he is not a genius who can perform uncommon feats, nor is he possessed of unusual powers of foresight. He is a person of normal intelligence who makes prudence a guide for his conduct.... He acts in accord with general and approved practice." But this standard often becomes a distant memory once the starter's gun for the trial is fired.

Finally, adding to the swirling confusion is the fact that doctors and nurses feel guilty for our errors (even when there was no true fault), often blaming ourselves because we failed to live up to our own expectation of perfection. This is natural—healthy, actually. Who would want a doctor so hardhearted that she didn't feel remorse when a patient died on her watch?

Just as naturally, what person would not instinctively lash out against a provider when faced with a brain-damaged child or spouse? It is to be expected that families or patients will blame the party holding the smoking gun, just as they would a driver who struck their child who ran into the street to get a ball. Some bereaved families (and drivers and doctors) will ultimately move on to a deeper understanding that no one is to blame—that the tragedy is just that. But whether they do or do not, write Merry and Smith, "It is essential that the law should do so."

Tort law is fluid: Every society must decide how to set the bar regarding fault and compensation. By mating the recompense of the injured to the finding of fault, tort systems inevitably lower the fault-finding bar to allow for easier compensation of the sympathetic victims. It is our thesis that this is problematic—and it would be even if we didn't care about the sensibilities or morale of physicians.

But we should care, even if only for selfish reasons. Physicians are increasingly demoralized and depressed, and providers in this sour mood are unlikely to be enthusiastic patient safety leaders—and not because of spite. At the root of it all is a basic paradox. Tort law is adversarial by nature, while a culture of safety is collaborative. In a safety-conscious culture, doctors and nurses willingly report their mistakes as opportunities to make themselves and the system better. An overly litigious environment devalues this learning and turns earnest caregivers striving for improvement into sitting ducks.

A malpractice culture also forces doctors to view every patient as a potential litigant. Only half-joking, one highly competent, empathic obstetrician we know says that the joy he used to get from bringing new life into the world has been nearly quashed by the worry that he'll be sued if the child doesn't get into Harvard. This defensive mindset changes clinical strategy from "What is the best for this patient?" to "How can I do what's needed without creating liability?" It ratchets the health care standard down from an ever-increasing quest for excellence to an ass-covering fandango.

This is not to say—as some do—that the malpractice system has done nothing to improve patient safety. Some of the defensive measures taken by doctors and hospitals make sense. Anesthesiologists now continuously monitor patients' oxygen levels, creating a trip wire for problems in surgery that might have gone undetected before. Nurses and physicians keep better records (judges and juries place a lot more stock in judgments made at the time than in self-serving "recollections" made after the fact). Informed consent laws, while still largely perfunctory, at least give patients the opportunity to think twice about procedures and ask some relevant questions. In these and other ways, the malpractice threat has served like the warning labels on cigarettes, or that boring but occasionally handy safety briefing you get from flight attendants before taking off.

In other ways, though, "defensive medicine" is a shameful waste, particularly when there are so many unmet needs. A 1996 study by Mark McClellan, now Commissioner of the U.S. Food and Drug Administration, estimated that limiting pain and suffering awards would trim health care costs by 5–9 percent by reducing unnecessary and expensive tests, diminishing referrals to unneeded specialists, and so on. This would save over $100 billion annually— enough to fund a major prescription drug benefit plan or provide health insurance to most of America's uninsured citizens without jeopardizing quality care.

In the last analysis, though, it is the way in which our legal system misrepresents medical errors that is its most damning legacy. By focusing attention on sharp-end first stories, it lets blunt-end second stories find refuge in institutional inertia and hidebound tradition: A successful lawsuit creates the illusion of making care safer without actually doing so. The malpractice system causes us to view medical mistakes through a lurid keyhole, which blocks the broad vistas where true solutions may be found. The system doesn't even appear to have any actual deterrent effect, which shouldn't really surprise us. Doctors in Canada are five times less likely to be sued than American doctors, but there is no evidence that they commit fewer errors.

What people often find most shocking about America's malpractice system is that it doesn't serve the needs of injured patients, either. Despite stratospheric malpractice premiums, generous settlements, big awards by sympathetic juries, and an epidemic of defensive medicine, many patients with "compensable injuries" remain uncompensated. In fact, less than 3 percent of patients who experience injuries associated with negligent care file claims. Given America's litigious climate, how can this be?

One reason is that the malpractice system behaves like any other mature market. You enter it only when the potential rewards exceed the cost of doing business. Many error-caused injuries are just too small to trigger the interest of malpractice attorneys who, it may surprise you, are the ones who really decide when and if to litigate—not the patient, or even the patient's family. This is because nearly all malpractice attorneys work on a contingency basis: They charge the client no fee, but take a generous portion of any award, typically 30 to 40 percent. The formula they use to test a case's "trial worthiness" was developed by the legendary judge Learned Hand in a 1947 case involving a runaway tugboat in New York Harbor. Using the Hand Formula, the attorney compares the expected value of the award, adjusted for the probability of winning, to the costs of bringing the action, which must be borne by the law firm: legal research, discovery and deposition costs, expert witness fees, and so on. And while some cases are a slam-dunk for the plaintiff (those seldom go to trial anyway—the defendant usually settles), a victory for an injured patient is not guaranteed. In fact, a 2003 survey showed that defendant physicians won 61 percent of the time. But when they lose, they lose big.

All of this puts a lot of pressure on a plaintiff's attorney to gauge the likely award accurately. While the costs of a patient's injury or degree of disability—along with the victim's age and future earning potential—can be assessed with some accuracy, the really big bucks lie in "pain and suffering." Here, a sympathetic—or just sympathetic-looking—plaintiff (plus a grieving family) can be worth his weight in gold. And, oh yes, plaintiff's lawyers also evaluate the nature and degree of the physician's alleged negligence; but as we'll discuss a little later, the actual presence or absence of "malpractice" is usually not the deciding factor to sue— nor does it predictably tip the verdict.

In addition to the plaintiff's injury and "attractiveness," plaintiffs' attorneys also scrutinize the defendant-physician's medical specialty, looks, and personality. Some doctors are more likely to be sued because of the nature of their jobs: Obstetricians and neurosurgeons, for example, run the highest risk. But even within these higher-liability specialties, the practitioner's personality can make a big difference. A 2002 Vanderbilt study showed that the number of complaints against individual docs (for bad attitude, inattention to patients, and so on) logged by the hospital's patient relations department was tightly correlated with their risks of being sued. Nine percent of the doctors received half the patient complaints—and these doctors were much more likely to be sued than doctors with better bedside manners. Another study found that doctors avoided suits and did better in malpractice proceedings if they had good communication skills and a sense of humor. Of course, this is only logical: Patients make less trouble for physicians they like and are more apt to give them the benefit of the doubt; though suing a good doctor because he's rude or a bit cold seems kind of like using a sledgehammer to hit a thumbtack.

Another reason most errors aren't brought to court or to the negotiating table is that many of the un-or undercompensated claimants are on government assistance—the very poor or very elderly—and lack the resources, personal initiative, or social clout to seek redress. Thus some worthy malpractice claims go begging while others go forward for a host of reasons that have nothing to do with the presence or degree of negligence. It is an awfully capricious way to run a justice system.

Finally, even when injured patients' cases do make it through the malpractice pachinko machine to a trial or settlement, it is astounding how little money actually ends up going to the victims and their families. After deducting legal fees and expenses, the average plaintiff sees about forty cents for every dollar paid by the defendant. If the intent of the award is to help families care for a permanently disabled relative or to replace a deceased breadwinner's earnings, this 60 percent overhead makes the malpractice system a uniquely wasteful business.

Since the late 1980s, the studies of Harvard lawyer-physician Troy Brennan and his colleagues have convincingly proved that our "ugly social system" of malpractice litigation leaves much to be desired. Lead author of the Harvard Medical Practice Study from which the now-famous IOM death toll was derived, the brilliant

Brennan—jocular and irreverent, with thinning red hair and a lanky frame—looks as if he'd be equally at home in an Irish pub as at the podium of a Cambridge lecture hall, where he teaches as a professor at Harvard's medical, law, and public health schools. He and his group are the source of virtually all we know about medical malpractice and its connection to medical errors.

Brennan's studies of malpractice claims in three states show that doctors have a more than 1-in-100 chance of being tagged with a lawsuit after a patient has an adverse event, even when the doctor has done nothing wrong. Although this may not sound like an excessive "risk" of a lawsuit, when you consider all the patients who suffer adverse events (e.g., medication side effects, complications after surgery), this rate adds up to a lot of suits. Over a career, the average doctor can nearly count on being sued at least once, and far more than that in the riskier specialties.

What types of cases trigger the most malpractice suits and yield the biggest awards? Brennan and his group found that the magnitude of the patient's disability was by far a better predictor of victory and the size of the award than was mere proof that there was breach of some ephemeral "standard of care." In other words, the American malpractice system rations compensation not according to the degree of malpractice, but degree of injury.

This is not altogether surprising, since malpractice trials are generally heard by juries composed of ordinary citizens who tend to be highly sympathetic to people like them who have been harmed. The defendant's talk about standards of care and probabilistic outcomes are a tough sell when stacked up against a dead or horribly disabled plaintiff. Defense attorneys know that they go to bat with two strikes against them when a patient is badly injured—particularly a young patient with a family. "In a case like this," says attorney Frank Dean, who represented Dr. Andrea Harris in the Cynthia Taylor lawsuit, "involving a patient who was already in the hospital, who has an arrest and anoxic [brain damage], one of the very significant perceptual issues we have to consider... is the fact that there was a catastrophic outcome, and to some jurors, catastrophic outcomes may equate with 'somebody must have messed up.'"

Despite expert testimony that Harris's decision to postpone intubation was medically sound—it passed the Johnston Substitution Test—Dean advised his client to settle out of court, which she did. According to him, the jury's sympathy for the patient would overwhelm any inclination it might otherwise have to weigh her actions against those of a "reasonable practitioner"; and the potential for an adverse judgment against the doctor alone was so huge that it could easily exceed her malpractice insurance coverage (which, for most physicians, averages $3 million), driving her into bankruptcy. These are familiar circumstances, so settling the case—even when the physician feels she was anything but negligent—is distressingly common, which further feeds the malpractice beast.

Of course, while awards or settlements help bring closure for patients and families, their effects can linger for physicians. Dr. Harris's insurance premiums immediately went up and she must now report the settlement every two years when she renews her clinical privileges at the hospital. At that time, her supervising physician is asked to certify that she is competent to practice medicine safely, a stain that lives on in perpetuity. The case is also reported to the federal National Practitioner Data Bank (NPDB), which is checked every time the physician applies for a new job—much like sex offenders are obliged to register with the local police every time they move. Physician lobbying groups have successfully fought to keep NPDB data confidential—available only to the hospitals that use it for credentialing—but consumer and patient advocacy groups mount continual counterpressure to "open it up." Knowing how easy it is for many undeserving physicians to wind up on the list, we're not sure which public interest would be served by this.

As we see, the malpractice system carries out its essential function in ways that are, in Brennan's words, "both lopsided and mismatched." Brennan's law school colleague Paul Weiler likens the system to a traffic officer who randomly tickets drivers, giving reams of citations to slow-pokes while too many speeders fly by unscathed.

But of all this talk about justice aside, a more practical—and political—issue presently dominates the malpractice debate: the cost of awards, and of coverage. The average medical malpractice judgment runs about one million dollars—and twice that for cases related to childbirth. It has doubled since 1997. Dr. Cheryl Edwards, forty-one, closed her obstetrics practice in Las Vegas when her malpractice premium jumped from $37,000 to $150,000 per year, leaving thirty pregnant women to find a new doctor. ("Get a lawyer to deliver your baby" has become the battle cry of her specialty in many states.) In south Florida, some obstetricians and neurosurgeons now pay $200,000 per year for malpractice coverage, and increasing numbers of Florida physicians are "going bare"—carrying no insurance at all. This may sound suicidal, but if deep pockets create tempting targets, the assets of a typical doctor pale in comparison to a plump insurance policy. Across the U.S., doctors now spend over $6 billion per year for malpractice coverage, and hospitals and nursing homes spend billions more. This is a lot of money that could go into preventing slips and mistakes rather than paying for them after the fact.

Naturally, this "malpractice crisis" has made physicians mad as hell, and many of them aren't taking it anymore.

Beginning in 2002, a series of rolling work stoppages broke out around the country, leading to the temporary closure of Las Vegas's major trauma center. Similar mini-strikes occurred in Pennsylvania and New Jersey. "Physicians are generally very independent," said one New Jersey gastroenterologist, taking a day off from his duties to donate blood. "If you get the physicians united, you know this is a crisis."

The causes of the massive rate hikes are complex. Some insurance companies lost their shirts in the bear stock market and jacked up rates to make up the difference. In states without limits on pain and suffering awards, juries sometimes see awarding huge judgments as a humane way of helping grieving families, using money extracted from the deep, bureaucratic pockets of insurance companies. These awards ultimately bubble back to the doctors in the form of higher insurance rates (and, since physician payments for clinical services are generally fixed by payers, the extra dollars come directly out of the physicians' bottom line).

But sadly, some of the spike in malpractice costs is undoubtedly due to the increased focus on medical errors in the post-IOM era. Even though the IOM tried mightily to steer the conversation toward systems-thinking rather than individual blame, when it came to malpractice (a topic curiously ignored in the IOM report) the new attention has backfired. Ironically, says Troy Brennan, "our own proselytizing about medical injuries is going to change the way an average jury looks at a medical injury claim, and that then changes the perception of the value of claims by plaintiffs' attorneys."

The present "malpractice crisis" (they seem to hit every decade or so) has led, once again, to spasmodic attempts to pass malpractice reform legislation, most of them aimed at the U.S. Congress. The debate in 2003 was over proposals to cap "pain and suffering awards"—the highest paying ticket in the malpractice lottery. Typical proposals aimed to limit any awards beyond actual damages or computable economic losses to between $250,000 and $500,000. California has had such a cap since 1976 (for once, the doctors outmaneuvered the trial lawyers), and it has moderated the spiraling increases in malpractice premiums to one-third the national average.

Predictably, the legislative process became a circus as soon as this emotionally laden subject hit the docket. Mary Rasar visited Capitol Hill in March 2003, three Republican senators at her side, to describe in heartrending terms her father's death after a car accident brought him to a Las Vegas emergency room. He died there—"a tragic, tragic story," said Nevada Senator John Ensign—because the ER's trauma center was forced to close when doctors could no longer afford to pay malpractice premiums. Score one for the reformers. But the rebuttal witness was Linda McDougal, the Minnesota woman who mistakenly underwent a mastectomy when a pathologist mixed up her breast biopsy specimen. The message: How can we justify caps on pain and suffering awards when there are cases like McDougal's? Back to deuce. Americans love a dramatic story, but such stories don't always make good public policy.

Given the lunacy of our present malpractice system, pain-and-suffering caps make sense as a way of at least moderating insurance premiums and keeping doctors in business. But they don't solve the fundamental problem. What physicians worry about most is not the cost of the settlement, but the costs—both financial and psychic—of the process. If a patient comes to us with a headache and, after a conscientious workup, we conclude it is almost certainly not a brain tumor—the odds are, say, 1 in 2,000—we reassure the patient on that score and look for other diagnoses. However, if one out of every two thousand times the patient *does* have a brain tumor and we did not order a CAT scan, we can count on being sued. In that case, the expense and emotional costs—time lost to depositions, hand-wringing and demoralization, sleepless nights, and suppressed anger over the inherent unfairness of it all—is the same for us whether the payout is for $400,000 or $2 million. As doctors, our decision making is driven more by the potential for being sued than by the cost of losing a judgment.

Malpractice judgments are the archetype of the "blame and shame game." The finger-pointing embodied in every case is a giant step backward from a more rational—and safer—systems approach to errors. A "systems view" of tort reform would look past the usual debates about award categories and dollar amounts and focus instead on true justice (weeding out and punishing the bad apples); it would compensate *all* victims of serious, preventable errors—not just those who are attractive to lawyers and jurors; and it would make changing deficient health care practices a goal of any error-related judgment. In the case of Mrs. Taylor, it would shift the focus from the sharp-end intubation judgment call by Dr. Harris to the blunt-end issues of how sick patients are monitored overnight and how ICU transfers are handled.

A 1990 study by Troy Brennan demonstrated an almost total disconnect between the malpractice process and efforts to improve quality in hospitals. Of eighty-two cases handled by risk managers (due to the possibility of a lawsuit) in which quality problems were involved, only twelve (15 percent) were even *discussed* by the doctors at their departmental quality meetings or M&M conferences. As Dr. Harris later recalled about the Cynthia Taylor case, "To my knowledge, it was never discussed with any of the physicians... I don't really know the risk management people... I know they exist, but [I don't know] who they are and their role and function in a situation like this... despite the fact that I spend up to 120 hours [per week] in the hospital, this is just not discussed...." Brennan sees this as more evidence of a "complete and utter mismatch between the malpractice system and efforts to improve patient safety."

Some have argued that the malpractice system has gone to the dogs because medicine has done such a poor job policing itself. One malpractice historian writes, "From the public's point of view... halting efforts to guarantee standards among various subsets of physicians themselves proved quickly and utterly ineffectual... The only alternative for patients was to try to hold individual practitioners, one at a time, to whatever standards they or their lawyers, one at a time, wanted to impose." Although we don't believe that this is cause and effect (a more robust self-policing system wouldn't change any of the forces that have tilted the malpractice scales), we (on behalf of our profession) do plead at least partially guilty to the charge of harboring underperforming doctors. Medicine's inability to confront its bad apples is not unique. Big institutions—from the Catholic Church to Wall Street brokerage houses—are notoriously inept at policing their own ranks.

We have come to believe that the right way to reform malpractice is to either fully or partly de-link compensation and blame through some sort of no-fault system—we'll have more to say about this in the last part of the book. But a move in this controversial direction must be coupled with a more aggressive process of medical credentialing and licensing—of identifying and weeding out the truly bad apples. As Professor Ian Kennedy, chair of an inquiry into error-related infant deaths in an English hospital, said: "Health care professionals and patients must be more grown up about errors and mistakes. We need a system which recognizes that accountability is not the same as blame. Blame is a serendipitous weapon used to pillory someone who happens to be caught in its sights."

The malpractice system is all about blame. So let us turn our attention, finally, to the meaning of health care accountability.

CHAPTER 17: ACCOUNTABILITY

Punishment is now unfashionable... because it creates moral distinctions among men, which, to the democratic mind, are odious. We prefer a meaningless collective guilt to a meaningful individual responsibility.

—Thomas Szasz, *The Myth of Mental Illness* (1961)

Scott Torrence, a thirty-six-year-old resident of a small town in New Mexico, spent his weekdays behind a desk at an insurance company and his weekends hanging out with his buddies. Each Sunday they played hoops at a neighborhood park until mid-afternoon, then headed for a local sports bar for a few beers, big-screen football, and some laughs. Scott, a former Marine, was in decent shape, despite a receding hairline and the fact that his "six pack" abs now were visible only in fading snapshots.

Today's game was a blast. Scott was so hot that he started hamming it up—he made some outside jumpers and a few behind-the-back passes that amazed his pals. Scott was also aggressive going for the rebounds—he snagged a bunch, but one took a funny bounce off the rim and struck him in the side of the head. His teammate joked, "Hey man, you ain't playin' soccer!" but Scott didn't laugh. He got a strange look in his eye, and dropped to one knee for a few seconds, but then got up and finished the game.

Still not feeling quite right, he passed on the ritual trip to the bar and went home. Getting out of the shower, he told his girlfriend he felt queasy and had a terrible headache. He had barely gotten into a clean set of sweats before he turned ashen and slumped onto the couch. She called an ambulance, which responded promptly and drove Scott, lethargic but coherent, to nearby St. Mary's Hospital.

The family practice physician on call at St. Mary's ER that day was Dr. Jane Benamy. She took Scott's medical history and performed the best exam she could using the hospital's limited facilities. By now, Scott complained that, in addition to the headache and nausea, the room was beginning to spin. Dr. Benamy performed a standard neurological exam and found Scott to be "nonfocal" (neither side of his body was weaker than the other)—which was a bit comforting, since it made a major hemorrhage into one side of his brain less likely. She ordered some basic lab tests, which came back normal, and performed a spinal tap, which showed no evidence of meningitis or bleeding into the fluid around the brain.

Dr. Benamy was now worried that something more insidious—but equally dangerous—might be going on, but she had used all of the diagnostic arrows in tiny St. Mary's quiver. The nearest Big House was Regional Medical Center, 140 miles away, and she called the neurologist there. Benamy had bad vibes about Scott and thought he should be seen by a neurologist and probably get a CAT scan or an MRI soon. Neither the scanners nor the specialist was available at St. Mary's.

The on-call neurologist at Regional, Dr. Roy Jones, didn't agree. He felt that Torrence's neurological exam, lab work, and complaints were all consistent with "benign positional vertigo": a transient disorder in which the patient experiences a sense of the room spinning, usually when the head rapidly changes position. Still, Dr. Benamy wasn't satisfied.

"I had exhausted everything I could do," she later recalled. "This was more dramatic than any patient with benign positional vertigo I'd seen."

Working in the tiny St. Mary's ER was like swimming in a water hole. One misstep and you were in over your head, and—as a provider without the latest equipment—you always felt a little exposed. The ER nurses were concerned about Torrence too, and they, like Benamy, wanted him out of their little pond and into Regional. But according to the rules, they could not move the patient without authorization from an accepting physician, and Dr. Jones just wouldn't play ball. So Benamy admitted Torrence to the forty-five- bed St. Mary's—really more of a hospitalette than a hospital—for observation.

On Monday morning, Benamy saw Torrence again. He still complained of dizziness and headaches, which now seemed to bore through his skull. His nausea had not decreased—in fact, it had caused him to vomit several times. With the rising sun came another new symptom: Light made his eyes and brain hurt even more, so the shades were drawn and his room was kept as dark as possible. This "photophobia," she knew, often accompanied a collection of blood or pus in the lining of the brain.

Benamy called Dr. Jones at Regional with an update. Again, he refused her request for transfer. As Jones later recalled, "I told her that given a normal neurological exam and normal spinal tap, it was my opinion that very little would be learned from a CAT scan." Jones stood by his original long-distance diagnosis and said the worsening headaches were probably due to the spinal tap—although post-tap headaches are usually mild and last only a few hours. So Scott remained a prisoner at St. Mary's, getting pain medication for his headache and IV hydration for the fluid he had lost from vomiting.

Monday night, Scott's headaches seemed to peak. A covering physician wrote in the chart that it was, "the worst one yet... the patient was grabbing his head, crying out, and writhing on the bed in pain." Later that night, Scott lost consciousness, came around, then lost consciousness again.

Tuesday morning, Benamy called Regional again. Thankfully, Jones had finished his two-week stint on service and a new attending, an internist named Dr. Brad Soloway, was now manning the transfer beeper. Soloway agreed that Scott's case sounded terribly worrisome. He authorized the transfer by air ambulance and arranged for a priority CAT scan as soon as the patient arrived.

Soloway met the patient briefly on arrival at Regional's ER, prescribed some sedation, then had Scott taken to the scanner. Few tests have revolutionized medicine more than the CAT scan, which can peer into the brain and spot a wide range of disorders, including strokes caused either by ischemia (a blocked blood vessel) or bleeding (a ruptured blood vessel). Its one Achilles' heel, though, is the cerebellum—the part of the brain that controls balance and motor coordination. It is one of the prime suspects in any case of severe vertigo. But because it is tightly encased by bone—a smart idea from an evolutionary standpoint, since it protects this vital nerve center from damage—subtle cerebellar anomalies can be missed by the scanner. To help compensate for this, radiologists reading CAT scans in cerebellar cases are told to spend extra time scrutinizing this area. If the CAT scan fails to identify the problem, then an MRI usually follows, since the MRI's higher resolution gives a much better view of the cerebellum (we usually try the CAT scan first because it is significantly less expensive, and many patients become claustrophobic in the MRI scanner's "doughnut").

In this case, though, the radiologist wasn't told about Scott's unusual clinical history, so, to him, Scott Torrence was just another patient with a possible stroke. The radiologist thus approached his scan in the usual way and pronounced it "normal." Undoubtedly, had Soloway and the radiologist discussed the film together, the cerebellum would have received more attention—even an additional scan. But the two busy specialists were working at opposite ends of the building and never met. The results were dictated onto the hospital's stat radiology line, where Soloway heard them twenty minutes later. Reassured by the clean film, Soloway wrote in Scott's chart that the scan confirmed Dr. Jones's diagnosis of "benign positional vertigo with post-spinal headache." Case closed.

Still, there was something about the patient's appearance that gnawed at Soloway—he was badly flunking the "eyeball test," even though all of the clinical tests were cold-normal. He checked on Torrence again before leaving the hospital, and, although he found the patient restless, there were no changes in his neurological symptoms. So Soloway prescribed another sedative and, after wracking *his* brain to think of anything else this could be, called it a day.

That night the nurses phoned Dr. Soloway at home and said Scott Torrence was in severe pain, even more agitated ("awake, moaning, yelling"), and that he had to be restrained lest he injure himself. Soloway prescribed more sedation, plus some Demerol. A short time later, the nurses called again—the painkiller and sedation had had no effect. Soloway told them to increase the dosage. The nurses called twice again. Twice again, Soloway told them to torque up the palliatives. With a clean CAT scan and spinal tap, there was really nothing else to do.

Even though Wednesday was Soloway's day off, he came into the hospital to check on Scott Torrence. The patient was now completely disoriented. His pupils, which for the last two days had contracted briskly to a beam of light, now reacted sluggishly—a potential sign of serious brain damage. Dr. Jones, the neurology specialist, was back on duty and Soloway called him at home. Jones reassured Soloway that he "was familiar with the case and... the non-focal neurological exam and the normal CAT scan made urgent clinical problems unlikely." Jones went on to tell Soloway that "he would evaluate the patient the next morning and assume the patient's care." Astonishingly, Jones would say later, "I see a lot of patients with headaches, some very severe... Pain in itself does not concern me as much as a focal neurological deficit." Soloway remained puzzled about Torrence's pathology, but did not push Jones to rush in to examine the patient personally. After all, Jones was the neurologist—the specialist, *the man*—when it came to such cases, and he remained unconcerned.

Later that morning, Soloway was on the phone briefing Torrence's girlfriend back at home on the status of his treatment when a breathless nurse grabbed him.

"He's not breathing!" she cried.

Soloway and others dashed to the patient's room and began CPR. Torrence was revived and placed on life support. Jones now agreed to come in immediately. He examined the patient and determined that a portion of Scott's brain had swelled, causing it to extrude through a natural opening in the skull—like toothpaste being squeezed from a tube. This nightmarish condition, called *herniation*, is a dreaded complication of brain damage and instantly ends a person's ability to breathe by crushing the nerves that control respiration.

Jones and Soloway ran to radiology to review the previous day's CAT scan. As the image appeared, their jaws dropped. The abnormality was subtle but definite. The scan showed there was indeed a stroke in the cerebellum—signs of mild cerebellar swelling were already visible. Had it been recognized at the time, the growing pressure could have been relieved through a combination of medications and surgery. Left untreated, however, the swelling continued until there was simply no more space in Scott's skull to hold the edematous tissue.

Three days after his admission to his local ER, Scott Torrence was pronounced dead. An autopsy revealed that the head trauma from the errant rebound had ripped a small artery that supplies the cerebellum with blood, an unusual but known complication from a head injury. The tear led to a blood clot, the clot led to a stroke, the stroke led to swelling, and the swelling led to herniation—a cascade of falling dominoes that could have been stopped at any stage by correct diagnosis and treatment.

Although we favor moving toward a no-fault system to compensate people for medical injuries, we must admit that cases like this are tough for no-faulters to defend. Certainly there are systems problems here: One can envision decision support, for example, that automatically prompts radiologists to recommend an MRI if a CAT scan is unrevealing in patients with cerebellar symptoms, or a videoconferencing system connecting St. Mary's and Regional—it's hard to believe that one glance at the patient (or of Dr. Benamy pleading) wouldn't have convinced Dr. Jones to accept the patient in transfer.

Yet at its core, this case seems less like one of bad systems than of bad doctoring. Dr. Jones's refusal to transfer a young man with obviously profound symptoms of *something* neurological smacks more of hubris than the voice of experience trying to calm an anxious patient and reassure a small town physician. And once Scott Torrence was at Regional Hospital, Jones's refusal to come in and examine him was, at best, a bad call; and at worst, lazy and sloppy.

Cases like these, while tragic, shouldn't surprise anyone. Despite years of training, doctors are as vulnerable as anyone to all the maladies that can beset any professional in a high-demand, rapidly changing profession: creeping obsolescence, alcoholism, procrastination, drug abuse, depression, burnout, or just failing to care enough. How can we reconcile the need for accountability for these human failings with our desire to shift from "blame and shame" to a new focus on system safety?

We asked Dr. Lucian Leape, the legendary surgeon who sounded the first alarms about medical errors back when few people were willing to listen. Now seventy-three years old, Leape remains handsome and elegant, with a warm smile and hearty laugh that make him singularly charming and approachable. Leape laments:

> There is no accountability. When we identify doctors who harm patients, we need to try to be compassionate and help them. But in the end, if they are a danger to patients, they shouldn't be caring for them. A fundamental principle has to be the development and then the enforcement of procedures and standards. We can't make real progress without them. When a doctor doesn't follow them, *something* has to happen. Today, nothing does, and you have a vicious cycle in which people have no real incentive to follow the rules because they know there are no consequences if they don't. So there *are* bad doctors and bad nurses, but the fact that we tolerate them is just another systems problem.

The struggle between accountability and professional freedom, between bad systems and bad apples, may be the most vexing problem of all when it comes to patient safety. Whenever these issues come up, discussions turn into arguments, opinions become polarized, and rationality gives way to elliptical and hyperbolic thinking—case making, not case solving.

It is undeniable that hospitals *do* have a tendency to protect their own, sometimes at the expense of patients. Hospital "credentials committees," which certify and periodically recertify individual doctors, are toothless tigers. Most committees rarely limit a provider's privileges, even when there is stark evidence he presents a clear and present danger to patients. Instead, they assign a committee member to "have a chat" with the physician in question, perhaps gently suggesting he or she shouldn't do a particular procedure anymore. They might even ask another physician, not on the committee but in a similar specialty, to "keep an eye on old Doug" and let them know if he continues to screw up, even if patients or other staff members don't report it. If alcohol or drug abuse is the problem, the physician may be ordered to enter a "diversion" program—the same way car thieves or muggers who steal property to buy drugs are "diverted" from society into rehab until they can get their act together. This is a noble idea, but one that sometimes errs on the side of protecting the interests of the dangerous provider over an unwitting public.

Our profession is also flummoxed by those physicians (or nurses) for whom God handed out more than the usual dose of carelessness. As we've described, slips are human, but there *are* some people who commit far more than their fair share—and when these absentminded professors end up in detail-oriented specialties like pathology, sparks can fly. In situations like this, James Reason recommends aggressive career counseling, along the lines of, "Don't you think you would be doing everyone a favor if you considered taking on some other job within the company?" "This is the way," says the world's expert in human error, only partly tongue-in-cheek, "management acquires some of its most distinguished members."

It is not that hospital credentials committees *never* take action. They do—removing a physician's privileges at a hospital or recommending to the state board that a doctor's license be suspended—when there is clear, repetitive evidence of gross negligence and incompetence. But when this happens—and it is really rare—it comes only after an orgy of soul-searching, hand-wringing, buck-passing, second-guessing and second chances that is painful, and sometimes embarrassing, to watch. In most cases, committee members just swallow hard and—unless the physician is under felony indictment or is so stewed that he can't walk down a corridor without banging into both walls—the credentials are rubber-stamped.

There are several reasons our self-policing is so inept and ineffectual.

One undoubtedly pertains to the "Fraternity of Medicine" idea—though we doubt that any conscientious physician, on or off a credentials committee, puts the good of the fraternity ahead of any patient's well-being, at least consciously. But just as the malpractice jury—a "jury of peers"—tends to side with the sympathetic patient, credentials committees are also reluctant to sanction *their* peers.

Another reason is practical. It takes nearly a decade to train even a general practitioner, and much longer if the doctor wants to practice in a rarified specialty such as brain surgery or transplantation. Committees are understandably reluctant to cancel somebody's ticket after the community has invested so much time, effort, and money to train them.

A third reason is simply that doctors aren't very good organizational managers. Their people skills are usually confined to bedside chats and working with colleagues and support staff in task-oriented jobs; they aren't particularly adept at managing conflicts and confrontations, so they avoid them. This is a pretty dumb reason to let an error-prone doctor continue to prowl the hospital wards, but because litigation (slander, defamation, and the like) lurks behind any challenge to professional competence (and committee members are only partially shielded from liability), many physicians are reluctant to go into that particular swamp unless the trail is awfully solid.

So we usually cop out. Life goes on and mistakes continue—many of them by the usual suspects. Dr. Atul Gawande sees in this recurring scenario something quite understandable, even a tad noble. When it comes to disciplining a basically good but troubled doctor, "no one," he says, "really has the heart for it." He writes:

> When a skilled, decent, ordinarily conscientious colleague, whom you've known and worked with for years, starts popping Percodans, or becomes preoccupied with personal problems, and neglects the proper care of patients, you want to help, not destroy the doctor's career. There is no easy way to help, though. In private practice, there are no sabbaticals to offer, no leaves of absence, only disciplinary proceedings and public reports of misdeeds. As a consequence, when people try to help, they do it quietly, privately. Their intentions are good; the result usually isn't.

One patient advocate, Dr. Sidney Wolfe, director of Ralph Nader's Public Citizen Health Research Group, is far less charitable than Dr. Gawande. Wolfe notes that from 1990 to 2002, just 5 percent of doctors were involved in 54 percent of the payouts reported to the National Practitioner Data Bank, the confidential log of malpractice cases maintained by the U.S. Government. Of the 35,000 doctors with two or more payouts, only 8 percent were disciplined by state boards. And among the 2,774 doctors who had made payments in five or more cases, only 463 (just one out of six) had been disciplined. One Pennsylvania doctor paid a whopping twenty-four claims, totaling $8 million, between 1993 and 2001, including a wrong-site surgery and a retained instrument case. Yet he had not been disciplined by the state licensing board.

"Amid the uproar about malpractice premium increases," Wolfe writes, "there is a deadly silence from physicians' groups on the crisis of inadequate discipline. The problem is not the compensation paid to injured patients, but an epidemic of medical errors."

That, of course, is more than a bit simplistic. In this group of multiply sued doctors are some superb obstetricians and neurosurgeons who have chosen—God only knows why, in the present environment—to take on the toughest cases in the specialties most likely to be sued. The average American obstetrician, for example, gets sued once every ten years, whether he deserves it or not, so a good fraction of Dr. Wolfe's "bad apples" are undoubtedly older practitioners who have just been in the queue longer than their younger counterparts. Does this really mean that obstetricians, as a breed, are worse doctors than pediatricians (who are sued far less often)?

And yet, Dr. Wolfe's enemies list undoubtedly *does* include some physicians that neither you nor we would want at the other end of a prescription pad or a scalpel—and we'd all be better off if these docs were surgically removed from the system. This will require more rational and explicit practice standards, better ways to measure whether doctors are meeting those standards (the increasing computerization of practice will help by making it much easier to tell whether docs are practicing high-quality, evidence-based medicine), and a shift in priorities: Local credentials committees and state licensing boards must see protecting patients as Job One.

Finally, critical safety rules simply must be enforced. We see no conflict between this tough love stance and the systems approach, since some errors—particularly willful and repeated violations of sensible safety rules—are indeed blameworthy. James Reason, too, sees the need to punish habitual rule-benders: "Seeing them get away with it on a daily basis does little for morale or for the credibility of the disciplinary system. Watching them getting their 'come-uppance' is not only satisfying, it also serves to reinforce where the boundaries of acceptable behavior lie... Justice works two ways. Severe sanctions for the few can protect the innocence of the many."

The balancing act is a tricky one—in our zeal to replace the malpractice system with another, more rational forum for accountability, we won't be doing ourselves any favors if we convert our licensing boards and credentials committees into Star Chambers. And, no matter what system (if any) eventually replaces our current dysfunctional methods of accountability, the underlying principles will remain the same. As Charles Bosk reminds us:

> The professional's last line of defense is a moral one because it is a proper moral performance alone that substantiates a claim to proper technical performance when events mock such a claim. It is not the patient dying but the patient dying when the doctor on call fails to answer his pages that makes it impossible to sustain a case of acting in the client's interest... Moral error breaches a professional's contract with his client. He has not acted in good faith. He has done less than he should have.

Ironically, for several decades the malpractice system has tormented providers who *have* acted in good faith—who have *not* done less than they should have, but have been standing at the sharp end of a bad medical outcome. Meanwhile, there has been virtually no reckoning for the blunt-end players—the politicians, the media, the CEOs, the managers—who have done much less than *they* should have to create a safe health care system. What they—and we—should do to help cure our epidemic of medical mistakes is the subject of the rest of this book.

PART IV: CURES

CHAPTER 18: ATTACKING A NEW DISEASE

In all science, error precedes the truth, and it is better it should go first than last.

— Hugh Walpole (1884–1941)

On August 13, 1998, the *Bay Area Reporter*, an exuberant San Francisco weekly known better for its dishy coverage of local political gossip than for hard news, ran a breathtaking banner on the front page:

"No Obits."

This headline was remarkable because for seventeen years, the *BAR*—newsweekly of the city's gay community—had served as both a forum for gay culture and a tombstone for its members. Beginning in 1981, when the first five cases of "pneumocystis pneumonia in homosexual men" were reported, it fell to the paper to chronicle the devastating toll the then-unnamed epidemic, later called AIDS, would take on the gay population. At the height of the AIDS epidemic, the newspaper devoted up to a quarter of its thirty-some pages to obituaries. Few of the dead had seen their forty-fifth birthday.

* * *

The nascent field of patient safety has the feel of a new disease. Its dynamics and sociology are all-too-similar to those early years of the AIDS epidemic. Both share the same sense of uncertainty and challenge, fear and hope—however desperate. Medical caregivers are groping for new models, new paradigms. They are reaching out for innovative solutions with one hand and covering their asses with the other—trying to make things better while also trying, in the meantime, not to make them worse. What sustains them is mainly blind faith in medicine's professional legacy: Given enough time and money, most problems get solved.

You may ask, quite reasonably, how a problem like medical errors can feel new when patients have been injured and killed at the hands of their caregivers since the time of Hippocrates—who, after all, admonished us to "first, do no harm," 2,500 years ago. It feels new because, until recently, the symptoms were hidden from view by caregivers and institutions racked with shame and fearful of consequences. In clinical medicine, new symptoms can signal the presence of a hidden disease: The jaundiced skin indicates a long-failing liver; the fever gives notice of a previously dormant parasite; purple welts in the lower abdomen expose the slow ooze of internal bleeding. The rash of clinical mistakes we call our "epidemic of errors" is simply the latest sign that something is dangerously wrong beneath the shining veneer of modern medicine.

And what a veneer! We point with pride to the miraculous new machines and heroic new procedures that grace our billion-dollar temples of healing. They are how we wish to be seen by the world; while in reality too much of our hidden, inner world resembles *The Picture of Dorian Gray*, where our secret sins fester out of sight. Such sins may go unreported, but they scar us just the same. The internal bleeding continues.

AIDS, of course, didn't stay hidden for long. The 1981 reports of young gay men succumbing to a devastating new illness immediately made front-page news, at least in urban centers like San Francisco, Los Angeles, and New York. We had no idea what was causing the terrible complex of symptoms: Was it an infection? A cancer? An environmental poison? Those of us on the front lines of care didn't even know if mere proximity was enough to transmit the disease, which, in those days, was a death sentence. Bob vividly recalls the 1984 day when one of his mentors, a prominent lung specialist at San Francisco General Hospital, stuck himself accidentally with a needle just used on an AIDS patient—a young man also jaundiced from hepatitis B. We all held our breath—we had no idea whether the chance of contracting AIDS from a needlestick was the same as with hepatitis (about one in five), far lower, or even higher (later studies by our UCSF colleague Julie Gerberding, now director of the federal Centers for Disease Control, determined the risk was actually one in 300). So ignorant were we of such basic answers that, when the lung specialist eventually came down with hepatitis but not AIDS, his case was written up in the *New England Journal of Medicine*.

The risk of needlestick transmission was only one of hundreds of questions that consumed us in those frenzied, early years of the epidemic. How could doctors and nurses care for diseased patients when we had no idea how the illness was acquired, spread, or treated? We agonized over containment strategies, many of which went against the political and social currents of the times. Should we push patients to modify their risky behaviors? Should hospitals separate AIDS patients until the disease's vector was known? Should cases— as they are with plague, smallpox and syphilis—be reported to health authorities? For that matter, what was the government's proper role in all of this? The answer, for years, was as little as possible.

So time marched on, and so did the *BAR*'s obits. Thousands died in those early years because so many caregivers and policymakers simply chose to avert their eyes. By the time an American president first publicly *mentioned* the disease (Ronald Reagan, in a 1987 speech), more than 25,000 AIDS victims had perished in the U.S. Federal funding was minuscule. Pharmaceutical companies, preferring to push existing drugs rather than risk money developing new ones, were hesitant to invest in research—where is the market in a rapidly fatal disease, particularly one so highly politicized? Academic medical centers and foundations—always more interested in basic research, new gadgets, and heroic surgeries than in public health—only reluctantly allocated resources to the new "twentieth-century plague." The late Dr. Jonathan Mann, visionary founder of the World Health Organization's AIDS program, said of those early years: "The dominant feature... was silence, for the human immunodeficiency virus (HIV) was unknown and transmission was not accompanied by signs or symptoms salient enough to be noticed.... During this period of silence, the spread was unchecked by awareness or any preventive action and approximately 100,000–300,000 persons may have been infected."

And yet, a decade and a half after this timid start, the newspaper at Ground Zero could finally report: NO OBITS. In less than a generation, the disease had garnered unprecedented media attention, generous federal funding, huge leaps in scientific understanding and medical therapies, enormous pharmaceutical investments, and new regulations that led to effective prevention and even acceleration of the FDA's normally glacial drug-approval process.

Two *billion* dollars a year now flows into AIDS-related research from the federal government alone. Coupled with additional funds from pharmaceutical companies and private foundations, this money has attracted thousands of researchers seeking or refining answers to questions that range from the mechanism of viral replication to the organization of long-term care for the infected. Substantial numbers in high-risk groups have changed their behaviors, leading to lower transmission rates.

The payoff has been breathtaking—not the long-sought cure, but conversion of AIDS from a mandatory death sentence to a "manageable chronic disease"—somewhat like diabetes and congestive heart failure. In the year 1995 alone, 51,000 Americans died of AIDS—slightly less than the total fatalities of the Vietnam War. Six years later, the death toll was down to 9,000—over an 80 percent drop in mortality. While AIDS continues to take a terrible toll globally, this experience gives us hope that when we Americans put our minds and money to it, we can eventually contain, if not cure, any epidemic.

This stunning about-face was made possible only because of public understanding and political pressure. What tactics can we borrow from the playbook used by AIDS activists and advocates, researchers and caregivers, to win our fight against medical mistakes in America?

One lesson is as old as the March of Dimes: the simple value of a human face—a "poster child"—a symbol of empathy to rally around. The first high-profile AIDS victim was a very reluctant hero: actor Rock Hudson, the very image of a Hollywood he-man, who died of the disease in 1985. Although Hudson had been gay all his adult life, the studio's code of silence and a cooperative press kept his secret hidden until the wasting illness (and several desperate trips to France for experimental treatment) made his plight all too public. At that point, Americans began to sense that, no matter what their moral or political beliefs about homosexuality, here was a disease that could strike anyone. By this time, too, AIDS had been associated with tainted blood supplies, further reinforcing the feeling that the disease knew no moral or cultural boundaries. Five years after Hudson's death, an eighteen-year-old all-American boy from Kokomo, Indiana—hemophiliac Ryan White—also died from AIDS, proving (if there was any doubt left) that even youth and "innocence" were no protection against this terrible killer.

Politically, Randy Shilts's 1987 bestseller, *And the Band Played On* (later an HBO movie) dramatically documented the epidemic's early years, society's indifference, and the extraordinary human toll they exacted. With the attention now of entertainment industry celebrities (who never appeared, it seemed, without red ribbons on their lapels or dresses), the pendulum began to swing the other way. Politicians soon fell in line, led by America's grandfatherly surgeon general, C. Everett Koop, who became the disease's Lincolnesque spokesperson during his years as "America's Family Doctor."

For AIDS, there was one more crucial ingredient. In 1987, the incendiary New York playwright Larry Kramer addressed a small community group in Greenwich Village. "Two-thirds of you will be dead in five years," he challenged the group—victims of not only a virus, but of a medical system that didn't care whether they lived or died. "If what you're hearing doesn't rouse you to anger, fury, rage, and action," he fumed, "gay men will have no future here on earth."

ACT UP was born. Within a few years, it joined with dozens of less strident AIDS groups to become the most powerful disease-oriented advocacy movement in history. By the mid-1990s, AIDS as a social phenomenon had come full circle. The outcast, outlaw disease and its caregivers had not just joined mainstream medicine, they—their agenda and their tactics—had begun to dominate it.

Which of these lessons drawn from the successful fight against AIDS might be transferable to our efforts to tackle medical mistakes?

Unfortunately, we lack a single, compelling figure—a Rock Hudson or Ryan White—to be an icon for this twenty-first-century disease. The Libby Zions, Betsy Lehmans, and Jesica Santillans all moved us for a news cycle or two, but their stories were quickly lost in the glare of the next tale of public dread: tainted meat, shark attacks, and—the apogee of angst—terrorism.

In a way, the very decentralized, diffuse, and nondenominational nature of medical errors is what makes the epidemic so hard to tackle. More people die in the U. S. each year of preventable medical mistakes than from AIDS and breast cancer combined, but you would never know it. The "disease" draws no celebrity pitchmen—no Jerry Lewis or Christopher Reeve or Betty Ford or Lance Armstrong. Patient safety advocates like Drs. Lucian Leape and Don Berwick are passionate crusaders and highly respected in medical circles, but they've hardly become household names. We have no Dr. Koop to make medical errors "his issue" and drive its message home during chitchats with Tim Russert.

When institutional leadership is lacking, patient-activists sometimes have to take the lead, as they did in the fight against AIDS. To date, a few patient safety groups have been organized, but most could fit around a good-sized kitchen table. None have the resources to organize a "million victim march" on Washington, say, or cover a major medical center with a huge, Christo-like Band-Aid, the way AIDS activists covered Senator Jesse Helms's house with a giant condom in 1991. These may be stunts, but stunts like these tell a complex story quickly and viscerally.

And so we paddle onward, doing what we can and waiting for the public to notice—really notice—just how bad this disease is, and how poised we are to save lives with the right approach and sufficient resources. Our destination is clear, but the far shore is not yet in sight. In the remaining chapters of this book, we will describe some of the ways we can make this journey faster, safer, and, most importantly—together.

CHAPTER 19: WHAT CAN POLICYMAKERS DO?

The art of politics is to be ahead of your time—about six months will do it. Any more than that, and people forget you were there.

— Gloria Steinem

Although we pride ourselves on American free enterprise and Yankee ingenuity, the fact is that government frames the way we address almost every major problem—social, economic, or scientific. It does this through law—civil and criminal codes—but also through administrative regulations; tax incentives, penalties, and subsidies; and direct spending for social and technical programs, including research.

Following a shamefully long period of bureaucratic inaction, the federal response to the HIV challenge ultimately became impressive and effective. After early moralizing focused on patients for their "deviant" behavior, federal laws protecting patient confidentiality encouraged HIV testing and reporting, and discouraged workplace discrimination. This has not only built a broad and reliable database about the epidemic and encouraged victims to seek treatment, but has also kept the problem visible to the public. While many people were uncomfortable, to say the least, with the idea that their office-mate might be battling HIV, they quickly learned that AIDS wasn't spread like a common cold. The cloud of stigma began to lift.

This transition from secrecy to openness has also come to characterize our approach to previously unmentionable diseases like breast cancer, colon cancer, and prostate cancer. In a similar way, we see the current taboo- and liability-laden atmosphere surrounding medical mistakes gradually dissipating. As medical errors (as opposed to culpable or criminal negligence) begin to shed some of their stigma, practitioners and patients will feel freer to report them, talk about them, and tackle them. Policymakers enter the equation here because of their vast power to provide forums for constructive dialogue, level the legal playing field through malpractice reforms, implement sensible and effective error reporting systems, and reach the media with a consistent—and scientifically correct—message.

Effective error prevention will take a lot of funding. The 1999 IOM report was paid for, in part, by federal funds. Tax dollars funded a 2001 report (which we edited) on evidence-based patient safety practices, now used by patient safety committees all over the country. Virtually none of the current research on medical errors would have been possible without federal funding. These studies— many of which we've described throughout this book—have revealed such fundamental insights as how often mistakes happen in various patient populations; the impact of information technology on error rates; ideas for reforming malpractice laws; how to decrease hospital-acquired infections; ways to improve pain management; how to make informed consent more meaningful, and so on.

And this funding does more than simply pay for the studies themselves. The massive infusion of dollars into AIDS research induced brilliant virologists, immunologists, field researchers, psychologists, and economists to shift their focus onto the disease, creating a "Manhattan Project"-type environment—the kind of shared mission that accelerates progress. Progress follows research the way day follows night; and researchers, like so many others in our capital-driven society, follow the money. The simple fact is that we need more talented people from many fields (medicine, ethics, law, psychology, engineering, information technology, group dynamics, to name a few) to devote themselves to the patient safety and quality movements—researching new ideas and testing them under battlefield conditions—and we'll only get them if we can offer the resources they need.

Unfortunately, on this score we still have a long way to go.

Overall federal research funding on medical errors flows through AHRQ, the Agency for Healthcare Research and Quality—the

"NASA" of the quality movement. Currently, this totals $60 million per year. In contrast, the budget of the National Institutes of Health is $27 *billion* per year. In other words, for every $500 we spend to come up with new diagnoses and treatments, we invest only one dollar on ways to deliver that care safely. When you consider that overall health care costs in the United States are approximately $1.5 *trillion* per year, we spend $25,000 for pills, procedures, and bedpans for every one dollar on patient safety.

This may seem like a fair exchange—modern medicine, after all, sometimes performs real miracles—until you realize that as powerful drugs proliferate, procedures become more complex, and more specialists come into being (making handoffs more frequent and precarious), these "improvements" in treating specific conditions may be significantly eroded by the risks inherent in delivering them. It does a lung-cancer patient no good to trade a low-risk X-ray for a higher resolution Magnetic Resonance scan if those powerful MRI magnets, when activated, turn a nearby oxygen tank or IV pump into a deadly unguided missile—don't laugh, such accidents have already happened.

We are not Luddites: Health care's technological progress is spectacular and worthwhile, but it is risky. In the eighteenth century, Voltaire wrote, "The role of the physician is to entertain the patient while nature takes its course." But that was then. Sir Cyril Chantler, Dean of London's Guy's Hospital, gave voice to our modern-day Faustian bargain. "Medicine used to be simple, ineffective, and relatively safe," he wrote. "Now it is complex, effective, and potentially dangerous."

The present level of federal funding devoted to reducing medical errors is not enough to do the job; though it has been effective at showing results are possible. Like AIDS research in the mid-1980s or the space program of the early 1960s, our funding must be significantly increased—doubling it would make a good start—if we are to make a dent in the epidemic. And, rather than making it a fixed sum, nearly certain to get chewed away in the next budget crunch, we'd favor a different funding method: Since medical errors accompany each advance in medical science, let's set aside a portion of the NIH budget—say, two-thirds of a percent each year—to abating the errors the system itself creates.

While government drives much of the system, policymakers in hospitals and clinics have roles to play as well. Unless administrators create and sustain systems that caregivers can adopt and use as their own, all the federal funding in the world will accomplish little. What we're talking about here is creating a culture of safety in places where safety, at best, has been an afterthought—the by-product of personal initiative and dumb luck.

Today, most hospitals pay at least lip service to the fledgling patient safety movement. In response to new regulations, they have created a few new job titles (often tacking "safety coordinator" onto the job description of existing employees performing other, primary duties) but few have invested any substantive resources in making patients safer. Effective safety programs will include broad portfolios of investments—computerized physician order entry (CPOE) and other IT solutions, teamwork training, reporting systems, and more. But until administrators hire trained professionals *whose job it is to promote and ensure safety*, these will only be stopgap measures.

To do more than the minimum in anything takes leadership, which can be hard to find in many bureaucracies. At most hospitals, CEOs or Boards are praised as dynamic and visionary when they are the first ones on their blocks to buy the latest and greatest positron emission scanners (even if they don't know exactly what they do) while resolutely "containing costs." From one perspective, it's hard to blame them. Even the operations of nonprofit hospitals are market-driven. If losing patients to a competitor downtown because they've won the high-tech "arms race" forces you to shut down a wing, you aren't doing your staff, or your current patients, any favors.

But too many of our leaders have become slaves to the market, and have sidestepped the true test of leadership: setting priorities. In the age of error epidemics, real leaders put their resources where they get the best results, not just the best billboards. If the chief measure of that success is the ratio of healthy patients leaving the hospital compared with the number of sick patients entering it, ensuring safe, high quality care *has* to be at the top of the list.

We'd love to tell you that this kind of thoughtful, decisive leadership is emerging at most hospitals, but plainly, it isn't. There are too many pressures on administrators to focus on other problems; too many professional and community groups who want to put their own issues first, even at the expense of the one issue all of them share: the need for an environment in which patients feel—and *are*—safe, regardless of their disease.

The only solution to this seemingly intractable problem is to apply a different kind of pressure, one that gets leaders to feel that they have more to gain by focusing on safety than by ignoring it. Where can this pressure come from?

Some of it might come from patients voting with their dollars—choosing providers with better safety records—but this is only part of the solution, and a minor one at that. Most patients don't choose their hospitals: Their doctors do. So until doctors and medical groups start shunning facilities with bad safety records—in general, or for specific procedures—administrators will have few incentives to, quite literally, clean up their acts. But even this pressure, if it comes to bear at all, will be limited: Most doctors are tightly linked to their hospitals and clinics; in few cases will safety concerns be enough to drive them away.

The broader market may play an even larger role. The most visible manifestation of the fledgling market movement is the business consortium known as the Leapfrog Group, founded in 2000, partly in response to the IOM report. Leapfrog members, all of them Fortune 500 companies, have been using their collective muscle to force changes to the systems and institutions providing services to their employees through financial incentives and efforts to shift market-share by touting both "safe" and "unsafe" hospitals. The effort is starting to bear fruit.

Regulators are also beginning to get into the game. As we've described, the Joint Commission on the Accreditation of Healthcare Organizations (JCAHO) has begun to call safety "balls and strikes." But JCAHO is a voluntary organization—hospitals aren't required to be accredited—and most of JCAHO's resources come from the hospitals themselves. This makes JCAHO a key player in the patient safety crusade, but one that may be inclined to back off when hospital administrators cry, "Kill the ump!"

The steps by Leapfrog and JCAHO are the beginning of an important trend: real pressure being brought to bear on health care organizations to prioritize safety. But if the history of reforms in any field tells us anything, it's that pressure for change must be focused and unremitting. This is especially true when we are trying to overcome not only culture and history, but also powerfully entrenched special interests, as we are when we try to reform our dysfunctional malpractice system.

* * *

As we described in Chapter 16, the fundamental problem facing malpractice reform is the conflict between fair compensation for the injured and the moral stain of fault attached to providers who, while responsible (in whole or in part) for error, are not liable in the sense of traditional tort law. Until this imbalance is removed, meaningful improvements in patient safety will be stunted.

In a series of articles stretching back to the early 1990s, Troy Brennan and his colleagues have made a strong case for scrapping the entire adversarial malpractice approach and replacing it with a no-fault system modeled on workers' compensation. Under this scheme, a no-fault pool is created from insurance premiums (and investments) from which awards would be made following the simple establishment of harm to the patient at the hands of the medical system. There would be no adversarial action—and no need to prove that the caregiver was negligent or the care was substandard. In other words, it creates a system based on reality, not wishful thinking or opportunism.

Of course, many will not find the notion of a new system that functions like "workers' comp" terribly comforting. But think about this: Since there would be no effort needed to find fault, billions of dollars that currently go to lawyers, expert witnesses, and discovery procedures would be largely saved. Remember, these expenses currently cost injured patients (not just the doctor or hospital paying them) more than *half* of all funds awarded, so this would be a staggering victory for patients. (For the record, workers' comp has an administrative cost of about 20 to 30 percent of total payouts, while Social Security Disability has overhead costs as low as 5 percent, although it, too, is criticized for bureaucratic inefficiency.)

Another advantage of a no-fault system is that it conserves one resource that is often singularly valuable to injured patients and their families: *time*. The path from injury to payout is vastly shorter under a no-fault system; and the great majority of injured patients who don't meet lawyerly tests for lucrative settlements or litigation would have prompt access to compensation previously denied them.

Last, but not least, a no-fault system would remove the single greatest barrier to an accurate and useful error reporting program. With the incentive to dissemble, avoid, or evade the whole topic of medical mistakes removed, safety issues would suddenly step into the sunshine, where their true dimensions could be measured, studied, and contained.

Of course, accepting a public policy conceptually and implementing it in the real world are two different things. Administration of a no-fault system must not only be squeaky-clean, it must avoid even the appearance of impropriety. Further, the threshold of compensation must be carefully set. If the bar is too low (say, compensation for minor and transitory gastrointestinal bleeding due to administration of aspirin—a common clinical side effect—while hospitalized), the system will go instantly bankrupt. Set the bar too high (restrict payouts only to page A-1 errors like wrong-site surgeries or retained objects), and we're right back where we started: with a selected few getting most of the benefits.

On moral terms, some might complain that no-fault secretly condones errors by simply paying off the victims, removing any incentive providers currently have to avoid malpractice suits. But Brennan's studies have proved that providers' biggest incentives under current malpractice laws are to avoid detection, deny responsibility, and resist even the most modest claims.

Finally, no-fault, if structured correctly, can give institutional policymakers incentives and new financial resources to actually improve their patient safety systems—the most important intervention of all. Investments in safety could be encouraged by what Brennan calls "experience rating" for hospitals and medical groups, whose insurance premiums would be reduced as their overall claims records showed improvement.

Is a 100 percent no-fault solution the way to go? And would it work in as litigious a place as the United States? Brennan has long been banging his head against these questions. He jokes, "I've been proselytizing about no-fault for the last ten years and I've managed to convince two or three people... and they all work for me!"

The two of us believe that no-fault is worth a try, but our precise recommendations differ slightly, probably due to our distinct upbringings. Kaveh, a Canadian by birth, feels that our present malpractice system is so dysfunctional that we would be best off with a completely no-fault system—scrapping the right to sue—coupled with a rededication of our institutions and providers to improving safety. The latter would need to be helped along by stronger regulations and tighter accountability. He argues that it is better— morally and financially—to let a few "bad apples" go unpunished than to unjustly penalize tens of thousands who don't deserve it, creating a rancid atmosphere all the while. This perspective is in keeping with the communitarian view of public policy held by many Canadians and Western Europeans, whose countries have all adopted universal government-sponsored health care based on the same instincts.

Bob, born in the United States, favors a conditional no-fault system that is much more selective about who gets off and who gets tagged. Some review process—an administrative process, not malpractice proceedings—would establish in each case whether an error is a slip (or unlucky judgment call) or a real, blameworthy mistake. The vast majority, we believe, will be the former—in these cases, there would be no-fault payouts based on a predetermined formula (death is worth a certain amount, loss of a limb some fraction of that, and so on). But he takes the more American point of view that the right to sue should be retained, with limitations on the dollar value of the awards and the raising of the malpractice bar to include only egregious, patently negligent errors. He thinks that Americans' passion for individual accountability would ultimately torpedo a system that could not assign fault (and with it the duty of compensation) on truly blameworthy errors. The errors committed by Dr. Roy Jones—who refused on several occasions to even examine Scott Torrence despite the young man's intractable vertigo and headache—would fall into this negligent, and thus blameworthy, category. On the other hand, Dr. Andrea Harris's judgment call to intubate Cynthia Taylor in the ICU rather than on the medical ward would result in a no-fault payment to the patient's anguished family—perhaps not the spoils of the Florida lottery, but a reasonable sum that would be paid relatively quickly, without rancor, and without 60 percent of the dollars being siphoned off the top.

A no-fault system for medical mistakes is not a brand-new idea. In fact, it has been tried in other countries, and their experiences reveal both opportunities and challenges.

New Zealand, for example, switched to a no-fault system for *all* personal injuries, including medicine, in 1972. Since then, it has discovered that a totally "no-fault" society can create its own problems—many locals now consider the compensation scheme too expensive and cumbersome. Whenever medical errors appear on the Auckland nightly news, for example, activists and politicians immediately begin clamoring to reinstate some kind of fault-based system for at least the more egregious errors. Even some of the promised savings of a totally no-fault system failed to materialize. Although the system dispensed with a well-entrenched corps of tort lawyers, judges, and expert witnesses, it substituted in their place, writes New Zealand anesthesiologist Alan Merry, "an army of administrators and case managers... and at least some of the saved legal activity, perhaps most of it, has been taken up by appeals or actions arising from disputes between injured people and the [system] itself."

In contrast, after two decades of no-fault experience in Sweden, the system remains effective and highly popular. If America adopted Sweden's limits on compensable injuries (medical injuries, to qualify, must have been "avoidable"; and eligible patients must have spent at least ten days in the hospital or endured at least thirty sick days), Brennan's group showed that overall costs of compensating patients would be no more, and probably far less, than our present malpractice system, while achieving all of the other benefits of a nonadversarial process.

The questions are complex and no solution is perfect, and so the status quo drags on. Are the American people and their political representatives truly ready to tackle medical errors with the seriousness of purpose the problem deserves—and, in doing so, overcome the special interests vested in the present system? As James Reason wryly observes: "Societies, just like the operators of hazardous systems, put production before protection... Safety legislation is enacted in the aftermath of disasters, not before them... [so] every society gets the disasters it deserves."

CHAPTER 20: A CULTURE OF SAFETY

Culture: the cry of men in face of their destiny.

— Albert Camus (1913–1960)

If we do succeed in getting our health care institutions to focus—really focus—on patient safety, the next question will be what precisely they should do. Since the medical specialty of patient safety is so new, we have few models to guide us.

Of course, there are parallels in other high-stakes, high-tech industries, such as aviation and nuclear power; but as we've seen, medical practitioners have their own view of the world, sometimes for good reason. We should be open to what we can learn from these other fields, but mindless adoption—"we'll take one from Column A, two from Column B"—that fails to account for medicine's unique attributes is doomed to fail.

There are also a few parallels in health care itself that offer some useful lessons. After studying these parallels, we believe that every hospital should have a core of clinicians—doctors, nurses, pharmacists, and others—trained in modern safety principles. Their special mission would be to help prevent mistakes by implementing effective safety systems, and by helping to create a culture of safety.

An early success story in this field comes from infection control. Yes, all doctors and nurses know that they should remove unnecessary catheters, wear sterile gowns, clean their hands often, and prescribe appropriate antibiotics. But experience has taught us that *all* of these things happen better and more predictably, and hospital-acquired infections are much fewer, if a clinician-leader and trained staff (called "infection control officers") are on the payroll and on the job. Infection control officers are also plugged into larger networks of infection tracking and prevention systems, such as state and local health departments and the federal Centers for Disease Control (CDC), so they're used to working with outsiders and using standardized reporting systems. These systems have been used effectively to combat and contain emerging infections like SARS and West Nile virus, and to "benchmark" the performance of individual hospitals against like institutions. Although the methods aren't perfect, they show that a concerted effort, built around a dedicated core of specialist-advocates, can do some great things.

Hospital-acquired infections are only one very specific quality and patient safety issue—there are dozens of others, as you've seen. Few institutions have teams in place to deal with these broader sets of problems. Creating that broad umbrella, we feel, is the logical place to start. Each hospital should have a Patient Safety Director—and preferably two: one a physician and one a nurse or pharmacist—with the clout, independence, and resources to measure errors, conduct routine audits of error-prone areas, coordinate detailed investigations, and follow them up by making sure solutions are implemented. Administratively, these people and their unit must be on par with—not under the thumb of—the other key hospital departments, and must be budgeted to be effective. Just as the work of infection control officers is facilitated by links to the CDC, which makes outbreaks in one area known to all the others, a similar national reporting system for medical errors, protected for confidentiality, would help local doctors determine their own "hot spots"—and do something about them—before a local problem becomes regional, or a regional problem, national.

Of course, all of this infrastructure will be worthless unless frontline caregivers in all specialties invest sufficient time, energy, and discipline to tackle the problems the core team identifies. This means the error abatement system, whatever form it eventually takes in any particular facility, must be "owned" by the people who use it. In aviation, certain safety experts specialize in "failure mode and effects analysis" (FMEA)—determining how things can go wrong and why, in a general sense—but they aren't experts in everything (aerodynamics, structures, engines, electrical systems, and so on). FMEA activity really takes place—and pays off—within various engineering specialties, where those general problem-solving methods are applied to specific pieces of equipment and circumstances. The same will be true in medicine.

One place to begin this interdisciplinary approach is through a standardized computerized physician order entry program that would be familiar to any doctor and any pharmacist in any hospital or clinic. Such a system would go a long way almost immediately toward reducing patient identification and medication errors. Remembering some of the CPOE debacles we chronicled earlier, the program needs to begin with research to determine the best ways to implement CPOE—and not just at a handful of major academic centers. Once the parameters for such a system are set, policymakers should aggressively prepare regulations, incentives, and funding to ensure that hospitals of all sizes obtain and use the information technology they need. Developing, installing, testing, and employing such systems—accompanied by robust clinical decision support programs—at every U.S. hospital should be achievable within ten years after political leaders give the go-ahead.

Some legislation already exists requiring hospitals to implement information technology, but these are generally unfunded or under-funded mandates. For example, California passed a law, SB 1875, that requires all nonrural hospitals to have computerized order entry by January 1, 2005, but no funding was provided. The federal Patient Safety Improvement Act of 2003, H.R. 877, was passed by the House of Representatives in March 2003, but is awaiting action in the Senate as this is written. This bill would provide $50 million in grants over two years for information technology implementation *nationally*. Note, however, that some large hospitals are already planning to spend this much *each* on IT, and there are *six thousand* acute care hospitals in the country. In other words, the proposed federal allocation is a rounding error compared with the scope of the task. Instead of medical errors, close your eyes and call our disease "terrorism," "blackouts," or even "cancer," and you'll get a sense of how inadequate the commitment has been—and continues to be.

Compare this to another unfunded state legislative mandate, a law that requires earthquake retrofits of all hospitals in California over the next twenty-five years. This mandate will cost California hospitals some $40 billion to meet. In the past *century*, fewer than 100 hospitalized patients have died in California earthquakes— including the Big Ones in 1906 and 1989—the same number that die of preventable errors in California hospitals *each week*. While we're the last people to advocate ignoring seismic safety in our notoriously shaky part of the world, how we ration scarce system dollars—to the benefit of the most patients—should always be first in mind. Wiring America's hospitals should be a national priority, and it will require more research, sensible regulations, and help for hospitals that simply don't have the money.

Money, org charts, and technology are only parts of the safety equation. Remember the old business adage that culture eats strategy for lunch—the creation of a safety culture will be perhaps the most vital step. Physicians should be out in front of this charge, but our independent streak represents an important obstacle. We are trained to believe that every patient and illness is unique and that our decisions must be tailored to their idiosyncrasies. We speak of the "art of medicine" the way other people talk about Van Gogh and Beethoven. Teamwork, checklists, standard operating procedures, systems thinking—none of it comes naturally to us. That kind of stuff may be OK for nurses, technicians, and clerks, but not for us. We're *doctors*.

If you detect a whiff of hubris, elitism, and wishful (if not magical) thinking in such attitudes, congratulations. You've just discovered why creating a culture of safety in a profession that considers itself a tad superhuman will be such a Herculean task.

But not impossible. Other occupations have suffered from the same malady and gotten over themselves. Recall the tales of the first astronauts, the push-the-envelope types like Chuck Yeager and his fellow fliers, chronicled so vividly by Tom Wolfe in *The Right Stuff*. Their brand of flying, which worshipped virtuosity and derring-do, saw pinheaded corporate rules as obstacles to be avoided as surely as mist-shrouded mountains. It was rollicking fun, macho, immensely satisfying (the tradition was "Flying & Drinking and Drinking & Driving")—and frequently fatal. The early test pilots had a mortality rate of one in four.

Ultimately, as aircraft—then spacecraft—became more complex and involved more people both in the air and on the ground, pilots had to learn to think as much like "systems managers" as goal-oriented, swashbuckling jet jockeys. Some of the pioneering astronauts fought this paradigm shift like wind shear. They were particularly incensed by NASA's tendency to regard the astronaut as "a redundant component" whose main function was to remain inert under stress. "An experienced zombie would do fine," wrote Wolfe of NASA's philosophy. "In fact, considerable attention had been given to a plan to anesthetize or tranquilize the astronauts, not to keep them from panicking but just to make sure they would lie there peacefully with their sensors on and not *do something* that would ruin the flight."

Over time, aviators of all stripes came to terms with the new reality. Their sense of dedication and professional pride remained intact, but came to be tempered by the absolute necessity of working within a system, whether that involved a cockpit team, a network of traffic controllers, or the sophisticated navigational aids and other high-tech equipment that got them safely back to base. And with this change in attitude, ultimately the Chuck Yeagers of the world were replaced by the John Glenns, the Sunday school-teaching, Eagle Scouting, family-man types.

Notwithstanding September 11 and the space shuttle crashes, both airplanes and spaceships have become manyfold safer over the last forty years. Although some of the advances relate to better equipment and training, much of the improvement can be traced to the increased use of protocols, algorithms, checklists—and teamwork. With the passing of the *Top Gun* era, flying has become more boring, but also one hell of a lot safer. It turns out that, in the end, neither passengers nor patients care very much about how much fun their doctors and pilots are having. They just want a safe journey.

Like those early pilots who failed to make the transition to the jet age, many physicians are dead set against giving up their "seat of the pants" autonomy to what they call "cookbook medicine." Some doctors continue to forswear standard procedures altogether, even when those procedures demonstrably cut risks and save lives. Too many of us, for example, still fail to order evidence-based therapies—those described in medical journals following extensive clinical trials—for common diseases, preferring instead to trust our own experience (which may be very atypical) and intuition (which may be hubris masquerading as good judgment). Some of us can't be bothered to wash our hands before examining patients.

When checklists are available for a surgical procedure, some physicians purposefully ignore them or follow them halfheartedly, assuming that *real* doctors don't need such memory aids, the way a proud octogenarian "forgets" to wear his hearing aid. Some of this resistance is practical. You can carry around only so many laminated cards for the hundreds of situations you might encounter—and until such information is made available in a more convenient format, such as on hand-held computerized devices, physicians are unlikely to embrace them.

Still, practice and principle *ought* to be the same thing. In a safety culture, they are. Tomorrow's physicians will be a lot more like today's airline captains than yesterday's *Right Stuff* heroes. Why? Not because they will be any less confident, skilled, or self-reliant, but because the tools available will not only support a more collegial and systematic approach—they will demand it.

Our biggest challenge, perhaps, in achieving a medical culture of safety is making our service still *feel* personal to the patient while meeting modern standards of evidence and delivering our care as an integrated team. As airline passengers, we *know* there are three or four people in the cockpit crew and maybe a half-dozen more in the cabin who are trained and knowledgeable about the "safety features" of our aircraft and well prepared to use them in an emergency. Still, we like to hear our captain's calm and reassuring voice, especially just after a patch of rough air, pointing out the beautiful rainbow out of the left side of the aircraft.

You can't manufacture and bottle safety, but you can make it a prized possession—a cultural value that nobody wants to lose. This is a generational change in medicine, and it has just started to emerge.

CHAPTER 21: A SYSTEM OF SAFETY

They say you can't do it, but sometimes it doesn't always work.

— Casey Stengel (1890–1975)

James Reason tells a moving story about a Soviet academician, Valeri Legasov, the lead investigator at the 1986 Chernobyl disaster, where an accident at a large nuclear power plant irradiated hundreds of square miles, including a nearby town built to house employees. In April 1988, two years to the day after the accident, Legasov hung himself from the second-floor balustrade of his dacha.

He left behind a recorded suicide note, which said, "After being at Chernobyl, I drew the unequivocal conclusion that the accident was... the summit of all the incorrect running of the economy which had been going on in our country for many years." Reason agreed with Legasov's diagnosis, but not his radical cure. "Our main interest," he wrote, "must be in the changeable and the controllable."

The one option we *don't* have in patient safety is to give up, to throw up our hands because our system is chronically underfunded or chaotically organized, as it is likely to remain for some time. Our job is to do the best we can with what we have. Even if we had all the money in the world, we can't fix everything at once, and it would be foolish to try.

So where do we start?

High-risk activities—places where we know errors are the most severe or occur most often—are the obvious places to begin. Banks, for example, know that a lot of misdated checks will appear spontaneously every January. They can't say for sure which customers will make the mistake of forgetting that it's a new year, or precisely how many will make it or how long they will persist—although records of previous years' performance will help with those estimates. But banks *do* know that a certain percentage of customers, within a certain period of time, will make this particular mistake—the banking equivalent of a medical slip: competent people making an error because of automatic behavior. When we know such automatic behaviors exist, and we know what situations trigger slips, our new, safety-oriented systems need to be there to help prevent the errors or—if they happen anyway—to minimize any resulting damage.

Medication and handoff errors, in both the hospital and outpatient settings, are two of our health care "Januarys." The kinds of errors that can occur and the situations that trigger them are so well known that doing something about them can put a few quick, confidence-building points on the patient safety scoreboard in a fairly short time. To prevent medication errors, the "cure" will undoubtedly involve some form of CPOE and bar-coding, since those technologies and prototype systems already exist and users know about them—although some rank-and-file resistance is inevitable, as there is with any change. The biggest barriers to implementation are finding the will and the means to pay for widespread implementation of effective systems, but these by themselves are not insurmountable.

Curing handoff errors will be harder. We've already seen how, in the Golden Age of the general practitioner—when there were far fewer procedures, drugs, specialists, and options—"Marcus Welby" did everything because there was so much less to do. Those days are gone forever and, despite their advantages in continuity of care, we're better off.

The unfortunate side effect of specialization, of course, is that patients are increasingly seen as collections of body parts and symptoms, not people. Once specialists have "done their thing," they move onto the next case and the patient—with other needs, other treatable conditions, other medications, and so on—sometimes gets lost in the shuffle.

In addition to devising and following strict protocols and checklists for transitions and using read-backs for critical oral exchanges, part of this boundary-spanning effort will be to have site-based generalists—such as hospitalists—in every caregiving institution. In addition to caring for individual patients, these physicians can improve the overall integration of care between inpatient departments, and between the hospital and outpatient settings. Intensivists serve a similar role in the ICU. On the outpatient side, a new type of generalist—one with the training and resources to truly coordinate ambulatory care without being forced into the demeaning and futile role of an HMO gatekeeper who blocks patients from seeing appropriate specialists—will be a critical component to improving safety. Right now, our corps of outpatient generalists—general internists, family physicians, and pediatricians—is frustrated and demoralized, mainly because their services are undervalued by both patients and payers. This situation will need to be fixed or we will see a whopping primary care shortage in coming years—and that will harm quality, access to care, *and* safety.

Finally, we need to get started on the hard work of creating computer links that allow information to flow seamlessly from sector to sector of the health care system. The massive blackout of August 2003 showed the nation the consequences of neglecting our electronic infrastructure, yet few notice when our medical blackouts and voltage drops kill people—and they do it every single day.

If the patient safety "epidemic" can be said to have begun with the IOM report in 1999, then where do we stand after the first five years of the epidemic? Let's consider this question by first looking back at the AIDS epidemic on *its* fifth birthday.

In 1986, five years after AIDS was first identified as a disease, the cause of the illness—HIV—had just been discovered, the first international conference on the disease was held, and the first research study on a potentially effective therapy, AZT, was published. Physicians and nurses were just starting to get a handle on how to manage real and suspected cases, and a skilled corps of dedicated researchers was beginning to form based on seed money trickling in from the government and private foundations.

To us, the fight against medical errors is at this same, tenuous crossroads. Practitioners are beginning to sense there is, and should be, something they can do about the problem. Leadership is sprouting among blunt-end managers and sharp-end caregivers, but there is still more resistance than collaboration among misguided, misinformed—and just plain scared—providers. Systems thinking is no longer a completely foreign concept in health care circles. Some federal funds have been allocated toward error reduction, and this sum has increased modestly every year. We've made a promising start. Here are a few examples:

During the 1990s, for example, the huge Veterans Affairs system, previously known mainly for its medieval facilities and stolid bureaucracy, made a tremendous investment in patient safety, spurred partly by public reaction to Ron Kovic's autobiography, *Born on the Fourth of July* (and the subsequent Oliver Stone film). Today, VA hospitals lead the nation in installing CPOE and bar-coding systems and implementing teamwork training. This is already paying dividends in improved quality and patient safety.

The field of anesthesiology has also made great strides in integrating technology, teamwork training, and simulators into day-to-day care. This is at least partly responsible for the free-fall in death rates of patients undergoing general anesthesia over the past century. In 1900, the risk of dying from general anesthesia while in surgery was one in 2,000. By 1950, this had improved to one in 3,300, and it plummeted by the end of the twentieth century to one in 200,000. These gains have been made possible not just by better anesthetics and improved monitoring systems and techniques, but by systems and training specifically designed to eliminate common errors.

At our own institution, UCSF Medical Center, we've seen an impressive change in culture and safety since the late 1990s, with better collaboration between nurses, doctors, pharmacists, and administrators; a well-functioning computerized incident reporting system; practical limits on trainee work hours (with corresponding efforts to minimize handoff errors caused by more frequent shift changes); thriving hospitalist and intensivist programs; and a new culture in which residents speak openly about their mistakes and help devise solutions to the problems that caused them. No one is talking about cure, but the progress is unmistakable.

Yet—even after societies and institutions agree that attacking an epidemic is a high priority—the risk of losing this focus is real. With AIDS, the waning sense of urgency has brought an unfortunate resurgence of dangerous behaviors in high-risk groups, and stagnant funding for research and treatment. This is troubling, but AIDS has not been allowed to fall off the public's radar screen: the many patient advocacy groups, disease-oriented lobbies, and self-perpetuating research and governmental organizations made sure of that. Even certain pharmaceutical companies and some medical specialties have a special stake in the disease—so they often use their own funds to promote "issue awareness" and participate in advocacy campaigns. A similar clamor is being raised about breast cancer, prostate cancer, colon cancer, Alzheimer's disease, and diabetes.

One advantage these other health-issue groups all have—and which the patient safety movement lacks—is an existing identity and cadre of activists upon which to build their programs. For AIDS, the core group was gay rights activists. For breast cancer, it was the feminist movement. For Alzheimer's, AARP and the "senior citizen" lobby, which had long championed such issues as Social Security and Medicare, were already in place.

Medical errors lack this element of group identity, but there is some hope. Other high-profile illnesses like heart disease, diabetes, and strokes also cut across social and cultural lines; but they are so widespread and cause so much death and suffering that they have managed to galvanize patients, providers, and politicians. Here, perhaps, is where the patient safety movement will find its warmest response. Whatever ails you, you will eventually come into contact with America's medical establishment—and *that's* where your risk of becoming an error victim begins.

The business case for individual hospitals and doctors is also wanting in patient safety. When the media picks up the scent, hospitals act—as they did after the Duke transplant mix-up. But there is as yet no "patient safety industry" to promote its wares by taking doctors on weekend seminars, nor to hand out glossy photos of "safety machines" for the hospital's next brochure. There is no foreign competition to jostle American hospitals out of their complacency and denial. Automobiles got safer in Detroit because foreign imports not only were better built and cheaper to own and operate, they began showing up with seat belts and roll bars. And, like airlines, hospitals seldom tout their safety records, even when they're excellent—in part because even a "safe hospital" will be home to many errors, and nothing makes a better lead for the six o'clock news than when an error at such an institution mocks its advertising campaign. And anyway, "What would they advertise?" asks health care journalist Michael Millenson. "Now killing fewer patients?"

Research in patient safety is also growing, but slowly. Talented researchers have begun to enter the pool, but they're paddling around at the shallow end. Top people don't get into career fields with hazy futures, and they avoid fields in which their discoveries—even when they are stupendously helpful—produce institutional yawns. And funding for patient safety research is limited and its future uncertain.

Federal and local hospital regulators are now much more safety conscious, but they are very sensitive to media and public pressure. Today, medical errors are on the tip of every regulator's tongue. But for how long? If we are lucky enough to go a year or two without any more Dukes, they're apt to drop the reins, lower the quirt, and we'll fall back into the pack—letting better organized health care "Seabiscuits" take the lead.

Need proof? Just remember all the cries of "never again" after the Challenger space shuttle explosion.

Taken together, we see that we've made a good start, but—despite the huge toll of medical mistakes on real people—safety is not very telegenic, and that fact alone puts it at high risk of being ignored once again. A healthy patient leaving a hospital on the mend after a successful procedure—with no side effects or complications—just isn't as exciting as a schoolgirl trapped in a well, or a desperately ill patient seeking a radical cure for a rare disease. We are basically asking policymakers and health care leaders to ante up for new systems and training that, quite literally, will result in a non-event: no accidents. Like Jerry's friend George on one famous *Seinfeld* episode, we are pitching a "show about nothing." He had no luck with network execs. Hopefully, we'll do better, for the sake of our patients.

If nothing else, all of these forces stacked against us will make our fight a long one. James Reason, again, perhaps says it best:

> Cognizant organizations understand the true nature of the "safety war." They see it for what it really is—a long guerilla struggle with no final conclusive victory. For them, a lengthy period without a bad accident does not signal the coming of peace. They see it, correctly, as a period of heightened danger and so reform and strengthen their defenses accordingly.... The conclusion of the safety war might be likened to the last helicopter out of Saigon rather than a decisive Yorktown, Waterloo, or Appomattox.... If eternal vigilance is the price of liberty, then chronic unease is the price of safety.

In more contemporary terms, the 2003 "victory" against SARS—the virulent respiratory disease that suddenly erupted out of Asia but was contained on every continent after a few harrowing months—is like the U.S. and British forces capturing Baghdad: quick, decisive, and thrilling. The patient safety "war" will be much more like the Iraqi aftermath: untidy and without obvious boundaries. We'll know *our* war is won when we no longer think of medical errors as an epidemic, but as a chronic condition we can manage. This will be an ephemeral moment, and you won't see it on CNN. We have no statue to topple.

CHAPTER 22: WHAT CAN PATIENTS DO?

Revolutions are the periods of history when individuals count most.

— Norman Mailer

If even doctor-patients and celebrities fall victim to medical errors—and if the solutions are largely to be found in refashioned systems of care—what can the layperson do?

The answer is that you can do more than you think, and in ways that might surprise you. Here are some things to think about:

The first rule is so obvious, it may be the last thing that would occur to you, but it's the cause of many serious medication problems. If you have a prescription, and you know it's for you and that the drug is the one your doctor intends, *take it*. You do yourself and the system no favors by intentionally or accidentally forgoing medication that can help you. Indeed, by not taking your pills (especially because you're afraid of a rare reaction or mistake), you just increase the chance you'll need more treatment later, and be subjected to more risks. So take your meds, but take them with your eyes open.

This is pretty straightforward stuff when the pills are coming from your own medicine cabinet, but a bit trickier in the hospital. There, although the prescription-writing and dispensing functions will take place outside your view, you *will* see the medication when it's brought to you. Before you take it, ask the nurse what it is and what it's for—even if you think you know. Back at home, make sure your meds are labeled clearly—don't put a new medication into an old container because it's easier to open or carry around. And don't mix medications by putting them all in one container (for ease, say, in travel) then try to sort them out when you take them. One reason for keeping your medications well marked and separate is so that if you *do* suffer a reaction, you or your partner or a relative (or even the paramedics) can quickly name and locate the offending drug. You'll also be able to ask your doctor or pharmacist any questions about the medication, its dosage, side effects, and risks—including possible drug interactions. As medications proliferate and our population gets older, this last one is becoming a more serious problem.

When you go to the doctor's office—particularly a specialist who is not your regular physician—or to the hospital, take a list of all of your current medications, including any over-the-counter medications (for allergies or pain relief, for example) and herbal remedies or dietary supplements that you use regularly.

During an office visit, most doctors hand you a written prescription when you leave. Check it before you walk out the door. You may not understand all the Latin, but letters are letters and if you can't make them out, the pharmacist might not be able to either. Be sure to read back the dosage as well as the name: Ones can look like sevens and eights can look like sixes. You have something of a backstop here, because the vast majority of drugs (especially initial prescriptions) are dispensed in a recommended clinical dose, and doses above that usually increase in some measured way—so a conscientious pharmacist is likely to question a "700" or "1,000" mg order when "100 mg" is the usual dose. But you don't need a safety net if you don't fall off the wire, so play it safe and confirm both the drug's name and dosage before you leave the office—and confirm it again when you pick up the prescription.

Fortunately for all of us, the U.S. Pharmacopeia has developed a list of abbreviations and shortcuts that are particularly likely to breed errors (Appendix II). For example, a patient who is supposed to receive 10 units of insulin should have the word "units" spelled out, since the shorthand "10U" has been mistaken for "100" on scores of occasions, sometimes fatally. In fact, be particularly alert if you are receiving *any* high-risk medication—like insulin, an oral diabetes drug, a blood thinner, chemotherapy treatment, or any of the notorious "sound alike" medications (Appendix III).

Handoff errors are likely to spawn more mistakes, and mistakes here can be even more serious. Although hospitals handle millions of transitions successfully each day, we consider them the soft underbelly of our current health care system. Here's what you can do:

First, introduce yourself (and reintroduce yourself) to anyone taking care of you during your hospital stay. This applies not just to doctors and nurses, but phlebotomists (the people who wake you up in the middle of the night to take your blood), orderlies, nurse's assistants, even meal deliverers—after all, you don't want that greasy Salisbury steak intended for the twenty-five-year-old appendectomy patient, six floors up, while he gets your "heart smart" salad and fruit cup. Orderlies and nurses' assistants often prep patients for procedures, too, such as shaving surgical sites. If you're not scheduled for an operation, don't let the process begin, even at this early, innocuous stage. Such mistakes sometimes trigger a cascade of further errors: The nurse from the cardiac cath lab comes to pick up the patient "who's just been shaved" and the floor nurse points to you!

And don't be cowed by the hospital's intimidating, class-oriented dress code. Just because you're in an ugly, backless hospital nightgown and the person addressing you is in a suit and tie or crisp white lab coat, your well-being is still the focus of his or her attention. Ask questions politely and persist until they're answered. If someone shows up with a gurney or wheelchair to take you to a procedure you don't know about, confirm it first with the floor nurse, the resident, or your doctor. If you are transported to a different location, ask the nurse if your chart will go with you and make sure your new caregivers are aware of your allergies, medications, and the condition for which you are being treated. Include with this your personal contact information, such as the names and telephone numbers of your spouse, adult children, or other responsible people: relatives, domestic partners, or neighbors. If you have an advance directive, like a DNR order, make sure you tell the nurse, the resident, and the attending physician.

While many people facing serious illness or major surgery feel unsociable or don't want to "impose" their problems on others, it helps to have visitors. This not only takes your mind off your illness, at least briefly, but it shows caregivers that other people are aware of your case, are interested in your well-being, and are going to check up on you. If you ever need one of these visitors to find out information or otherwise run interference on your behalf, they will at least be a familiar face to the hospital staff, who will therefore be a little more accommodating.

When you or a loved one are nearing discharge or transfer to a new facility (or to a different unit within the same hospital), recognize that you are approaching a danger zone. Like a raft entering white water, your risk will eventually pass, but while you're in transition, it helps to stay alert. Get a list of your current medications (they may be different in the hospital from your prescriptions at home) and make sure the caregivers at your new location know about them. If you are hooked to an IV line or urinary catheter, ask if it is supposed to be removed before transfer. Don't assume that any advance directive (a DNR or the name of your proxy decision-maker) will automatically make the transition with you. Keep a copy of the directive with your personal, bedside effects—magazines, book, hairbrush, or whatever. Oddly enough, these sundries are sometimes successfully transferred when your official documents are left behind, since they are often put in a bag and placed on your lap, or in your bed, during transportation. If you are already in a nursing home or other group care facility, do the same thing, since a sudden trip to the hospital is always possible. And if you're at home, keep a copy of any DNR order or advance directive on the refrigerator door (this is where most paramedics will look first; some states or communities have different protocols for storing important medical records—if so, follow these).

As of this writing, nearly all of these records are kept on paper, so between medications and directives and doctors' and relatives' names and numbers, you can accumulate quite a stack. Don't let that deter you from keeping the information available when and where you might need it. In the future, this information may be available through secure Internet connections, or on "smart cards" where your records (including EKG readings and X-ray or scanner images) can be stored digitally on a computer chip—but we're a few years away from that.

Finally, be an informed consumer. While most of us depend on referrals for physicians, specialists, surgeons, and hospitals—or these things are dictated to us by our doctors or medical insurance plans—you are not a prisoner of someone else's system. When possible or if you suspect a problem, ask about the methods your caregivers and institutions are using to prevent medical errors. For a hospital, start with the Web site (many have a "Frequently Asked Questions" (FAQ) area) or the Patient Relations or (if they have one) Quality departments. If you don't get answers, or the answers are unsatisfactory, bump up your inquiries to the Medical Director or CEO. While most busy staffers won't have time for an extended discussion of safety in general, they certainly should be able to answer—quickly and accurately—questions like these:

- Do you have a computerized physician order entry system? If not, when?
- Do you track patients and prescriptions using bar-coding?
- Do you have an incident reporting system? Is it computerized? How many reports do you process each month? What is done with the reports? How many Root Cause Analyses have you completed in the past year?
- Do you have a Patient Safety Officer? Does he or she get paid to do this job? If so, who is it and what are that person's qualifications?
- Does the ICU have a trained intensivist on duty?
- Do the medical wards have trained hospitalists who care for inpatients and help drive patient safety efforts?
- Are the physicians who will care for me board certified in their specialties?

- What is the patient-to-nurse ratio? (It should be no higher than 2:1 in the ICU, and about 6:1 on the regular ward)

- What percentage of the floor nurses are RNs (as opposed to lesser-trained nurses like LVNs)?

- Is a clinical pharmacist available on my floor to help me understand and organize my medications?

- Does the hospital run simulator or teamwork-training exercises?

- What procedures are used to prevent handoff errors (between shifts, during transport to procedures, during transport to other wards, during discharge)?

- What patient safety initiatives have you started in the past year? How many have you completed in the last three years? Which ones are you proudest of?

At the back of this book (Appendix IV), you'll find an expanded list of questions to ask your caregivers in specific areas, including advice on how to interpret the answers. Above all, remember that *you are the reason the hospital exists*. Your well-being is, and should be, everyone's highest concern.

CLOSING THOUGHTS

In the face of the hellish errors we've introduced you to, it may seem Pollyanna-ish to end by looking at the bright side, but we will. As we walk down the corridors of our own hospital, we see patients being readied for discharge from the regular wards who, only a decade ago, would have required the services of the ICU. And twenty years ago, they would have been dead. If you thumb quickly through the procedures we've discussed in this book—cardiac electrophysiology, embolization of cerebral aneurysms, treatment for severe sepsis, heart-lung transplants—you'll be struck, as we were, by how many of them were simply impossible when we were children, and unfathomable a generation before. Modern medicine has a dark side only because its light side shines so brightly. The more we do, the more we *can* do—so our doctor's bag gets bigger and deeper and more full of wonder drugs and wondrous machines. We can only lament at how the human beings who use them must struggle to keep up, and avoid pulling out the wrong pill.

When the first steam locomotive was invented in the early nineteenth century, scientists believed that if it ever got above 35 mph, the human body wouldn't withstand it. Thank goodness we didn't stop fiddling with transportation devices after the first train wreck or airplane crash. The art and science of medicine are no different. We do what we do because it gives the vast majority of us a better life—and in many cases, a longer life as well.

Like death and taxes, errors will always be with us; they are the shadow cast by every human being who stands up and takes a risk. But at the high noon of our endeavors—when our achievements are at their zenith—that shadow should be very small. We're not there yet, but we can be—and that's something that should give us comfort.

Ultimately, understanding medical mistakes means we must understand human nature. The error-free doctor will come along as soon as we have the error-free pilot, astronaut, schoolteacher, electrician, lawyer, and football player. Of course, accepting human frailty can be frustrating—especially when the error happens to, or is caused by, us.

But together, we can assemble a system that is stronger and more reliable than the sum of its parts: not perfect, but much better. It will be a system in which books like this will be a charming relic of the "days of the giants"—an era of rugged individualists, of gunslinging malpractice lawyers, and of Doctor Deities who look much better receding in the rearview mirror than approaching us in the headlights.

So we feel confident ending this book on an optimistic note. Physicians realize (even if not all of them are ready to admit it) that they are not captains of a ship, but quarterbacks of a team. The media knows that while sensationalism sells, even newspaper reporters and TV correspondents (and malpractice attorneys) get sick—and nobody wants to be tomorrow's headline. Policymakers never have enough money for all of the important things they want to do, but they always have money to fix mistakes after they happen. Let's put those resources to better use. As Albert Einstein said, "Insanity is doing the same thing over and over again and expecting a different result."

In the coming decade, we will attack our epidemic of medical mistakes with better systems, more training, and more resources. We will succeed not because we think our system and our practitioners are perfect, but because we know they're fallible. We will exchange knowledge about our mistakes not in courtrooms, but in classrooms—including that great virtual classroom called the Internet. We will find ways to compensate every victim of a significant medical injury without turning the health care system into a giant game of Lotto. We will develop machines, programs, and procedures that do not replace people, but give them a longer reach and surer touch. As healers and as patients we will all be more compassionate with—and more understanding of—each other. We are all in this together.

AFTERWORD

Now this is not the end. It is not even the beginning of the end. But it is, perhaps, the end of the beginning.

— Winston Churchill (1874-1965)

Of all the cases in *Internal Bleeding*, perhaps the one that resonated most deeply with readers was the one in Chapter 12, in which a young doctor confidently — but mistakenly — terminates a patient's resuscitation when he discovers a "DNR" (do not resuscitate) order on the patient's chart. Only after the patient dies do the nurses realize that the brash but well-intended doctor pulled the wrong chart from the rack, and that the decision to call off the Code Blue was a tragic mistake.

After *Internal Bleeding* was published, clinicians and hospital leaders from all over the world told us that all of our cases, no matter how improbable or outlandish, were far from unique. ("How did you know we had *that?*" several told us in e-mails or after lectures. "Were you hiding under a rock at our hospital?") Such is the nature of medical errors: because so much stands in the way of sharing our experiences and insights, nobody knows that their mistakes are the products of universally-broken systems rather than singular acts of boneheadedness.

And that's how we learned that our "Wrong DNR" case was not the only one in which confusion about a patient's resuscitation status led to a death. You'll be glad to know that many hospitals, once they recognized the frequency of this particular blunder, were prompted to assess whether they could fall prey to it — and those that kept their DNR orders in patients' charts stacked in the nurses' station quickly recognized that they could. How could this particular system be made foolproof?

You may remember that, in the hospital where the "Wrong DNR" case occurred, the idea of marking the patient's DNR status on his or her hospital wristband was rejected by the nurses, who worried that DNR wristbands would stigmatize patients. But if the wristband was simply color-coded to indicate the DNR status, patients or visitors wouldn't be the wiser and tragic errors might be averted. Yes, that was the answer!

But once it became a candidate for color-coding, the wristband – previously a bland white totem of hospital bureaucracy adorned only with the patient's name and hospital number – now became fair game for identifying all sorts of safety threats. If we're going to use one color for DNR, people thought, why not other colors to give the docs and nurses a heads-up about other risks: perhaps blue for the demented patient who might fall out of bed, pink for the stroke patient unable to speak and swallow, green for the patient on powerful blood thinners?

Before long, some patients' wrists began to resemble Benetton ads. And you will not be surprised to learn that no two hospitals used the same colors, so doctors and nurses had no easy way to remember what any particular color stood for. More chaos.

The final straw came when some hospitals settled on yellow wristbands for their "Do Not Resuscitate" patients. In 2004, the Lance Armstrong-inspired "LiveStrong" yellow wristband became a mega-trend, with 30 million sold in 60 countries, including to U.S. presidential candidates George W. Bush and John Kerry and nearly every celebrity appearing on *Entertainment Tonight*. Oops. "Before you wear your cool yellow LiveStrong wristband at the hospital," warned the *St. Petersburg Times*, "think twice." One Florida hospital administrator, whose facility asked patients to either remove the yellow bracelets or cover them with white tape, lamented, "It could be confusing, particularly in the situation of a code or a cardiac arrest where people have to think very quickly. We wouldn't want to mistake a Lance Armstrong bracelet [for a DNR order] and not resuscitate someone we're supposed to." Luckily, as of this writing, no one has died from this particular goof.

Yet.

*   *   *

November 29, 2004 marked the fifth anniversary of the famous report *(To Err is Human)* by the Institute of Medicine, the one from which the "jumbo jets crashing" analogy was drawn (Chapter 3). We recently asked a group of 400 practicing "hospitalists" (physicians who focus on caring for hospitalized patients and therefore must cope with the anarchy of modern hospitals every day) whether they believed that safety had improved, stayed the same, or worsened since 1999. The results were instructive and somewhat reassuring: 45 percent said safety had improved, 38 percent saw no difference, and 17 percent regarded it as worse. They were more hopeful about the future: two-thirds thought care would be even safer five years from now.

Patients are less convinced. In a recent survey, more than one-third of patients reported that they or a close family member had been the victim of a medical error. Forty percent thought the quality of U.S. health care had worsened in the past five years, while only 17 percent thought it was better.

Part of the problem is that we have no way of being sure who's right. The studies that gave rise to the 44,000-98,000 deaths per year estimates were conducted in 1984 and 1992; they were sufficiently expensive and time-consuming that they are unlikely to be repeated. So the sobering fact is that we really don't know whether we're still killing the equivalent of a jumbo jet full of people each day. Perhaps we're down to a 727. Or maybe even a commuter plane.

On this one, we tend to side with the glass-is-half-full types. We believe that health care has become a bit safer over the past five years, and the enthusiastic reception this book received – from doctors, nurses, and hospital boards and administrators – further convinced us that there are a lot of good people out there trying to make a difference. To give you a better sense of the progress that we *have* made, but also to indicate the areas in which we still have a long way to go, let's examine (and grade our efforts in) five major areas: regulation, error reporting systems, information technology, the malpractice system and other vehicles for accountability, and workforce and training issues.

REGULATION. *Grade: A-minus*

In the last few years, hospitals have managed to implement a number of simple procedural improvements, like "read-backs" of important verbal communications, "Sign Your Site," and the team huddle ("time out") before the start of the surgery. We can thank regulators, particularly the Joint Commission on Accreditation of Healthcare Organizations (JCAHO), for the rapid adoption of these safeguards.

Why has regulation been so crucial? Just recall what happened when some well-meaning orthopedic surgeons started signing their surgical sites with an "X" – some doctors signing the leg to be operated on, and others signing the one to leave alone – before JCAHO forced everybody to use one, and only one, procedure. Sort of reminds you of colored wristbands, doesn't it?

JCAHO has also helped matters by revamping its accreditation methods. In the old days, the inspectors came and hospitals exhumed a huge stack of dusty policy manuals, few of which had any bearing on what really happened on the wards. Now, JCAHO inspectors follow the course of patients – from the ER to the ward, to the ICU and then to radiology – to see how care is actually delivered. It's not perfect, but it's much better. And beginning this year – God bless their cold regulatory hearts – the inspectors will start making unannounced visits, hopefully prompting hospitals to be on good behavior all the time, rather than on perfect behavior for one week every 3 years, after which the kids go back to throwing chalk and erasers for the next thousand days.

Regulation has been particularly important in overcoming the dominant tradition of physician autonomy – the "Chuck Yeager Syndrome" we described in Chapter 20 – and its resultant tendency to customize nearly everything. A commercial airline pilot we know recently spent a day in the operating rooms of one of America's most renowned hospitals. We asked him for his impressions. "I had two main ones," he said. "First, the people are marvelously trained, highly committed, and the technology is simply fantastic. But when I asked a nurse something simple, like 'how do you set up the operating room for a hip replacement,' or 'how do you get informed consent from a patient before the surgery,' I always heard the same answer. 'For Dr. Smith, we do it *this* way, and for Dr. Jones we do it *that* way.' I was stunned, because it would be like me walking into a cockpit of a 767 and expecting things to be set up my own special way. That would be unthinkable – it would be too unsafe."

But as important as regulation has been in jump-starting our fledgling safety efforts, it has its limits. You can't use regulation to develop a culture of safety, or control whether doctors and nurses respect each other, or influence how a busy ER physician decides whether a patient's vague left arm pain might be a heart attack. Moreover, the history of regulation is beset with examples of overreaching and unintended consequences, both of which can ultimately hamper flexibility and innovation. Accordingly, we think that much of the low-hanging fruit will be picked soon and that other ways of promoting patient safety will become increasingly important.

ERROR REPORTING SYSTEMS. *Grade: C*

A recent article in *The New York Times* bemoaned the fact that many New York hospitals were not reporting all of their errors to the state, despite the fact that the law insists that they do so. Nowhere in this article was there any discussion about what was being done with all the reports that *were* submitted. As we've already seen, this is the Achilles heel of error reporting systems: the flawed notion that reporting has any intrinsic value, in and of itself. The problem is not limited to government reporting systems, but is also seen within hospitals, where a growing database of incident reports is often taken as proof that safety is improving (because it is seen as evidence of a healthy "reporting culture"), although there is no persuasive evidence that supports this association.

Error reporting systems *can* be powerful tools when the reports are used to improve systems or educate providers. After all, the book you're holding is, in essence, the product of an error reporting "system" — namely, cases that came to our attention, which we've tried to turn into learning tools. Contrast this with the state health department that proudly touts its "100,000 error reports" as evidence that it is protecting patients from medical mistakes. With few exceptions, it isn't.

As Dr. Don Berwick, president of the Institute for Healthcare Improvement, has said, "I'm distressed at the amount of attention that [reporting] is getting... You can't improve safety without transparency. That's absolutely clear. But a reporting system is just a small step toward progress." Ultimately, we need new ways of thinking about error reporting and to apply far more resources than we currently do toward turning such reports into action if we are going to prevent reporting from being a vast and expensive waste of time and good will.

INFORMATION TECHNOLOGY. *Grade: B-minus*

As you've seen from our earlier discussion (Chapter 4), we believe that information technology (IT) will play an important role in reducing many kinds of medical mistakes, but that it, like error reporting, has been oversold as *the* solution. Remember that most of the studies demonstrating the value of computerized physician order entry or electronic medical records have come from a few institutions with decades of commitment to IT and robust, homegrown systems. Your local community hospital that enters the 21st century by plunking down $10 million to buy an off-the-shelf computer system often comes to a sobering realization after the shrink wrap is removed: most of these systems are clunky at best and useless at worst. Why? Well, until recently so few hospitals were buying clinical computer systems that IT companies operating in the health care "space" were being perfectly rational when they focused their R&D efforts on finding better ways to generate bills, not to prevent medical mistakes.

Thankfully, this is beginning to change. After decades of wondering when local hospitals would become as wired as local supermarkets, health care computerization is finally getting some traction. The systems are improving, and many hospitals are beginning to see good results, particularly in decreasing medication errors. But the dark side remains (though few like to talk about it, for the same reason that you never told anyone that you never quite figured out how to program your VCR. Maybe the TiVo will be easier...). You'll remember some of the "train wrecks" that we described earlier, including those at Cedars-Sinai Medical Center in Los Angeles (where the plug was pulled on a relatively user-unfriendly homegrown system after a physician rebellion) and Boston's Beth Israel-Deaconess Hospital (where one researcher's data caused a massive system to crash for several days, leading to the memorable *Boston Globe* headline, "Got Paper?"). More worrisome are reports of multiple errors actually *introduced* by IT systems themselves, including one patient whose heart attack may have been caused by easy access to an outdated computerized medication list, and another who was listed by the computer as having been moved from one hospital room to another before he was actually moved, leading to a near-disastrous drug error.

Notwithstanding these cautionary notes, the experience of the Veterans' Administration (who could have dreamed a decade ago that the VA – yes, *that* VA – would be the nation's patient safety leader? It just shows what a real system and a little leadership can do) and other IT pioneers demonstrates that clinical systems can be made to work, and that doctors and nurses can be taught to use (and like) them if they are well-built and implemented.

Most importantly, in 2004 health care IT finally penetrated the Washington Beltway, beginning with President Bush's mention of it in his January 2004 State of the Union speech ("By computerizing health records, we can avoid dangerous medical mistakes, reduce costs, and improve care."). A few months later, the president appointed Dr. David Brailer as the nation's IT Czar (more formally, the "National Health Information Technology Coordinator"). Brailer – a physician, PhD health economist, and entrepreneur whose baby face belies his brilliance and street-smarts – seems the ideal person for the job, which is why it was doubly disappointing that in November 2004 Congress denied his office the $50 million in start-up funding it had been promised. Although Brailer gamely termed this a "bad bounce," it is clear that the federal goal of computerizing most American hospitals in the next decade cannot be met without stronger and more consistent federal support.

The reason this support is so important is that the business case to invest in computers – particularly at your doctor's office, where a complete transformation from paper to computer records would cost $50,000-$100,000 (purchase, installation, archiving old records, and lost productivity) – is still insufficient to make it happen by itself. With some thoughtful investments, adoption of universal computer standards so that information can be moved seamlessly around the system, and a bit of public pressure, we believe that most of U.S. health care can be computerized within a decade. That would be a very good thing.

Interestingly, although doctors – worried that computers would slow them down or lock them into practicing "cookbook medicine" – have traditionally stood in the way of computerizing hospitals, their attitudes may be changing. Many young (and even some not-so-young) physicians find it increasingly bizarre to come home and check their e-mail over a wireless network, make a plane reservation on Orbitz, and "IM" with their child at Penn, but drive each morning to their time-capsule of a hospital, where they scratch out their orders and notes with pen and parchment. It is when they raise their voices and demand computers with the same vigor that they demand a choice spot in the doctor's parking lot and a new MRI scanner that health care IT will really take flight.

THE MALPRACTICE SYSTEM AND OTHER VEHICLES FOR ACCOUNTABILITY.

Grade: D-plus

As we discussed in Chapter 16, the malpractice system – while horribly broken and fundamentally unfair – is not the main culprit when it comes to medical mistakes, although many physician advocacy groups would have you believe otherwise. Moreover, the political mud wrestling over tort reform has centered on caps on pain-and-suffering awards, which, whatever their merits, would not fundamentally alter the dynamics of the malpractice system in terms of patient safety. The reforms that *might* actually make a difference in safety – the switch to a no-fault system for compensating victims of medical errors and the change to an "enterprise liability" model (in which malpractice lawsuits would be directed at organizations such as hospitals rather than providers) – were never seriously discussed in last year's presidential contest, even in the no-stone-unturned blogosphere.

In contrast to malpractice, we believe that the lack of account-ability for poor performance *does* harm patient safety. In fact, of all the wonderful feedback we received about *Internal Bleeding*, the issue of how we dealt with bad apples was the one in which the critiques were the most pointed, and perhaps correct. We remain steadfast in our belief that our traditional "blame and shame" approach will not mend our broken system, but we have to acknowledge that there is some incompetence – or worse – out there and it must be dealt with more effectively.

In visiting hospitals across North America to talk about the book, we met hundreds of incredibly committed, competent, and passionate doctors and nurses. But we also heard painful stories – from hospital administrators, patients, and clinicians themselves – about doctors or nurses who simply should not be working, and of a system that lacked the capacity to do anything about it. Many lawyers, of course, claim that our dysfunctional malpractice system must be preserved since the health care system is so inept in weeding out unsafe providers. But those same lawyers, or their colleagues, eagerly race to sue a doctor or hospital that tries to take away a dangerous physician's license to kill. We can't have it both ways.

Of all the stories we heard about problem clinicians, perhaps the most flabbergasting was about "Code Orange," the method by which some hospitals deal with a physician having a raging temper tantrum. What happens when a nurse calls a Code Orange? Every available nurse comes running and simply surrounds the doctor and stares at him, like the final scene in the movie *Witness*, in which all the unarmed Amish villagers encircle the armed villain and save Harrison Ford and his Amish hosts from a bloody death. That a Code Orange might ever be necessary in a place of healing is astonishing.

Unfortunately, our tools to ensure accountability have, if anything, become more limited in the past year. Medical staff peer review committees, which were designed to allow physician peers to evaluate their colleagues' competence and recommend disciplinary action (including loss of licensure) for truly incompetent physicians – never particularly effective – are now under even greater threat. As part of new "patient safety" legislation, the Florida electorate passed a law in November 2004 that stripped the presumption of confidentiality from the peer review process. If this half-baked measure holds up, the chance that any group of physicians will willingly take on one of its colleagues, even a dangerous one, will fall from slim to none.

WORKFORCE AND TRAINING ISSUES. *Grade: B*

Here, we're doing a bit better, mainly through our deeper understanding of the importance of manpower and training in patient safety, and a few examples of action.

The dominant workforce issue has been the national nursing shortage, particularly in acute care environments, and the increasingly persuasive research demonstrating that patients die when there are too few nurses, nurses' hours are too long, or nurses are under-trained. Partly driven by these data points, California has mandated minimum nurse-to-patient ratios, and other states may follow suit. The jury is still out on whether these mandated ratios improve safety – while having more nurses seems like a good thing, some hospitals have been forced to close whole wards because they are unable to meet the ratios, and others have fired key ancillary personnel (like physical therapists and patient transporters) in order to free up dollars to meet the ratios. As of this writing, the state is in the process of relaxing the ratio requirements slightly, although this change is being contested by the California Nurses Association.

Physician training has also been rocked by the safety movement. In 2003, the Accreditation Council for Graduate Medical Education (ACGME), the group that blesses the nation's residency programs, began enforcing limits on residents' duty hours (maximums of 80 hours per week or 30 hours per shift). Although one recent study found that ICU residents working shorter shifts committed fewer errors (and, as a nice two-fer, they were less apt to fall asleep at the wheel on their drive home), it is worth noting that this study took place at a hospital with an unusually strong group of residents and a state-of-the-art IT system. Whether the study's results play out at the 99 percent of other teaching hospitals that lack both of these attributes will be interesting to watch. We continue to believe that resident work-hour regulations probably harm safety in the short-term by increasing the number of handoffs, but will ultimately improve safety because better rested residents will be less prone to slips and because hospitals are now, finally, putting their weight behind systems to improve the reliability of handoffs.

These work-hour regulations are only the start of a new emphasis on trainees as key players in safety programs, not only in terms of working conditions, but also in terms of how they are trained and tested. This increased emphasis on competency assessment is likely to extend beyond the formal training period; more and more specialty medical boards are requiring periodic recertification, though the requirements for physicians remain far less stringent than those imposed on pilots.

As we described in the book, another aspect of medical education that has been neglected is teamwork and simulation training, and these strategies are receiving much more attention. The best known model is one drawn from aviation ("Crew Resource Management"), in which participants are trained to tamp down hierarchies, use checklists and other redundancies, and communicate clearly, particularly in crises. Emerging research supports the premise that such training (sometimes using simulators), if thoughtfully adapted to clinical situations, can improve both performance and safety.

Unfortunately, there is a huge gap between the promise of teamwork and simulator training and their actual use. Despite the fact that patient outcomes are increasingly determined by how well teams function under pressure (for example, how quickly a patient with a stroke is given a powerful blood thinner or a patient with a heart attack has a cardiac catheterization and placement of a stent), no teamwork training is yet required of providers, and few medical and nursing schools include it in their curricula. Simulator training, because it is more expensive and complex to deliver, is even less well developed: even institutions known as "simulator centers" generally use the machines to train medical students or discrete specialists such as anesthesiologists, not all their rank-and-file clinicians.

In the end, all of the regulations, computers, and reporting in the world won't allow us to claw our way out of the patient safety mess if we don't change the way doctors and nurses are trained and how they relate to each other and to their patients. As more studies demonstrate the best models for teamwork training and simulation and prove that such training does change clinical practices and culture, we simply must push to make this training a standard part of education and practice. There is no shortcut to culture change.

*   *   *

The past five years have demonstrated that patient safety resonates deeply with the public, that attacking medical mistakes effectively takes new mental models, research, technologies, and training, and that investments in safety can save lives. At this point, we give the American health care system's efforts an overall grade of C-plus, with striking areas of progress tempered by clear opportunities for improvement. That's better than the D-minus we began with in 1999, but you can be sure that both of us would have stern chats with our children if they brought home report cards with C-plusses. Our guess is that you would too.

The problem continues to be one of focus and priority. The federal commitment remains insufficient and tentative. After the IOM Report, the Agency for Healthcare Research and Quality (AHRQ), the federal agency charged with improving safety, was given $50 million to begin a patient safety research enterprise. A few years later, this program was abruptly cut back just as it was bearing fruit, replaced mostly with a set of projects narrowly focused on computerization. Similarly, few hospitals have made major investments in safety (such as for paid safety officers, or in teamwork or simulator training), particularly outside of IT. It is difficult to "blame" hospitals for this: most lack the funds that would allow them to make such investments without harming other important clinical initiatives or their ongoing revenue streams. Yet these examples demonstrate that the business case for patient safety, though more compelling than it was before 1999, remains inadequate to the size of the task. In fact, the most important question going forward is this: what is the right mix of financial, educational, research, regulatory, organizational, and cultural activities and forces to catalyze the far-greater investment (in money, time, and attention) that will be needed to make health care significantly safer?

From the mundane — what color should the wristband be? — to the almost overwhelming — how to change several generations of ingrained culture in doctors and nurses, or how to computerize one-seventh of the American economy — plenty of work remains to be done. Five years after *To Err is Human*, we have reached the end of the beginning. Our patients clearly do not think that we are finished.

Nor do we.

BIBLIOGRAPHY

Books on Medical Errors and Errors More Generally

1. Berwick, D.M. *Escape Fire: Designs for the Future of Health Care*. San Francisco: Jossey Bass, 2003.

2. Bogner, M.S.E. *Human Error in Medicine*. Mahwah, N.J.: Lawrence Erlbaum Associates, 1994.

3. Bosk, C.L. *Forgive and Remember: Managing Medical Failure*. Chicago: University of Chicago Press, 1979.

4. Casey, S.M. *Set Phasers on Stun: And Other True Tales of Design, Technology, and Human Error*. Santa Barbara: Aegean Publishing Company, 1993.

5. Columbia Accident Investigation Board. *Report of the Columbia Accident Investigation Board*, August 2003.

6. Cook, R.I., Woods, D.D., Miller, C. *A Tale of Two Stories: Contrasting Views of Patient Safety*. National Patient Safety Foundation at the AMA: Annenberg Center for Health Sciences, 1998.

7. Gawande, A. *Complications: A Surgeon's Notes on an Imperfect Science*. New York: Metropolitan Books, 2002.

8. Gibson, R., Singh, J.P. *Wall of Silence: The Untold Story of the Medical Mistakes that Kill and Injure Millions of Americans*. Washington, D.C.: Lifeline, 2003.

9. Helmreich, R.L., Merritt, A.C. *Culture at Work in Aviation and Medicine: National, Organizational, and Professional Influences*. Aldershot, Hampshire, U.K.: Ashgate, 1998.

10. Kahneman, D., Slovic, P., Tversky, A. *Judgment Under Uncertainty: Heuristics and Biases*. Cambridge: Cambridge University Press, 1987.

11. Merry, A., Smith, A.M. *Errors, Medicine, and the Law*. Cambridge: Cambridge University Press, 2001.

12. Millenson, M.L. *Demanding Medical Excellence. Doctors and Accountability in the Information Age*. Chicago: University of Chicago Press, 1997.

13. National Quality Forum. *Safe Practices for Better Healthcare. A Consensus Report*. Washington, D.C.: National Quality Forum, 2003.

14. Paget, M.A. *Unity of Mistakes: A Phenomenological Interpretation of Medical Work*. Philadelphia: Temple University Press, 1993.

15. Paget, M.A. *Reflections on Cancer and an Abbreviated Life*. Edited by Marjorie L. DeVault. Philadelphia: Temple University Press, 1993.

16. Perrow, C. *Normal Accidents: Living with High-Risk Technologies. With a New Afterword and a Postscript on the Y2K Problem*. Princeton, N.J.: Princeton University Press, 1999.

17. Reason, J.T. *Human Error*. New York: Cambridge University Press, 1990.

18. Reason, J.T. *Managing the Risks of Organizational Accidents*. Aldershot, Hampshire, U.K.: Ashgate, 1997.

19. Robins, N.S. *The Girl who Died Twice: Every Patient's Nightmare: the Libby Zion Case and the Hidden Hazards of Hospitals*. New York: Delacorte Press, 1995.

20. Rosenthal, M.M., Sutcliffe, K.M., eds. *Medical Error. What Do We Know? What Do We Do?* San Francisco: John Wiley & Sons, 2002.

21. Sagan, S.D. *The Limits of Safety: Organizations, Accidents and Nuclear Weapons*. Princeton, N.J.: Princeton University Press, 1993.

22. Sharpe, V.A., Faden, A.I. *Medical Harm: Historical, Conceptual, and Ethical Dimensions of Iatrogenic Illness*. New York: Cambridge University Press, 1998.

23. Shojania, K.G., Duncan, B.W., McDonald, K.M., Wachter, R.M., eds. *Making Health Care Safer: A Critical Analysis of Patient Safety Practices*. Evidence Report/ Technology Assessment No. 43 from the Agency for Healthcare Research and Quality: AHRQ Publication No. 01-E058; 2001. Available at http://www.ahrq.gov/ clinic/ptsafety/.

24. Spath, P.L. *Error Reduction in Health Care: A Systems Approach to Improving Patient Safety*. San Francisco, Chicago: Jossey-Bass Publishers and AHA Press, 1999.

25. Stewart, J.B. *Blind Eye: How the Medical Establishment Let a Doctor Get Away with Murder*. New York: Simon & Schuster, 1999.

26. Tenner, E. *Why Things Bite Back: Technology and the Revenge of Unintended Consequences*. New York: A. A. Knopf, 1996.

27. Vaughan, D. *The Challenger Launch Decision: Risky Technology, Culture, and Deviance at NASA*. Chicago: University of Chicago Press, 1997.

28. Wiener, E.L., Kanki, B.G., Helmreich, R.L. *Cockpit Resource Management*. San Diego: Academic Press, 1993.

The Institute of Medicine (IOM) Reports on Medical Errors and Healthcare Quality

1. Kohn, L., Corrigan, J., Donaldson, M. *To Err Is Human: Building a Safer Health System*. Washington, D.C.: Committee on Quality of Health Care in America, Institute of Medicine. National Academy Press, 2000. ["The IOM Report"]

2. Committee on Quality of Health Care in America, IOM. *Crossing the Quality Chasm: A New Health System for the 21st Century*. Washington, D.C.: National Academy Press, 2001.

3. Aspden, P., Corrigan, J.M., Wolcott, J., Erickson, S.M. *Patient Safety: Achieving a New Standard for Care*. Washington, D.C.: National Academy Press, 2004.

Journal Articles on Medical Errors

1. Altman, D.E., Clancy, C., Blendon, R.J., "Improving patient safety – five years after the IOM report," *NEJM* 351 (2004), pp. 2041–3.

2. Ash, J.S., Berg, M., Coiera, E., "Some unintended consequences of information technology in health care: the nature of patient care information system-related errors," *Journal of the American Medical Informatics Association* 11 (2004), pp. 104–12.

3. Baker, G.R., Norton, P.G., Flintoft, V., et al., "The Canadian Adverse Events Study: the incidence of adverse events among hospital patients in Canada," *Canadian Medical Association Journal* 170 (2004), pp. 1678–86.

4. Barenfanger, J., Sautter, R.L., Lang, D.L., et al., "Improving patient safety by repeating (read-back) telephone reports of critical information," *American Journal of Clinical Pathology* 121 (2004), pp. 801–3.

5. Barger, L.K., Cade, B.E., Ayas, N.T., et al., "Extended work shifts and the risk of motor vehicle crashes among interns," *NEJM* 352 (2005), pp. 125–34.

6. Bates, D.W., Gawande, A. "Improving safety with information technology," *NEJM* 348 (2003), pp. 2526–34.

7. Berwick, D.M. "Disseminating innovations in health care," *JAMA* 289 (2003), pp. 1969–75.

8. Berwick, D.M., "Errors today and errors tomorrow," *NEJM* 348 (2003), pp. 2570–2.

9. Blendon, R.J., DesRoches, C.M., Brodie, M., et al. "Views of practicing physicians and the public on medical errors," *NEJM* 347 (2002), pp. 1933–40.

10. Brennan, T.A., Leape, L.L., Laird, N.M., et al. "Incidence of adverse events and negligence in hospitalized patients. Results of the Harvard Medical Practice Study I," *NEJM* 324 (1991), pp. 370–76.

11. Brennan, T.A. "The Institute of Medicine report on medical errors—could it do harm?" *NEJM* 342 (2000), pp. 1123–25.

12. Chassin, M.R., Galvin, R.W. "The urgent need to improve health care quality. Institute of Medicine National Roundtable on Health Care Quality," *JAMA* 280 (1998), pp. 1000–05.

13. Chassin, M.R. "Is health care ready for Six Sigma quality?" *Milbank Quarterly* 76 (1998), pp. 565–91, 510.

14. Cook, R.I., Render, M., Woods, D.D. "Gaps in the continuity of care and progress on patient safety," *BMJ* 320 (2000), pp. 791–94.

15. Frankel A, Graydon-Baker, E., Neppl, C., et al., "Patient Safety Leadership WalkRounds," *Joint Commission Journal of Quality and Safety* 29 (2003), pp. 16–26.

16. Forster A.J., Murff, H.J., Peterson, J.F., Gandhi, T.K., Bates, D.W., "The incidence and severity of adverse events affecting patients after discharge from the hospital," *Ann Intern Med* 138 (2003), pp. 161–7.

17. Forster, A.J., Asmis, T.R., Clark, H.D., et al., "Ottawa Hospital Patient Safety Study: incidence and timing of adverse events in patients admitted to a Canadian teaching hospital," *Canadian Medical Association Journal* 170 (2004), pp. 1235–40.

18. Gaba, D.M. "Structural and organizational issues in patient safety: a comparison of health care to other high-hazard industries," *California Management Review* 43 (2000), pp. 1–20.

19. Gaba, D.M., Howard, S.K. "Fatigue among clinicians and the safety of patients," *NEJM* 347 (2002), pp. 1249–55.

20. Gallagher, T.H., Waterman, A.D., Ebers, A.G., et al. "Patients' and physicians' attitudes regarding the disclosure of medical errors," *JAMA* 289 (2003), pp. 1001–07.

21. Gandhi, T.K., Weingart, S.N., Borus, J., et al., "Adverse drug events in ambulatory care," *NEJM* 348 (2003), pp. 1556–64.

22. Gawande, A.A., Studdert, D.M., Orav, E.J., Brennan, T.A., Zinner, M.J., "Risk factors for retained instruments and sponges after surgery," *NEJM* 348 (2003), pp. 614–21.

23. Kuperman, G.J., Gibson, R.F. "Computer physician order entry: benefits, costs, and issues," *Ann Intern Med* 139 (2003), pp. 31–39.

24. Landrigan, C.P., Rothschild, J.M., Cronin, J.W., et al., "Effect of reducing interns' work hours on serious medical errors in intensive care units," *NEJM* 351 (2004), pp. 1838–48.

25. Leape, L.L., Brennan, T.A., Laird, N., et al. "The nature of adverse events in hospitalized patients. Results of the Harvard Medical Practice Study II," *NEJM* 324 (1991), pp. 377–84.

26. Leape, L.L. "Error in medicine," *JAMA* 272 (1994), pp. 1851–57.

27. Leape, L.L, "Reporting of adverse events," *NEJM* 347 (2002), pp. 1633–8.

28. Leape, L.L., Berwick, D.M., Bates, D.W. "What practices will most improve safety? Evidence-based medicine meets patient safety," *JAMA* 288 (2002), pp. 501–07.

29. Localio, A.R., Lawthers, A.G., Brennan, T.A., et al. "Relation between malpractice claims and adverse events due to negligence. Results of the Harvard Medical Practice Study III," *NEJM* 325 (1991), pp. 245–51.

30. Marshall, M.N., Shekelle, P.G., Leatherman, S., Brook, R.H. "The public release of performance data: what do we expect to gain? A review of the evidence," *JAMA* 283 (2000), pp. 1866–74.

31. Mazor, K.M., Simon, S.R., Gurwitz, J.H., "Communicating with patients about medical errors: a review of the literature," *Arch Intern Med* 164 (2004), pp. 1690–97.

32. Millenson, M.L. "Pushing the profession: how the news media turned patient safety into a priority," *Quality and Safety in Health Care* 11 (2002), pp. 57–63.

33. Pierluissi, E., Fischer, M.A., Campbell, A.R., Landefeld, C.S., "Discussion of medical errors in morbidity and mortality conferences," *JAMA* 290 (2003), pp. 2838–42.

34. Poon, E.G., Blumenthal, D., Jaggi, T., et al., "Overcoming barriers to adopting and implementing computerized physician order entry systems in U.S. hospitals," *Health Affairs (Millwood)* 23 (2004), pp. 184–90.

35. Pronovost, P.J., Weast, B., Holzmueller, C.G., et al., "Evaluation of the culture of safety: survey of clinicians and managers in an academic medical center," *Quality and Safety in Health Care* 12 (2003), pp. 405–10.

36. Pronovost, P., Berenholtz, S., Dorman, T., et al., "Improving communication in the ICU using daily goals," *Journal of Critical Care* 18 (2003), pp. 71–5.

37. Pronovost, P.J., Weast, B., Bishop, K., et al., "Senior executive adopt-a-work unit: a model for safety improvement," *Joint Commission Journal of Quality and Safety* 30 (2004), pp. 59–68.

38. Pronovost, P.J., Nolan, T., Zeger, S., Miller, M, Rubin, H., "How can clinicians measure safety and quality in acute care?" *Lancet* 363 (2004), pp. 1061–7.

39. Samore, M.H., Evans, R.S., Lassen, A., et al. Surveillance of medical device-related hazards and adverse events in hospitalized patients. *JAMA* 291 (2004), pp. 325–34.

40. Schuster, M.A., McGlynn, E.A., Brook, R.H. "How good is the quality of health care in the United States?" *Milbank Quarterly* 76 (1998), pp. 517–63, 509.

41. Shojania, K.G., Wald, H., Gross, R. "Understanding medical error and improving patient safety in the inpatient setting," *Medical Clinics of North America* 86 (2002), pp. 847–67.

42. Shojania, K.G., Duncan, B.W., McDonald, K.M., Wachter, R.M. "Safe but sound: patient safety meets evidence-based medicine," *JAMA* 288 (2002), pp. 508–13.

43. Studdert, D.M., Thomas, E.J., Burstin, H.R., et al. "Negligent care and malpractice claiming behavior in Utah and Colorado," *Medical Care* 38 (2000), pp. 250–60.

44. Studdert, D.M., Brennan, T.A. "No-fault compensation for medical injuries: the prospect for error prevention," *JAMA* 286 (2001), pp. 217–23.

45. Thomas, E.J., Studdert, D.M., Burstin, H.R., et al. "Incidence and types of adverse events and negligent care in Utah and Colorado," *Medical Care* 38 (2000), pp. 261–71.

46. Thomas, E.J., Brennan, T.A. "Incidence and types of preventable adverse events in elderly patients: population based review of medical records," *BMJ* 320 (2000), pp. 741–44.

47. Vincent, C. "Understanding and responding to adverse events," *NEJM* 348 (2003), pp. 1051–56.

48. Wachter, R.M., "The end of the beginning: Patient safety five years after 'To Err is Human'," *Health Affairs (Millwood)* 2004 Nov 30; [Epub ahead of print].

49. Wachter, R.M., Shojania, K.G., "The faces of errors: a case-based approach to educating providers, policymakers, and the public about patient safety," *Joint Commission Journal of Quality and Safety* 30 (2004), pp. 665–70.

50. Weingart, S.N., Wilson, R.M., Gibberd, R.W., Harrison, B. "Epidemiology of medical error," *BMJ* 320 (2000), pp. 774–77.

51. Wu, A.W., Folkman, S., McPhee, S.J., Lo, B. "Do house officers learn from their mistakes?" *JAMA* 265 (1991), pp. 2089–94.

52. Zhan, C., Miller, M.R., "Excess length of stay, charges, and mortality attributable to medical injuries during hospitalization," *JAMA* 290 (2003), pp. 1868–74.

Quality Grand Rounds series, Annals of Internal Medicine
[Editors, Robert M. Wachter, Kaveh G. Shojania]

1. Wachter, R.M., Shojania, K.G., Saint, S., et al. "Learning from our mistakes: Quality Grand Rounds, a new case-based series on medical errors and patient safety," *Ann Intern Med* 136 (2002), pp. 850–52.

2. Chassin, M.R., Becher, E.C. "The wrong patient," *Ann Intern Med* 136 (2002), pp. 826–33.

3. Bates, D.W. "Unexpected hypoglycemia in a critically ill patient," *Ann Intern Med* 137 (2002), pp. 110–16.

4. Hofer, T.P., Hayward, R.A. "Are bad outcomes from questionable clinical decisions preventable medical errors? A case of cascade iatrogenesis," *Ann Intern Med* 137 (2002), pp. 327–33.

5. Gerberding, J.L. "Hospital-onset infections: a patient safety issue," *Ann Intern Med* 137 (2002), pp. 665–70.

6. Cleary, P.D. "A hospitalization from hell: a patient's perspective on quality," *Ann Intern Med* 138 (2003), pp. 33–39.

7. Lynn, J., Goldstein, N.E. "Advance care planning for fatal chronic illness: avoiding commonplace errors and unwarranted suffering," *Ann Intern Med* 138 (2003), pp. 812-18.

8. Brennan, T.A., Mellow, M.M. "Patient safety and medical malpractice: A case study," *Ann Intern Med* 139 (2003), pp. 267–73.

9. Goldman, L, Kirtane, A. "Triage of patients with acute chest pain and possible cardiac ischemia: the elusive search for diagnostic perfection," *Ann Intern Med* 139 (2003), pp. 987–95.

10. Pronovost, P.J., Wu, A.W., Sexton, J.B., "Acute decompensation after removing a central line: practical approaches to increasing safety in the intensive care unit," *Ann Intern Med* 140 (2004), pp. 1025–33.

11. Redelmeier, D.A., "The cognitive psychology of missed diagnoses," *Ann Intern Med* 142: (2005), pp. 115-20.

12. Gandhi, T.K., "Fumbled hand-offs: one dropped ball after another," *Ann Intern Med* 142 (2005), pp. 352–58.

Websites on Medical Errors

Agency for Healthcare Research and Quality (AHRQ): Medical Errors & Patient Safety: http://ahrq.gov/qual/errorsix.htm

AHRQ WebM&M: Morbidity and Mortality Rounds on the Web. Available at: http://www.webmm.ahrq.gov/ [Editors: Robert M. Wachter, Kaveh G. Shojania]

AHRQ Patient Safety Network (PSNet). Available at: http://www.psnet.ahrq.gov [Editors: Robert M. Wachter, Kaveh G. Shojania]

British Medical Journal Theme Issue on Medical Error: 18 Mar 2000 (Volume 320, Issue 7237). Available at: http://bmj.com/content/vol320/issue7237/

Effective Clinical Practice Theme issue on Medical Error: November/December 2000 http://www.acponline.org/journals/ecp/pastiss/nd00.htm

FDA Patient Safety News. Available at: http://www.fda.gov/cdrh/psn

Institute for Safe Medication Practices: http://www.ismp.org/

Leapfrog Group for Patient Safety: http://www.leapfroggroup.org/

National Patient Safety Foundation: http://www.npsf.org/

Profiles in Patient Safety: case-based series of articles appearing in *Academic Emergency Medicine.* Available at: http://www.aemj.org/cgi/content/full/9/4/324

APPENDIX I

List of the Seventeen Individual Errors in the Wrong Patient Case (Chapter 1)

1. An unidentified person on the telemetry floor misdirected RN$_1$ by saying "patient Morrison" was not on the floor (when she was) and by saying that she had been transferred to oncology (6:15 A.M.).

2. An unidentified person on the oncology floor misdirected RN$_1$ by saying the patient she sought (Ms. Morrison) was on the floor when she was not (6:20 A.M.).

3. An unidentified person on the oncology floor told RN$_2$ to bring her patient (Ms. Morris, the wrong patient) to the electrophysiology laboratory (6:30 A.M.).

4. RN$_2$ took her patient to the electrophysiology laboratory despite (a) the patient's objections, (b) the lack of a consent form and order in the chart, and (c) lack of knowledge on her own part or that of her charge nurse that the procedure was planned (6:45 A.M.).

5. RN$_1$ failed to verify the patient's identity against the electrophysiology laboratory schedule when the patient arrived in the electrophysiology laboratory (6:45 A.M.).

6. RN$_1$ failed to recognize the significance of Ms. Morris's objections to undergoing the procedure (6:45 A.M.).

7. The electrophysiology attending physician failed to verify Ms. Morris's identity when he spoke with her by telephone, and he failed to understand the basis of her objections to the procedure (6:45 A.M.).

8. RN$_1$ failed to appreciate the significance of the lack of an executed consent form in the chart, especially given that the electrophysiology schedule stated that the correct patient (Ms. Morrison) had signed the form (6:45 to 7:00 A.M.).

9. The electrophysiology fellow failed to verify the patient's identity, failed to recognize the significance of the lack of pertinent clinical information in her chart, and failed to obtain consent that was informed (7:00 to 7:15 A.M.).

10. The electrophysiology charge nurse failed to verify the patient's identity (7:10 A.M.).

11. RN$_3$ failed to verify the patient's identity (7:15 to 7:30 A.M.).

12. The neurosurgery resident did not persist in obtaining a satisfactory answer to his question as to why his patient was undergoing a procedure about which he had not been informed (7:30 A.M.).

13. RN$_4$ failed to verify the patient's identity (8:00 A.M.).

14. The electrophysiology attending physician failed a second time to verify the patient's identity when he did not introduce himself to Ms. Morris at the beginning of the procedure (8:00 A.M.).

15. The electrophysiology fellow disregarded the fresh groin wound from Ms. Morris's cerebral angiogram the day before and started the electrophysiology procedure on the opposite side (8:00 A.M.).

16. A telemetry nurse (RN$_5$) and two electrophysiology nurses (RN$_3$ and RN$_4$) failed to verify the identities of the patients they discussed on the telephone (8:30 to 8:45 A.M.).

17. The electrophysiology charge nurse failed to persist in obtaining a satisfactory answer to her question of why no patient with the name Joan Morris appeared on the electrophysiology schedule (8:30 to 8:45 A.M.).

From Chassin, M.R., Becher, E.C. "The wrong patient," *Ann Intern Med* 136 (2002), pp. 826–33. Reproduced with permission. Not all of these mistakes are described in the text of this book.

APPENDIX II

Dangerous Abbreviations Used in Prescribing

ABBREVIATION	INTENDED MEANING*	COMMON ERROR
U	Units	Mistaken for a zero (0) or a four (4), resulting in overdose. Also mistaken for "cc" (cubic centimeters) when poorly written.
μg	Micrograms	Mistaken for "mg" (milligrams), resulting in overdose.
Q.D.	Latin abbreviation for every day	The period after the "Q" has sometimes been mistaken for an "I", and the drug has been given "QID" (four times daily) rather than daily.
Q.O.D.	Latin abbreviation for every other day	Misinterpreted as "QD" (daily) or "QID" (four times daily) rather than every other day (if the "O" is poorly written, it looks like a period or "I").
SC or SQ	Subcutaneous	Mistaken for "SL" (sublingual–given under the tongue, rather than injected under the skin, subcutaneous) when poorly written.
TIW	Three times a week	Misinterpreted as "three times a day" or "twice a week."
D/C	Discharge; also discontinue	Patients' medications have been prematurely discontinued when D/C (intended to mean "discharge") was misinterpreted as "discontinue" because it was followed by a list of drugs.
HS	Half strength	Misinterpreted as the Latin abbreviation "HS" (hour of sleep), resulting in the full strength of the drug being given at bedtime.
cc	Cubic centimeters	Mistaken as "U" (units) when poorly written.

ABBREVIATION	INTENDED MEANING*	COMMON ERROR
AU; AS; AD	Latin abbreviation for both ears; left ear; right ear	Misinterpreted as the Latin abbreviation "OU" (both eyes); "OS" (left eye); "OD" (right eye).

*In general, these errors can be prevented by spelling out the full word (e.g., "units," "micrograms") instead of using the abbreviation, or through the use of computerized physician order entry (CPOE). Adapted with permission of the National Coordinating Council for Medication Error Reporting and Prevention. © 1998-2003.

APPENDIX III

Examples of Easily Confused Sound-alike or Look-alike Drugs

Generic Drug Names*	Brand Names*
acetohexamide/ acetazolamide	Adderall/Inderal
amiodarone/amrinone § **	Alupent/Atrovent §
bupropion/ buspirone	Ambien/Amen
chlorpromazine/ chlorpropamide	Asacol/Os-Cal
clomiphene/clomipramine	Cardizem/Cardiem
cyclosporine/ cycloserine	Celebrex/Celexa/Cerebyx
daunorubicin/doxorubicin §	Dynacin/DynaCirc
dimenhydrinate/ diphenhydramine	Flomax/Fosamax; Flomax/ Volmax
dobutamine/dopamine §	Indinavir/Denavir
glipizide/glyburide §	Lamictal/Lomotil/Lamisil
hydralazine/hydroxyzine	Lanoxin/Lonox
methylprednisolone/ methyltestosterone	Levbid/Lopid/Lithobid
nicardipine/nifedipine §	Levoxyl/Luvox
prednisone/prednisolone §	Lovenox/Lotronex
sulfadiazine/sulfisoxazole §	Nizoral/Nasarel/Neoral
tolazamide/tolbutamide §	Remeron/Zemuron
vinblastine/vincristine §	Vioxx/Zyvox
	Zyrtec/Zyprexa

§ Drugs that not only have similar names but similar actions or usages (e.g., *glipizide* and *glyburide* are both used to treat diabetes).

* In 2001, the FDA began requiring pharmaceutical companies to use "tall man" lettering to help differentiate some of these sound-alike/look-alike medications (e.g., *ClomiPHENE* and *ClomiPRAMINE*; *ZyRTEC* and *ZyPREXA*).

** In 2000, the name *amrinone* was changed to *inamrinone* (eye-nam-ri-none) to prevent confusion.

Adapted from Cohen, M. Zyrtec-Zyprexa mix-up. *AHRQ WebM&M*, April 2003. Available at http://webmm.ahrq.gov/cases.aspx?ic=10 (last accessed March 2, 2005). Reprinted with permission.

APPENDIX IV

Questions You May Want to Ask Your Hospital, Medical Group, or Doctor, Along with Some Comments by the Authors*

Things You Can Do as an Outpatient

What to Do/Check	*Discussion/Recommendations*
Is your doctor board-certified in his/her specialty?	All else being equal, board certification indicates that your physician has demonstrated a certain level of competence.
Has your state licensing board issued any findings of misconduct against your doctor?	Most licensing boards require a high level of proof and relatively egregious infractions before sanctioning a licensed physician. Most infractions revolve around personal behavior (drug use, inappropriate sexual conduct); fewer involve quality of care concerns. The National Practitioner Data Bank, which lists malpractice judgments, is not accessible to individuals (and, as described in the book, is a highly imperfect indicator of quality or safety).
Label your medications clearly and keep them in their original bottles. Bring your medications with you to your doctor visits. Don't take a medication you can't identify— ask the doctor or pharmacist first. Be certain that the doctor's office has a correct list of your drug allergies.	These are just common sense.
Read your prescription before you leave the office to be sure you understand it and it is legible.	Be on the lookout for high-risk drug abbreviations (Appendix II). Be particularly alert if you are on high-risk medications like insulin, an oral diabetes drug, a blood thinner, chemotherapy, or a medication that has a sound-alike alternative (Appendix III).

Things to Check on If You're Having Surgery or Another Procedure

What to Do/Check	Discussion/Recommendations
If you're having a surgery on a symmetrical body part (like an arm, leg, or eye), check to find out what the hospital or clinic does to prevent wrong-sided surgery.	Hospitals and surgery centers should have "sign the site" programs, and should employ "time-outs" prior to the incision, during which the team huddles to agree on the intended surgical procedure and site.
Ask whether you should receive any treatments to prevent infections, blood clots, or heart problems.	Evidence-based strategies to prevent these complications are among the patient safety practices with the best supporting evidence. These practices include: • Appropriate use of prophylactic antibiotics to prevent surgical infections • Appropriate use of a blood thinner, mechanical leg compression, or early ambulation to prevent blood clots; and • Appropriate use of a medication called a beta blocker to prevent postoperative heart attacks.
How many of my surgery/procedures have been done in the past year, both by the individual surgeon/proceduralist and by the institution?	In general, more is better. The Leapfrog Group's website lists some volume thresholds in procedures for which evidence supports a volume-quality relationship (http://www.leapfroggroup.org/consumer_intro2.htm).

Things to Do to Prevent Errors in a Hospital or Nursing Home

What to Do/Check	Discussion/Recommendations
Before you are given a medication, ask what it is and what it's for.	
Before you get a medication, a transfusion, an X-ray, or a procedure, make sure the nurse confirms your name both by asking you and checking your wristband.	A few hospitals may supplement this through the use of bar-coding; for example, checking both your wristband and the bar code on a medication bottle.

What to Do/Check	*Discussion/Recommendations*
Make friends with your nurses, phlebotomists, and other hospital personnel. Make sure they address you by name.	
Before being taken off the floor for a procedure, ask what it is and be sure you understand where you are going and why.	
Be sure your family members' contact information is available to the hospital or nursing home personnel.	It is not a bad idea to have a card with your family members' contact information by your bedside, as well as in the chart.
Before being transferred floor-to-floor in a hospital, or from one institution to another, check to be sure all catheters and other paraphernalia that should be removed have been.	In one study, one out of three physicians were unaware whether their patient had a urinary catheter. These catheters are sometimes necessary, but pose a risk for infection. Remind your doctors and nurses that your catheter is still in and ask whether it needs to be.
If you have an Advance Directive (and you should), keep a copy with you, make sure your family has one, give one to your nurse or doctor to place on your chart, and be certain it is transferred from site to site.	

Being an Informed Consumer: Patient Safety Questions for the Hospital's Patient Relations or Quality Departments

What to Do/Check	*Discussion/Recommendations*
Does the hospital have computerized physician order entry (CPOE) and bar-coding? If not, when do they plan to have them?	It would be great if they had them and they were up and running. If they say they have a CPOE system, ask what percent of MD orders are written on the system (if it is less than half, then the docs are still kicking the tires and the system is not really implemented). If CPOE and bar-coding are not in place, and are not budgeted to be in place within 3–5 years, worry.

What to Do/Check	*Discussion/Recommendations*
Is there a functioning, preferably computerized, incident reporting system?	The computerized systems make reporting, and dissemination of the information, much easier. So it would be good to hear, "yes we do."
How many incident reports are logged each month?	Although it might seem counterintuitive, the more the better: If a midsized (200–300 beds) facility doesn't receive at least 50–75 reports a month, then the hospital lacks a reporting culture—workers aren't sharing errors and near-misses, either because they worry about blame or are convinced it won't do any good.
What is done with these incident reports?	You'd like to know that they go to the relevant managers in the area (the catheterization lab, the OR), who are expected to respond to them. Also, there should be an über-manager who watches for trends (an uptick in patient falls, bed ulcers, or medication errors, for example).
How many detailed root cause analyses have been done in the past year?	Like the incident reports, you might think that "zero" would be a great answer since it would mean there were no major errors. But trust us, there were. So we'd expect that the average 200–300 bed hospital will have done 5–8 full-blown RCAs in the past year.
Is there a Patient Safety Officer who is compensated for this role? What are his or her qualifications?	Many hospitals will not have a paid Patient Safety Officer yet, but all midsized and large hospitals should in the next 3–5 years. This guarantees that it is someone's job to be concerned about safety. It should be a respected physician, nurse, or pharmacist with some additional training in human factors, systems engineering, quality improvement and similar areas.
Is there an active Patient Safety Committee that meets at least monthly?	The answer must be yes.

What to Do/Check	Discussion/Recommendations
Are there trained intensivists in the critical care units (ICUs) and hospitalists on the medical wards?	There is strong evidence that the on-site presence of intensivists, at least during the day, is associated with better ICU outcomes. For small hospitals without intensivists, linking the ICU electronically to trained intensivists who remotely monitor the patients may be the next best thing. The evidence supporting the value of hospitalists caring for general medical and surgical patients is not quite as strong, but two studies did show lower death rates. We believe that the on-site presence of physicians who specialize in overseeing and coordinating patients' hospital care is almost certain to improve safety.
Are the physicians who will care for you board-certified in their specialty?	See earlier answer.
What is the patient-to-nurse ratio, and what percentage of the nurses are registered nurses (RNs)? Also, what fraction of the RNs hold bachelor's degrees?	Ratios of more than 6:1 or 7:1 on the medical and surgical wards are associated with a higher risk of errors, as is more than 25–30 percent of care being delivered by non-RNs (i.e., licensed practical nurses or nurses' aides). In the ICU, all the nurses should be RNs, and the ratio should be no more than 2 patients for every nurse. Finally, a recent study found that hospitals with higher proportions of RNs with bachelor's degrees had lower postoperative mortality rates. On this score, aim for 50 percent or more.
Are there clinical pharmacists on the hospital wards who can help you understand and organize your medications?	There is good evidence that the involvement of clinical pharmacists, particularly in the discharge process, improves safety.

What to Do/Check	Discussion/Recommendations
Does the hospital run simulator or other specific teamwork training?	Ideally, the hospital would require simulator training for people working in high-risk areas like the OR, ER, and on Code Blue teams. In addition, specific teamwork training (Crew Resource Management) may be helpful. Few hospitals do this yet, but more will over time, particularly if the evidence of the benefit of this kind of training accumulates in health care settings.
What does the hospital do to prevent handoff errors?	We would want to know, at the very least, that verbal orders are read back and checklists are completed before patients move from one unit to another (like from the ICU to the floor, or from the floor to a nursing home).
What patient safety initiatives has the hospital undertaken in the past year?	They should have at least one or two that they can describe proudly, preferably with results they can tell you about.

* Appendices II, III, and IV are reproduced at www.ruggedland.com/ InternalBleeding, and can be printed from that site.

ENDNOTES

Abbreviations used in Endnotes and Bibliography:

Am J Med = *American Journal of Medicine*
Ann Intern Med = *Annals of Internal Medicine*
Arch Intern Med = *Archives of Internal Medicine*
BMJ = *British Medical Journal*
JAMA = *Journal of the American Medical Association*
JGIM = *Journal of General Internal Medicine*
LAT = *Los Angeles Times*
NEJM = *New England Journal of Medicine*
NYT = *New York Times*
WSJ = *Wall Street Journal*
WP = *Washington Post*

A NEW EPIDEMIC

20   heart attack was Kaveh Shojania: Unlike many instances of medical mistakes, these two stories had happy endings—but only after a big dose of "pain and suffering" for both the patients and doctors involved. Carlos survived his overdose and Bob his nail-biting ambulance ride. He never took ambulance priority codes for granted again. The young programmer recovered too. He did, in fact, sue Kaveh, the supervising physician, and the hospital—an action that was settled, as many such cases are, without a trial. During this time, Kaveh seriously considered quitting medicine, but was talked out of it by numerous colleagues who assured him that his diagnosis in this very unusual case had been reasonable (it turned out that the patient had a history of a very high cholesterol, but had avoided treatment and missed many scheduled doctor's appointments). However, this brush with fate served mainly to motivate Kaveh to learn more about the nature of medical mistakes, with it ultimately ending up as his professional focus.

21   "postmortems of medical errors...": Weick, K. "Reduction of medical errors through mindful interdependence," in Rosenthal, M.M. and Sutcliffe, K.M., eds., *Medical Error: What Do We Know? What Do We Do?* (San Francisco: Jossey-Bass, 2002), p. 187.

23   are drawn from published accounts: Cases drawn from published reports (in which real names and locations are used) are the Ramon Vasquez prescription mix-up (Chapter 4), the Betsy Lehman chemotherapy error (Chapter 4), Willie King's wrong leg amputation (Chapter 7), Dr. Arbit's two wrong-sided brain operations (Chapter 7), the Canadian woman with the retained surgical retractor (Chapter 8), and the Jesica Santillan transplant mix-up at Duke (Chapter 14). All other cases are original—these cases use pseudonyms and other changes in details that don't alter the fundamental medical error issues. Of these, several (the wrong patient (Chapter 1), the insulin-heparin switch (Chapter 5), the failure to transfer the advance directive from the nursing home to the hospital (Chapter 10), and the intubation judgment call that resulted in a malpractice suit (Chapter 16)) have been previously presented in our Quality Grand Rounds series in the *Annals of Internal Medicine*. The case of the patient who

misunderstood the discussion about resuscitation (Chapter 13) was presented in our patient safety journal, *AHRQ WebM&M*. The remaining cases have not been previously published.

23   are privileged to edit: *Quality Grand Rounds* (sponsored by the California HealthCare Foundation and published in the *Annals of Internal Medicine)* and *AHRQ WebM&M* (a web-based medical errors journal, modeled on traditional Morbidity and Mortality conferences; it is sponsored by the federal Agency for Healthcare Research and Quality and freely available at http://webmm.ahrq.gov).

CHAPTER 1: THE WRONG PATIENT

31   to meet the bottom line: The jam-packed hospital is a relatively new phenomenon. Many hospitals had lots of unfilled beds in the '70s and '80s, a by-product of that era's cushy health care marketplace. A half-empty hospital is a monument to inefficiency, but no one cared very much as long as hospitals and doctors simply sent in their bills, and insurance companies (or the government) coughed up the dough. But by the late 1980s, with health care experiencing tremendous inflation, fears surged that the costs of care would bankrupt our country, just as military costs did the Soviet Union. The market became the method: Hospitals belt-tightened first by cutting costs, then by merging and finally, reluctantly, by closing if they couldn't stay afloat. Throw in the aging of the population and you see why patients today often have to wait in the ER overnight before their bed upstairs opens, and why there was so much post-9/11 angst about whether hospitals could handle busloads of bioterror victims. (They can't, by the way; see Inglesby, T.V., Grossman, R., O'Toole, T. "A plague on your city: Observations from TOPOFF,"*Clinical Infectious Diseases* 32 (2001), pp. 436–45).

An important milestone was when the Big Three automakers discovered they were spending more on their employees' health care (and that of their dependents) than on steel (while trying to compete with Japan on price and quality, even though Japan's health care costs were half those in the U.S.). The result was the growth in managed care, the withering of the capacity of American hospitals, and the marked decline in reimbursements to hospitals and doctors. Since hospitals (like airliners) have crippling fixed costs (there needs to be an operating room, a cafeteria, and an accounting department whether the hospital is half-full or full), the only way to survive economically is to run packed.

Although we do believe that the packed hospital and the resulting emphasis on throughput is an important cause of errors, it is worth noting that one of the seminal and shocking studies of deaths due to medical error was conducted in 1984, before the dramatic, market-driven changes of the late '80s and early '90s. Other early studies had found similarly high rates of mistakes even in the "good old days" of leisurely hospital stays.

32   to allow it to be otherwise: Because of these regulations and San Francisco's propensity for fog, the FAA nixes parallel landings at San Francisco International Airport (SFO) about 30 percent of the time, which immediately halves the landing capacity of the airport and makes SFO one of the major bottlenecks in the U.S. air transit system.

33   but you'd be wrong: But perhaps not for long. An experimental system at the Massachusetts General Hospital is using GPS technology to track patients and providers.

Fitzgerald, T. J. "Cart 54, where are you? The tracking system knows," *NYT* 30 Oct 2003, p. G7.

33   (like Pena and Pineda): Astonished by the frequency of these accidents-waiting-to-happen, we went on to review the hospital's medical service over a three-month period and discovered that at least one pair of patients with the same last name was admitted on nearly one-third of the days.

41   listed in Appendix I): Chassin, M.R., Becher, E.C. "The wrong patient," *Ann Intern Med* 136 (2002), pp. 826–33.

CHAPTER 2: IT'S THE SYSTEM, STUPID

43   everywhere but medicine: Reason, J. *Human Error* (Cambridge: Cambridge University Press, 1990).

44   speed above everything else: Schlosser, E. *Fast Food Nation: The Dark Side of the All-American Meal* (Boston: Houghton Mifflin, 2001).

44   "Human fallibility...": Reason, J. *Managing the Risks of Organizational Accidents* (Brookfield, Vt.: Ashgate, 1997), p. 25.

45   at an earlier step: Reason, *Managing the Risks*, p. 9.

46   how the message is interpreted: Xiao showed that skilled and well-practiced trauma teams communicate actively, often by using nonverbal cues. Xiao, Y., Mackenzie, C.F., Patey, R., et al. "Team coordination and breakdowns in a real-life stressful environment," *Proceedings of the Human Factors and Ergonomics Society (HFES) 42nd Annual Meeting* 42 (1998), pp. 186–190. See also Birdwhistell, R.L. *Kinesics and Context: Essays on Body Motion Communication* (Philadelphia: University of Pennsylvannia Press, 1970); and Mehrabian, A. *Silent Messages: Implicit Communication of Emotion and Attitudes* (Belmont, Calif.: Wadsworth Publishing Co., 1971).

46   "We suspect that these physicians": Chassin, "The wrong patient."

46   "why did they do what they did?": The "first story/second story" model was described by medical researchers Richard Cook and David Woods; it aims to counter investigators' tendencies to adopt the "first story" of malfeasance at the sharp end of a process or procedure. See Cook, R.I, Woods, D.D., Miller, C. *A Tale of Two Stories: Contrasting Views of Patient Safety* (Chicago: National Patient Safety Foundation at the AMA: Annenberg Center for the Health Sciences; 1998). An even more robust model for applying standard procedures when investigating errors was proposed by Yale organizational theorist Charles Perrow. Perrow favors using the acronym DEPOSE (Design, Equipment, Procedures, Operations, Supplies and materials, and Environment). According to Perrow, a structured accident investigation—whether of a medical error, a nuclear power plant accident, or a crash of a space shuttle—ought to look for contributing factors in each of these categories before conveniently concluding that a particular warning system misfired, a particular protocol was flawed, or an individual operator

was incompetent. See Perrow, C. *Normal Accidents: Living with High-Risk Technologies. With a New Afterword and a Postscript on the Y2K Problem* (Princeton, N.J.: Princeton University Press, 1999). A popular alternative framework for accident investigations, particularly in health care settings, was developed by English psychologist Charles Vincent. It is described in Vincent, C., Taylor-Adams, S., Stanhope, N. "A framework for the analysis of risk and safety in medicine," *BMJ* 316 (1998), pp. 1154–57, and summarized in Vincent, C. "Understanding and responding to adverse events," *NEJM* 348 (2003) pp. 1051–56. The elements of the Vincent framework are: Institutional, Organization and Management, Work Environment, Team, Individual Staff Member, Task, and Patient.

47 goal of national safety: *Joint Inquiry into Intelligence Community Activities Before and After the Terrorist Attacks of September 11, 2001.* (Washington, D.C.: Government Printing Office, 2003).

48 contributed to the accident: Vaughan, D. *The Challenger Launch Decision: Risky Technology, Culture, and Deviance at NASA.* (Chicago: University of Chicago Press, 1996).

49 "We'll blow another one...": ibid., p. 421–22.

50 "that were in effect...": *Report of the Columbia Accident Investigation Board*, Aug 2003, pp. 101, 197.

50 "one in which you had to prove...": Schwartz, J. "Inspections were lacking, shuttle panel member says," *NYT* 29 May 2003, p. A18.

50 "If eternal vigilance...": Reason, *Managing the Risks*, p. 37.

50 "When things are going right...": Weick, K.E. "Reduction of medical errors through mindful interdependence," in Rosenthal, *Medical Error*, p. 190. On July 15, 2003, NASA announced that it would establish an agency-wide safety arm, with a staff of about 250 engineers and other professionals, empowered to abort launches. Leary, W.E. "NASA, in response to Columbia panel, plans an agency-wide safety center," *NYT* 16 July 2003, p. A13.

51 "So if these flaws...": Schwartz, J. "Inspections were lacking, shuttle panel member says," p. A18.

51 completely obvious in hindsight: Described in Fischhoff, B. "Hindsight does not equal foresight: the effect of outcome knowledge on judgment under uncertainty," *Journal of Experimental Psychology: Human Performance and Perception* 1 (1975), pp. 288–99.

51 but led nowhere: Gladwell, M. "Connecting the dots. The paradoxes of intelligence reform," *The New Yorker* 10 Mar 2003, pp. 83–88.

51 at the time of the terrorist attacks: *September 11 and the Imperative of Reform in the U.S. Intelligence Community. Additional views of Senator Richard C. Shelby, Vice Chairman, Senate Select Committee on Intelligence.* 10 Dec 2002, p. 72.

52   the rule fundamentally *un*safe: The growing complexity of modern work has only added to the catch-22s. Reason describes a hypothetical company that began delivering passengers and mail a century ago. The founders would have bought a stagecoach and some horses, and hired men to drive the coaches. Their work would have exposed them to many hazards, including hostile locals, rock-strewn tracks, and bad weather. Some of these dangers could be anticipated, while others would be learned through painful experience. Over time, the drivers would be given maps, guns, perhaps even escorts, and they'd learn quickly how to make their trips safer. The feedback was direct and immediate. In those pioneering days, writes Reason, if disaster struck, the fault "lay almost entirely with the people on the spot. A driver could ignore local warnings and select a dangerous route, or overturn his coach by taking a bend too fast; the guard's gritty Winchester rifle could jam, or run out of ammunition, or he could simply fail to shoot straight." (Reason, *Managing the Risks*, p. 13).

But the modern incarnation of this company would be as a multinational behemoth, chock-full of breathtakingly complex systems for managing people and equipment, bursting at the seams with checks and cross-checks to catch human error before it could harm people or packages. "In these complex systems," writes psychologist Jens Rasmussen, "many errors and faults made by the staff and maintenance personnel do not directly reveal themselves by functional response from the system. [Conversely], humans can operate with an extremely high level of reliability in a dynamic environment when slips and mistakes have immediately visible effects and can be corrected. Survival when driving through Paris during rush hours depends on this fact." (Rasmussen, J. "Interdisciplinary workshops to develop a multi-disciplinary research programme based on a holistic system approach to safety and management of risk in large-scale technological operations," Paper commissioned by the World Bank, Washington, D.C. (1988) pp. 3–4). In the unsettling view of one group of organizational theorists (the "Normal Accident" school), the paradoxical fragility and the ever-increasing opacity of "safe" but complex systems makes another shuttle crash, Three Mile Island or, worse, an accidental nuclear war, all but inevitable. See Perrow, C. *Normal Accidents: Living with High-Risk Technologies* (New York: Basic Books, 1984).

CHAPTER 3: JUMBO JETS CRASHING

55   The IOM's history is described in Berkowitz, E.D. *To Improve Human Health: A History of the Institute of Medicine* (Washington, D.C.: National Academy Press, 1998). The dietary reference report is *DRI: Dietary Reference Intakes For Calcium, Phosphorus, Magnesium, Vitamin D, and Fluoride.* Standing Committee on the Scientific Evaluation of Dietary Reference Intakes. Food and Nutrition Board, Institute of Medicine (Washington, D.C.: National Academy Press, 1999). The stem cell report is *Stem Cells and the Future of Regenerative Medicine.* Committee on the Biological and Biomedical Applications of Stem Cell Research, Board on Life Sciences, National Research Council, Board on Neuroscience and Behavioral Health, Institute of Medicine (Washington, D.C.: National Academy Press, 2001).

55   Kohn, L.T., Corrigan, J.M., Donaldson, M.S., eds. *To Err Is Human: Building a Safer Health System* (Washington, D.C.: National Academy Press, 2000). The report is usually referred to as "the 1999 report" because it was released in November 1999.

56   media feeding frenzy: Dentzer, S. "Media mistakes in coverage of the Institute of

Medicine's error report," *Effective Clinical Practice* 3 (2000), pp. 305–8.

56   best to handle the release: Millenson, M.L. "Pushing the profession: how the news media turned patient safety into a priority, "*Quality and Safety in Health Care* 11 (2002), pp. 57–63.

56-7   spate of congressional hearings: Kaiser Family Foundation (1999). *LAT* 30 Nov 1999. *Time* Magazine 13 Dec 1999.

57   "…public media hit hard on it": The studies from which the IOM numbers were loosely derived are Brennan, T.A., Leape, L.L., Laird, N.M., et al. "Incidence of adverse events and negligence in hospitalized patients: Results of the Harvard Medical Practice Study I," *NEJM* 324 (1991), pp. 370–76; and Thomas, E.J., Studdert, D.M. Burstin, H.R., et al. "Incidence and types of adverse events and negligent care in Utah and Colorado," *Medical Care* 38 (2000), pp. 261–71. The seminal review, largely ignored at the time, is Leape, L.L. "Error in medicine," *JAMA* 271 (1994), pp. 1851–57. Dr. Lundberg's confession about burying the Leape paper in the pre-Christmas edition of *JAMA* is in Lundberg, G.D., Stacey, J. *Severed Trust: Why American Medicine Hasn't Been Fixed* (New York: Basic Books, 2000), pp. 169–72.

59   armory was compelling: The history of this effort is reviewed in great detail in Millenson, M.L. *Demanding Medical Excellence: Doctors and Accountability in the Information Age.* (Chicago: University of Chicago Press, 1997). The extensive research on procedures and geographic variation is summarized in Birkmeyer, J.D., Sharp, S.M., Finlayson, S.R., et al. "Variation profiles of common surgical procedures," *Surgery* 124 (1998), pp. 917–23. The improved surgical outcomes in high-volume centers is in Birkmeyer, J.D., Finlayson, E.V., Birkmeyer, C.M. "Volume standards for high-risk surgical procedures: potential benefits of the Leapfrog initiative," *Surgery* 130 (2001), pp. 415–22. On aspirin and beta blockers, Jencks, S.F., Cuerdon, T., Burwen, D.R., et al. "Quality of medical care delivered to Medicare beneficiaries: A profile at state and national levels," *JAMA* 284 (2000), pp. 1670–76. The literature on colorectal screening is summarized in Schuster, M.A., McGlynn, E.A., Brook, R.H. "How good is the quality of health care in the United States?" *Milbank Quarterly* 76 (1998), pp. 517–63, and Chassin, M.R., Galvin, R.W. "National Roundtable on Health Care Quality. The urgent need to improve health care quality: Institute of Medicine National Roundtable on Health Care Quality," *JAMA* 280 (1998), pp. 1000–05. A more recent indictment of quality is McGlynn, E.A., Asch, S.M., Adams, J., et al. "The quality of health care delivered to adults in the United States," *NEJM* 348 (2003), pp. 2635–45.

59   1 percent had made a change: Taylor, H., Leitman, R. "Health Care News," *Harris Interactive* 2 (2002), p. 1.

61   "Talk about overuse…": Altman, L.K. "The doctor's world: Getting to the core of mistakes in medicine," *NYT* 29 Feb 2000, p. D1.

62   The report is Committee on Quality of Health Care in America of the Institute of Medicine. *Crossing the Quality Chasm: A New Health System for the 21ˢᵗ Century* (Washington, D.C., National Academy Press, 2001). Regarding why it failed to get the attention of IOM I, health care journalist Michael Millenson blamed, in part, the dullness of the exposition: "The

report contained few human interest stories, had a complicated 'plot' (unlike 'tens of thousands of dead patients'), and led off with a long executive summary whose core consisted of list after list of possible actions." Millenson, "Pushing the Profession."

62   highlights in an endnote for those who are interested: In the mid-1970s, California was besieged by a "malpractice crisis," with soaring insurance rates and seemingly endless litigation (a crisis reprised in 2002–2003, for all the same reasons). The California Medical Association and California Hospital Association commissioned a study to learn how many patients are injured by medical care. They found that about 5 percent of Californians hospitalized in the mid-1970s were injured from medical care, and nearly 1 percent had an injury that led to permanent disability or death (California Medical Association. *Report of the Medical Insurance Feasibility Study* (San Francisco: California Medical Association, 1977)).

Ten years later, researchers from the Harvard School of Public Health launched a similar but more ambitious study. The Harvard team reviewed more than 30,000 medical charts in fifty-two New York hospitals. Although the public perception of the Harvard Medical Practice Study (HMPS) was entirely shaped by the mortality statistics, the study was actually focused on sorting out the relationship between medical injuries and malpractice litigation, like the earlier California study (Hiatt, H.H., Barnes, B.A., Brennan, T.A., et al. "A study of medical injury and medical malpractice," *NEJM* 321 (1989), pp. 480–84).

The HMPS chart reviewers were charged with slogging through hundreds of thousands of cryptic handwritten notes in these dusty medical records to find evidence of *adverse events*, which the researchers defined as injuries caused by medical care as opposed to the disease process itself. The results were striking. The HMPS found that 3.7 percent of hospitalized patients in New York in 1984 suffered a medical injury during their hospitalization, and about one-seventh of these were fatal (Brennan, T.A., Leape, L.L., Laird, N.M., et al. "Incidence of adverse events and negligence in hospitalized patients: Results of the Harvard Medical Practice Study I," *NEJM* 324 (1991), pp. 370–76). In other words, if you checked into a New York hospital in 1984, you had a one in 200 chance of dying because of a medical injury. Extrapolating these numbers to all hospitalizations in New York State, the authors estimated that about 100,000 New Yorkers were injured by hospital care in 1984, and 14,000 died from these injuries. To answer criticisms regarding the methods and update the data in the era of managed care, the Harvard investigators performed a similar analysis of 15,000 medical records in Utah and Colorado in 1992 (Thomas, E.J., Studdert, D.M., Burstin, H.R., et al. "Incidence and types of adverse events and negligent care in Utah and Colorado," *Medical Care* 38 (2000), pp. 261–71). They found a comparable rate of medical injuries (2.9 percent, compared with 3.7 percent in the New York study) but a somewhat lower death rate (7 percent of injuries resulted in death, vs. 14 percent in New York).

The IOM's decision to extrapolate the New York and Utah-Colorado statistics into yearly national death rates and highlight them in the report led to a curious and spirited interchange in the normally buttoned-down medical journals. Several authors defended the HMPS methodology and stated that, if anything, the IOM mortality numbers were an *underestimate* since, a) they came from chart reviews; no doctor wants to air his dirty laundry, so one need not be unduly cynical to believe that some doctors will document a patient's demise in a way that shines the best possible light on their care and b) both the

HMPS and the Utah-Colorado study looked at hospital errors only, and omitted the unknown (but non-trivial) number of deaths from outpatient errors (see Leape, L.L. "Institute of Medicine medical error figures are not exaggerated," *JAMA* 284 (2000), pp. 95–97).

The opposing team focused first on the source of the mortality estimates. Although the IOM loosely stated that "98,000" was derived from the New York study and "44,000" from the Utah-Colorado study, their precise derivation was never specified, making this a striking example of Immaculate Extrapolation (Sox, H.C., Woloshin, S. "How many deaths are due to medical error? Getting the number right," *Effective Clinical Practice* 3 (2000), pp. 277–83).

Even more remarkably, the numbers were also attacked by one of the HMPS's own lead investigators, Troy Brennan, a Yale-trained MD, JD, and MPH. Brennan argued that while the methodology of the Harvard studies was unassailable, he and his team were counting "preventable adverse events," not necessarily errors. Lucian Leape sees it differently, and cites a follow-up HMPS paper, which does cite rates of "errors": Leape, L. L., Brennan, T. A., Laird, N., et al. "The nature of adverse events in hospitalized patients: Results of the Harvard Medical Practice Study II," *NEJM* 324 (1991), pp. 377-84. In either case, the HMPS and Utah-Colorado studies clearly characterized an episode of postoperative bleeding that resulted in a patient being brought back to the operating room as a "preventable adverse event," even though there was no blunder by the surgeon and hemorrhages like this just happen sometimes even despite flawless technique (Brennan, T.A. "The Institute of Medicine report on medical errors—could it do harm?" *NEJM* 324 (2000), pp. 1123 25).

A similar argument was advanced by Dartmouth's Elliott Fisher and Gilbert Welch, who wrote:

> To most of us, an error is a screw-up. The word connotes unambiguous culpability: Someone is to blame... The term adverse event, on the other hand, probably has no immediate meaning to most people. It is perhaps best translated as "something bad has happened." Although error and adverse event mean different things, the terms are often muddled in the error movement, and the public may be led to believe that eliminating errors will eliminate adverse events. Let's be clear: It won't.
>
> The reason is that many adverse events are expected—that is, the use of diagnostic tests, medications, and surgical interventions all lead, at a predictable rate, to false-positive results, adverse reactions, complications, and death. It is true that some of these events—the so-called preventable adverse events—might have been prevented if something different been done... [However,] most of the preventable adverse events in medicine bear no resemblance to the big screw-ups that are typically held up as examples of errors (amputating the wrong leg in surgery, administering 10 times the normal chemotherapy dose) (Fisher, E.S., Welch, H.G. "Is this issue a mistake?" *Effective Clinical Practice* 3 (2000), pp. 290–93).

This distinction between "preventable adverse events" and "errors" is crucial, and the conflation of these two ideas is one of the most persuasive critiques of the IOM's mortality statistics.

Moreover, problems with hindsight bias also make us see errors in retrospect when the care was reasonable at the time (Caplan, R.A., Posner, K.L., Cheney, F,W. "Effect of outcome on physician judgments of appropriateness of care," *JAMA* 265 (1991), pp. 1957–60).

The final assault on the IOM numbers came from Clement McDonald and colleagues at Indiana's Regenstrief Institute, who noted that even the lower of the IOM's death estimates exceeded America's yearly death toll from car crashes, but:

> Motor vehicle occupants do survive their ride if collisions are avoided. Unlike most people who step into motor vehicles, most patients admitted to hospitals have high disease burdens and high death risks even before they enter the hospital... Of course, medical errors are never excusable, but the baseline death risk has to be known and factored out before drawing conclusions about the real effect of [errors] (McDonald, C.J., Weiner, M., Hui, S.L. "Deaths due to medical errors are exaggerated in Institute of Medicine report," *JAMA* 284 (2000), pp. 93–95).

Even more directly, Dartmouth's Fisher and Welch added:

> All deaths are not the same. Talking about death in the context of airplane crashes or car accidents engenders particularly poignant images—active, healthy people experiencing sudden, unexpected death. This is how the publicists communicate the magnitude of the medical error problem. Talking about death in the medical care system this way, however, is at best misleading. Many people die, most after contact with the health care system. Sometimes their death is hastened by medical care (unintentionally), and how often this happens is a subject of legitimate debate. But the impact of deaths from errors on overall life expectancy is small. To equate this cause of death with the traumatic death of healthy individuals is disingenuous (Fisher, "Is this issue a mistake?")

In the end, we are left like Goldilocks, not quite sure whether the IOM death statistics are too low, too high, or just about right. What is clear is that trying to figure out whether a clinical decision was an error is tricky, and that the assessments are tremendously influenced by things like the quality of the charting, the bias of the reviewer, and how the patient fared. We suspect that many of the problems in the estimates cancel each other out and thus the IOM estimates are probably in the right ballpark. In any case, whether the "right" answer is that 44,000 or 98,000 (or even 30,000 or 200,000) people a year die from medical errors, everyone agrees that this is a tremendous problem that was ignored in the pre-IOM era.

62   how everyone viewed medical errors: The forty-year-old women getting married Newsweek cover story (1986) was famously debunked in Susan Faludi's *Backlash: The Undeclared War Against American Women* (New York: Crown Publishers, 1991). For breast cancer risk, see Rensberger, B. "The misleading statistics of breast cancer," *WP* 8 Nov 1995.

62-3   the IRS—in customer satisfaction: Taylor, H. "For the second year running, there has been a dramatic increase in confidence in leadership of nation's major institutions," Harris Poll #9, 3 Feb 1999; and Lieber, R.B. "Now are you satisfied? The 1998 American Customer

Satisfaction Index," *Fortune* 137 (1998), p. 161.

63   has never been wider: Blendon, R.J., DesRoches, C.M., Brodie, M., et al. "Views of practicing physicians and the public on medical errors," *NEJM* 347 (2002), pp. 1933–40.

CHAPTER 4:
DOCTORS' HANDWRITING AND OTHER PRESCRIBING ERRORS

68   We asked 158 physician colleagues: At the 2002 "Management of the Hospitalized Patient" continuing medical education course, San Francisco.

68   split between the defendants: Prager, L.O. "Jury blames doctor's bad penmanship for patient death," *American Medical News* 22/29 Nov 1999; Hall, M. "Doctor held liable for fatal handwriting mix-up," *USA Today* 21 Oct 1999, p. 3A; Waters, R. "Precarious Prescriptions: Can your doctor's handwriting kill you?" *WebMD*, available at my.webmd.com/content/article/1691.50655 (last accessed October 4, 2003); Ricks, D. "Poison in Prescription: Illegible writing can lead to dangerous medication errors," *Newsday* 19 Mar 2001, p. A3. The jury apportioned the liability equally between the doctor and the pharmacist, blaming the doctor for the handwriting, and the pharmacist for not questioning the impossibly high dose of Plendil.

69   The handwriting study is Berwick, D.M., Winickoff, D.E. "The truth about doctors' handwriting: A prospective study," *BMJ* 313 (1996), pp. 1657–58.

69   "ClomiPRAMINE": Freeman, R.A. "Do spelling and penmanship count? In medicine, you bet," *NYT* 11 Mar 2003; Cohen, M.R. "Zyprexa-Zyrtec Mix-up," *AHRQ WebM&M* Apr 2003. Available at webmm.ahrq.gov (last accessed November 8, 2003). Appendix III of this book is an expanded list of sound-alike, look-alike medications.

72   often by dumb luck: Bates, D.W., Cullen, D.J., Laird, N., et al. "Incidence of adverse drug events and potential adverse drug events: Implications for prevention: ADE Prevention Study Group," *JAMA* 274 (1995), pp. 29–34. Rates of ADEs are even higher in outpatients; see Gandhi, T.K., Weingart, S.N., Borus, J., et al. "Adverse drug events in ambulatory care," *NEJM* 348 (2003), pp. 556–64.

73   that the organ is failing: Chertow, G.M., Lee, J., Kuperman, G.J., et al. "Guided medication dosing for inpatients with renal insufficiency," *JAMA* 286 (2001), pp. 2839–44.

73   tools for fighting infections: Evans, R.S., Pestotnik, S.L., Classen, D.C., et al. "A computer-assisted management program for antibiotics and other antiinfective agents," *NEJM* 338 (1998), pp. 232–38.

74   salaries for five years: Yearly RN salary estimate of $47,000 is from the 2000 National Sample Survey of Registered Nurses. An additional 20 percent has been added for benefits. The calculation is thus: $56,400 = one nurse's salary and benefits for one year. Accounting for an annual inflation rate of 3 percent, $30 million would fund 500 nurse FTEs, or 100 nurses for five years.

74   had functioning CPOE: Leapfrog Group, 2003.

75   hospitals were in the red: American Hospital Association Annual Survey, 2001.

78   the horror stories keep coming: Browne, M.W. "Is it a bird or is it a plane? Radar may not know, the source of confusion in the Iranian accident remains unclear," *NYT* 5 July 1988, pp. 5; 8(N), A10(L); Healy, M. "Aegis malfunctioned a month before the Iran Air disaster," *LAT* 8 July 1988, p. 10; Neumann, P.G. "Aegis Vincennes, and the Iranian Airbus," *Risks-Forum Digest* 8 (1989), p. 74; Lezard, T. "London Ambulance Service Computer fails again," Ibid. 2 (1992), p. 14; "Software cited in air traffic error," *NYT* 9 Dec 1998, p. B18(L), Noguchi, Y. "Phone Customers' Service Switched; Thousands 'Slammed' by Computer Error," *WP* 13 Dec 2001, p. E05; Kristof, K. "The Nation; Bank Says Deposits Went Uncredited; Glitch: Bank of America scrambles to correct a computer error that blocked payments to customers' accounts," *LAT* 17 Mar 2002, p. A-30; "$1.2 billion error found in county pension fund," *NYT* 9 Apr 1998, pp. A21(N), A23(L); "Bank's error, thieves' joy," *NYT* 9 Feb 1995, pp. A11(N), B9(L); Hansell S. "Bank says cash machine problems are fixed," *NYT* 7 Feb 1992, pp. C4(N), D4(L); Sawyer, K. "Computer error causes Hubble Space Telescope to shut down temporarily," *WP* 11 Dec 1991, p. A3; "Spacecraft 'bug' said to be fixed by NASA," *LAT* 18 Aug 1991, p. A13; Kuttner, R. "Missed phone connections," *Boston Globe* 28 Aug 2002, p. A23; Seelye, K.Q. "Florida seeks federal help in voting," *NYT* 18 Sept 2002; Mercuri, R. "Florida Primary 2002: Back to the Future," *Risks-Forum Digest* 24 (2002), p. 22; Barron, J. "Power surge blacks out Northeast, hitting cities in 8 states and Canada, midday shutdowns disrupt millions," *NYT* 15 Aug 2003, p. A1.

79   "Got paper? Beth Israel copes with computer crash," *Boston Globe* 26 Nov 2002, p. C1. A follow-up article describing the lessons of the BI Deaconess crash and the need for robust back-up systems in hospitals increasingly dependent on their computers is Kilbridge, P. "Computer crash—lessons from a system failure," *NEJM* 348 (2003), pp. 881–82.

79-80 The Cedars story is described in Chin, T. "Doctors pull plug on paperless system," *American Medical News* 17 Feb 2003, pp. 1, 4; Ornstein, C. "Hospital heeds doctors, suspends use of software. Cedars-Sinai physicians entered prescriptions and other orders in it, but called it unsafe," *LAT* 22 Jan 2003, p. B1. The point of view of the Cedars-Sinai administration is described in Langberg, M.L. "Challenges to implementing CPOE: A case study of a work in progress at Cedars-Sinai," *Modern Physician* Feb (2003), pp. 21–22.

80   define high-quality organizations: The Leapfrog Group got its name from the concept, promoted by health care quality guru Dr. Donald Berwick, that change in medicine must involve bold leaps, not timid, incremental advances. Leapfrog initially set 2004 as the target date for full CPOE implementation, but, not surprisingly, has pushed its deadline back to 2005 as it became clear that the vast majority of hospitals simply could not comply in time.

CHAPTER 5: THE FORGOTTEN HALF OF MEDICATION ERRORS

87   a fatal dose of insulin: This case is further analyzed in an article in our Quality Grand Rounds series: Bates, D.W. "Unexpected hypoglycemia in a critically ill patient," *Ann Intern*

Med 137 (2002), pp. 110–16. Bates notes that that identical heparin-insulin mix-up errors have occurred at other hospitals, resulting in at least two deaths.

88   particular error fall precipitously: Bates, "Incidence of adverse drug events and potential adverse drug events...," found that 48 percent of the errors at the ordering stage were intercepted, while none of the errors at the administration stage were intercepted.

91   "Errors are largely unintentional...": Reason, *Managing the Risks*, p. 154.

93   roll bars will protect us: Tenner, E. *Why Things Bite Back: Technology and the Revenge of Unintended Consequences* (New York: Knopf, 1996).

93-4 "people have no need...": Merry, A. and Smith, A.M. *Errors, Medicine and the Law* (Cambridge: Cambridge University Press, 2001), p. 54.

94   customers to follow suit: Wald, H. Shojania, K.G. "The use of bar coding to enhance patient safety," In: Shojania, K.G., Duncan, B.W., McDonald, K.M., Wachter, R.M., eds. *Making Health Care Safer: A Critical Analysis of Patient Safety Practices.* Evidence Report/Technology Assessment No. 43 from the Agency for Healthcare Research and Quality: AHRQ Publication No. 01-E058 (2001); Landro, L. "Blood mixups can be deadly, but are also easily prevented," *WSJ* 27 Feb 2003; McNeil, D.G. "To cut errors, FDA orders drug bar codes," *NYT* 14 Mar 2003, pp. A1, A16.

95   manually override the system: Pucket, R. "Medication-management component of a point-of-care information system," *American Journal of Health System Pharmacists* 52 (1995), pp. 1305–09.

95   intended and actual patient: Patterson, E.S., Cook, R.I., Render, M.L. "Improving patient safety by identifying side effects from introducing bar coding in medication administration," *Journal of the American Medical Informatics Association* 9 (2002), pp. 540–53.

95-7 Cook, R. "Potassium chloride's reappearance on the ward: A signal about coupling and failure," National Patient Safety Foundation listserv, message dated 19 Feb 2002.

97   under a microscope: You might think that celebrity patients, or physician-patients and their relatives, get better care than the average Joe, and, to a certain degree, that's true. But, like gravity, the law of unintended consequences works in this situation, too. Errors in VIP care occur because of the "too many cooks" problem—hordes of specialists descend on the patient, making handoff fumbles and miscommunications more likely; and it's hard for the regular staff—from floor nurses to orderlies—to function efficiently when everyone's walking on eggshells. See Otte, A., Audenaert, K., Otte, K., et al. "The dilemma of being a physician-patient," *Medical Science Monitor* 9 (2003), pp. SR20–22.

97-8 "The errors were not rare...": Berwick, D.M. *Escape Fire: Lessons for the Future of Health Care* (New York: The Commonwealth Fund, 2002).

100   ER-related malpractice suits: Rusnak, R.A., Stair, T.O., Hansen, K., Fastow, J.S. "Litigation against the emergency physician; common features in cases of missed myocardial infarction," *Annals of Emergency Medicine* 18 (1989), pp. 1029–34.

103   correctly diagnosed and hospitalized: Lee, T.H., Rouan, G.W., Weisberg, M.C., et al. "Clinical characteristics and natural history of patients with acute myocardial infarction sent home from the emergency room," *American Journal of Cardiology* 60 (1987), pp. 219–24. More recent estimates show some improvement, with about one in fifty patients with MI being discharged mistakenly: McCarthy, B.D., Beshansky, J.R., D'Agostino, R.B., Selker, H.P. "Missed diagnoses of acute myocardial infarction in the emergency department: Results from a multicenter study," *Annals of Emergency Medicine* 22 (1993), pp. 579–82; Pope, J.H., Aufderheide, T.P., Ruthazer, R., et al. "Missed diagnoses of acute ischemia in the emergency department," *NEJM* 342 (2000), pp. 1163–70.

103   white male than for the black female: Schulman, K.A., Berlin, J.A., Harless, W., et al. "The effect of race and sex on physicians' recommendations for cardiac catheterization," *NEJM* 340 (1999), pp. 618–26. Although the possibility of overt racism among some physicians is there, the phenomenon may be more subtle than that. A more recent study found that black patients did, in fact, receive fewer cardiac catheterizations than white patients, but this disparity held whether their physician was white or black. Chen, J., Rathore, S.S., Radford, M.J., et al. "Racial differences in the use of cardiac catheterization after acute myocardial infarction," *NEJM* 344 (2001), pp. 1443–49. Additional studies demonstrating clear racial differences in treatments or outcomes include: Bach, P.B., Cramer, L.D., Warren, J.L., Begg, C.B. "Racial differences in the treatment of early-stage lung cancer," *NEJM* 341 (1999), pp. 1198–1205; Moore, R.D., Stanton, D., Gopalan, R., Chaisson, R.E. "Racial differences in the use of drug therapy for HIV disease in an urban community," *NEJM* 330 (1994), pp. 763–68; and Schneider, E.C., Cleary, P.D., Zaslavsky, A.M., Epstein, A.M. "Racial disparity in influenza vaccination: Does managed care narrow the gap between African Americans and whites?" *JAMA* 286 (2001), pp. 1455–60. Medicine is just beginning to address this problem with educational initiatives and feedback to providers and health care systems, but there is a long way to go.

104   twice in their careers: Ting, H.H., Lee, T.H., Soukup, J.R., et al. "Impact of physician experience on triage of emergency room patients with acute chest pain at three teaching hospitals," *Am J Med* 91 (1991), pp. 401–08.

104   decisions of 119 physicians: Pearson, S.D., Goldman, L., Orav, E.J., et al. "Triage decisions for emergency department patients with chest pain: Do physicians' risk attitudes make the difference?" *JGIM* 10 (1995), pp. 557–64.

105   wounding himself in the process: The story is described in the Memorial Resolution for Amos Tversky, Stanford University. Tversky died tragically of malignant melanoma at age fifty-nine. In 2002, the Nobel Prize in Economics was awarded to Tversky's close collaborator, Princeton's Daniel Kahneman. Undoubtedly, Tversky would have shared the prize, but Nobels are never awarded posthumously.

105   "What *were* you thinking?": Author's interview with Dr. Donald Redelmeier, 6 May 2003.

106   fits the facts or not: Croskerry, P. "Achieving quality in clinical decision making: Cognitive strategies and detection of bias," *Academic Emergency Medicine* 9 (2002), pp. 1184–1204.

107   "Even after studying rationality...": Redelmeier, D.A. "Standing on the shoulders of giants (Memoriam for Amos Tversky)," *Medical Decision Making* 16 (1996) p. 423.

107   "Decisions about war...": Author's interview with Dr. Donald Redelmeier, 6 May 2003.

107   "consider young women with fever...": Redelmeier, D.A., Tversky, A. "Discrepancy between medical decisions for individual patients and for groups," *NEJM* 322 (1990), pp. 1162–64.

107-8 "People's beliefs about arthritis...": Redelmeier, D. A., Tversky, A. "On the belief that arthritis pain is related to the weather," *Proceedings of the National Academy of Sciences, USA* 93 (1996), pp. 2895–96.

108   demanding a decision: One choice, of course, is to do nothing. We call this the "test of time" and it is a common strategy for outpatients with nonspecific symptoms who otherwise seem well; but it is less useful for critically ill patients. The stakes are just too high and the hospital's meter—amounting to thousands of dollars each day for each admitted patient—is constantly ticking.

108   in a most uncertain world: One notable exception to this tendency toward professional hubris is seen in meteorologists. When your local weatherman says that the weather in your area will probably be good, he is probably right. The reason for this is that most forecasts are made with access to almost continuous, objective, near-term data as well as complex models based on decades of observations. Contrary to popular belief, most errors in weather forecasts are not for sunny days that turn rainy, but for very severe weather that never occurs. This is quite understandable, since the price of a bad call on tornados is comparable with a missed diagnosis of cancer, and no weather forecaster—or physician—wants to jeopardize their public by saying, "well, this probably won't happen" when there's a definite, if tiny, chance that it might. Thus both professions tend to err on the side of caution, but the necessity for such caution diminishes as the hard data gets better. See Murphy, A.H. and Winkler, R.L. "Approach verification of probability forecasts," *International Journal of Forecasting* 7 (1992), pp. 435–55. The interpretation regarding the accuracy of forecasters and its relationship to feedback was described by Fischhoff, B., in *Judgment Heuristics*, and in Griffin, D. and Tversky, A. "The weighing of evidence and the determinants of confidence," *Cognitive Psychology* 24 (1992), pp. 411–35.

109   "It can be argued...": Griffin, "The weighing of evidence..."

109-10 "...I capitalize it...": Nuland, S.B. *How We Die: Reflections on Life's Final Chapter*

(New York: Alfred A. Knopf, 1994), p. 248.

110   reasoning of dozens of clinicians: Kassirer, J.P., Gorry, G.A. "Clinical problem solving: A behavioral analysis," *Ann Intern Med* 89 (1978), pp. 245–55; Pauker, S.G., Kassirer, J.P. "The threshold approach to clinical decision making," *NEJM* 302 (1980), pp. 1109–17; and Kassirer, J.P. "Teaching clinical medicine by iterative hypothesis testing: Let's preach what we practice," *NEJM* 309 (1983), pp. 921–23.

112   very-low-risk group: In Bayesian terms, the test had a moderate rate of false-positives, and individuals most likely to have false-positive tests were those with a very low likelihood of being HIV infected. When applying the same test to a gay man, however, a positive test was much more likely to be true.

113   "A patient has no more right...": Cited in Cassem, N.H. "Treating the person confronting death," in *The Harvard Guide to Modern Psychiatry*. Nicholi, A.M., ed. (Cambridge: Harvard University Press, 1978), pp. 585–86.

115   Bleich, H.L. "The computer as consultant," *NEJM* 284 (1971), pp. 141–47.

115   Garry Kasparov: Hoffman, P. "Retooling machine and man for the next big chess faceoff," *NYT* 21 Jan 2003, pp. D1, D6.

116   computerized solutions have been largely ignored: Selker, H.P., Beshansky, J.R., Griffith, J.L., et al. "Use of the Acute Cardiac Ischemia Time-Insensitive Predictive Instrument (ACI-TIPI) to assist with triage of patients with chest pain or other symptoms suggestive of acute cardiac ischemia," *Ann Intern Med* 129 (1998), pp. 845–55, and Pozen, M.W., D'Agostino, R.B., Selker, H.P., et al. "A predictive instrument to improve coronary-care-unit admission practices in acute ischemic heart disease," *NEJM* 310 (1984), pp. 1273-78.

116   after the heartbreaking crash: Johnson, G. "To err is human; trust the machines," *NYT* 14 July 2002, pp. 1, 7.

117   but rarely get: Chassin, M.R., Galvin, R.W., and the National Roundtable on Health Care Quality. "The urgent need to improve health care quality," *JAMA* 280 (1998), pp. 1000–05.

117   Any doctor who could be replaced...: Slack, W.V. *Cybermedicine: How Computing Empowers Doctors and Patients for Better Health Care* (San Francisco: Jossey-Bass, 1997), p. 82.

117   diagnostic certainty is futile: Goldman, L., Kirtane, A. "Triage of patients with acute chest pain and possible cardiac ischemia: The elusive search for diagnostic perfection," *Ann Intern Med* 139 (2003), pp. 987–95.

119   operate on preconceived notions: Rosenhan's fascinating study is described in Gladwell, M. "Connecting the dots. The paradoxes of intelligence reform," *The New Yorker*, 10 Mar 2003.

119-20 "One uniquely distinguishing...": Croskerry, P. "Achieving quality in clinical decision making: cognitive strategies and detection of bias," *Academic Emergency Medicine* 9 (2002), pp. 1184–1204.

CHAPTER 7: OF LIFE AND LIMB

124 This foot-in-mouth...: Olson, W. "A story that doesn't have a leg to stand on (amputation of man's left leg rather than the right one may have been medically justified)," *WSJ* 27 Mar 1995, pp. A18(W), A20(E). Also see Cook, R., Woods, D., Miller, C. *A Tale of Two Stories: Contrasting Views of Patient Safety* (Chicago: National Patient Safety Foundation, 1998). Dr. Sanchez's subsequent chronology is drawn from several newspaper accounts, particularly those in the *Tampa Tribune* and the *Associated Press*.

125 twice in five years!: Bloom, M. "Scrambled surgery: a comic opera scenario at Memorial Sloan-Kettering has tragic repercussions," *Physician's Weekly* 16 May 1996; Steinhauer, J. "Surgeon treated wrong side of two brains, Albany says," *NYT* 1 Mar 2000, p. A1; Steinhauer, J., "Questions of competence: A special report; inquiry creates aura of doubt around doctor and hospital," *NYT* 12 Mar 2000, p. 43; Steinhauer, J. "So, the brain tumor's on the left, right? (Seeking ways to reduce mix-ups in the operating room; better communication is one remedy, medical experts say)," *NYT* 1 Apr 2001, pp. 23(N), 27(L).

129 a fact of medical life: Baseball's legendary Mickey Mantle got a lot of flack from fans and others for queue-jumping on the liver transplant line. Still, rank hath other, less visible medical privileges. Tversky disciple Dr. Don Redelmeier conducted a study showing that, among nominated actors, Academy Award winners on average live four years longer than losers. Kolata, G. "Transplants, morality and Mickey," *NYT* 11 June 1995, p. E5; Redelmeier, D.A., Singh, S.M. "Survival in Academy Award-winning actors and actresses," *Ann Intern Med* (2001), pp. 955–62.

129 out from a C-note: Of the $35,000, $10,585 was Dr. Arbit's surgical fee. It was all returned to the patient.

130 getting ready to repair: In the Ayyappan case, it is highly probable that the films brought into the OR were those of Mr. Gupta rather than those of Mrs. Ayyappan. Although the investigators are a bit unclear on this score, the weight of evidence suggests that Dr. Arbit consulted these films before surgery; if so, they only served to reinforce his belief that the tumor was on the right side, as indeed it was in the Gupta image. Of course, an X-ray switch, if it truly occurred, would have been only one of the many errors that took place in this case.

131 final check of the data: Meinberg, E.G., Stern, P.J. "Incidence of wrong-site surgery among hand surgeons," *Journal of Bone and Joint Surgery* 85-A (2003), pp. 193–97.

131 nearly one in thirty!: Kolata, G. "1-in-a-trillion coincidence, you say? Not really, experts find," *NYT* 27 Feb 1990, pp. v139;Bt(N)pCl(L).

132 share the same birthday: To calculate this probability, we begin by recognizing that the probability of at least two people sharing a birthday is equal to one minus the probability of no

one sharing a birthday. If there are two people, it's easy to see that the chance that the second will have a different birthday than the first is 364/365, since there are 364 available days other than the first person's birthday (ignoring leap years, of course!). If there are three people, there are still 364 available days for the second person, and 363 for the third, so the overall probability is: 1 - (364/365) * (363/365) = 1 - 0.992. In other words, there is about a 0.8 percent chance that two of the three will share a birthday. The general formula for 'n' people ends up being: 1 - ((365-1/365) * ((365-2/365) * ((365-3/365) * ... * ((365-n+1)/365). Converting this to less unwieldy factorials, this translates into: 1 - ([365!/((365-n)!*365^n)]. When n=23 (ie, there are 23 people in the room), this equals 50.7 percent (i.e., there is an even chance that two will share a birthday). Once there are 50 people, the chance is 97 percent.

132   surgeon entered the OR suite: One review of such wrong-sided surgery cases that resulted in malpractice claims showed that while half were deemed to have been caused primarily by the surgeon, the other half were the fault (the immediate, sharp-end fault) of the crew prepping and draping the wrong body part. See Meinberg, "Incidence of wrong-site surgery."

133   promise to get better: Risk Management Foundation of the Harvard Medical Institutions. "Did Wrong-Site Surgery Remedy Work?" Feb 1999; and *The American Academy of Orthopedic Surgeons, Academic News.* "'Sign Your Site' gets strong member support," 1999. Evidence of improved compliance comes from Meinberg.

CHAPTER 8: DID WE FORGET SOMETHING?

136   months and years earlier: Gibbs, V.C., Auerbach, A.D., "The retained surgical sponge," in: Shojania, *Making Health Care Safer.*

136   third were surgical instruments: Gawande, A.A., Studdert, D.M., Orav, E.J., et al. "Risk factors for retained instruments and sponges after surgery," *NEJM* 348 (2003), pp. 229–35.

136   three times a year at his hospital: Altman, L.K. "The doctors' world: The wrong foot, and other tales of surgical error," *NYT* 11 Dec 2001, p. F1.

138   one time out of every three: Thanks to our colleague, Charles McCullough, professor of Epidemiology and Biostatistics at UCSF, for walking us through this statistical maze.

140   even by skilled radiologists: O'Connor, A.R., Coakley, F.V., Meng, M.V., Eberhardt, S. "Imaging of retained surgical sponges in the abdomen and pelvis," *American Journal of Roentgenology* 180 (2003), pp. 481–89; and Choi, B.I., Kim, S.H., Yu, E.S., et al. "Retained surgical sponge: Diagnosis with CT and sonography," *American Journal of Roentgenology* 150 (1988), pp. 1047–50.

CHAPTER 9: PRACTICE MAKES PERFECT

143   *New England Journal of Medicine*: Luft, H.S., Bunker, J.P., Enthoven, A.C. "Should operations be regionalized? The empirical relation between surgical volume and mortaility,"

NEJM 301 (1979), pp. 1364–69.

143   what they do best: Halm, E.A., Lee, C., Chassin, M.R. "Is volume related to outcome in health care? A systematic review and methodologic critique of the literature," *Ann Intern Med* 137 (2002), pp. 511–20.

144   results might be just as good: That this kind of cooperation can lead to better outcomes was demonstrated in O'Conner, G.T., Plume, S,K., Olmstead, E.M., et al. "A regional intervention to improve the hospital mortality associated with coronary artery bypass graft surgery: The Northern New England Cardiovascular Disease Study Group," *JAMA* 275 (1996), pp. 841–46. Unfortunately, such cooperation across institutional boundaries is unusual.

145   nearer facility most of the time: Finlayson, S.R., Birkmeyer, J.D., Tosteson, A.N., Nease, R.F., Jr. "Patient preferences for location of care: Implications for regionalization," *Medical Care* 37 (1999), pp. 204–09. The evidence that shifting procedures to high-volume facilities would save thousands of lives each year is in Dudley, R.A., Johansen, K.L., Brand, R., et al. "Selective referral to high-volume hospitals: Estimating potentially avoidable deaths," *JAMA* 283 (2000), pp. 1191-93.

146   without adequate care: Statement by George Lynn, representing the American Hospital Association, before the U.S. Department of Justice and Federal Trade Commission Hearing, "Perspectives on Competition Policy and the Health Care Marketplace: Single Specialty Hospitals," 27 Mar 2003.

147   best candidates into RAF cockpits: Gough, M., Bell, J. "Introducing aptitude testing into medicine," *BMJ* 298 (1989), pp. 975–76.

147   changing them one iota: Wanzel, K.R., Ward, M., Reznick, R.K. "Teaching the surgical craft: From selection to certification," *Current Problems in Surgery* 39 (2002), pp. 573–659.

149   often raises costs: Legorreta, A.P., Silber, J.H., Costantino, G.N. "Increased cholecystectomy rate after the introduction of laparoscopic cholecystectomy," *JAMA* 270 (1993), pp. 1429–32.

149   rate seen after fifty cases: "A prospective analysis of 1,518 laparoscopic cholecystectomies. The Southern Surgeon's Club," *NEJM* 324 (1991), pp. 1073–78; Moore, M.J., Bennett, C.L. "The learning curve for laparoscopic cholecystectomy: The Southern Surgeon's Club," *American Journal of Surgery* 170 (1995), pp. 55–59.

150   administered by senior instructors: Thomas, E.J., Helmreich, R.L. "Will airline safety models work in medicine?" In Rosenthal, *Medical Error.*

151   lap choleys immediately afterward: Morino, M., Festa, V., Garrone, C. "Survey on Torino courses: The impact of a two-day practical course on apprenticeship and diffusion of laparoscopic cholecystectomy in Italy," *Surgical Endoscopy* 9 (1995), pp. 46–48.

152   150-degree movie screen: Seilberg, D. "War games: Military training goes high-tech." CNN.com 23 Nov 2001.

154   resident's four-year training period: Bridges, M., Diamond, D.L. "The financial impact of teaching surgical residents in the operating room," *American Journal of Surgery* 177 (1999), pp. 28–32.

155   fancy anatomical simulator: Matsumoto, E.D., Hamstra, S.J., Radomski,, S.B., Cusimano, M.D. "The effect of bench model fidelity on endourological skills: A randomized controlled study," *Journal of Urology* 167 (2002), pp. 1243–47.

155   converted to digital form: Zajtchuk, R., Satava, R.M. "How virtual reality is helping improve patient care in the form of advanced educational tools and theraputic options," *Communications of the Association for Computing Machinery* 40 (1997), pp. 63–64.

155   "eventually it will be standard procedure...": Dr. Fried presented his research on the ES3 at the Second Annual Patient Safety Conference held by the Agency for Healthcare Research and Quality, 2–4 Mar 2003, Arlington, Va..

156   "To study the phenomena...": Osler, W. Books and Men [Remarks made at the opening of the new building of the Boston Medical Library, January 12, 1901]. In: *Boston Medicine and Surgery Journal*. 17 Jan 1901, p. 2. A more recent article highlights the ethical imperative of promoting simulator training: Ziv, A., Wolpe, P.R., Small, S.D., Glick, S. "Simulation-based medical education: An ethical perspective," *Academic Medicine* 78 (2003), pp. 783–88.

156   removing brain tumors: Gladwell, M. "The physical genius: What do Wayne Gretzky, Yo-Yo Ma, and a brain surgeon named Charlie Wilson have in common?" *The New Yorker* 2 Aug 1999, p. 57. It may interest readers to know that Charlie Wilson, our colleague, was chair of UCSF's neurosurgery department (he has since retired from active practice) and was considered by many to be the finest technical neurosurgeon in the world.

156   very early age: Ericsson, K.A., Charness, N. "Expert performance: Its structure and acquisition," In: Ceci, S.J., Williams, W.M., eds. *The Nature-Nurture Debate: The Essential Readings: Essential Readings in Developmental Psychology* (Oxford: Blackwell, 1999), pp. 200–55; and Howe, M.J.A., Davidson, J.W., Sloboda, J.A. 1999. "Innate talents: Reality or myth?" ibid.

CHAPTER 10: HANDOFFS AND FUMBLES

159   placed in his nursing home chart: Karen Ann Quinlan and Nancy Cruzan made news in the 1970s and '80s when traumatic injuries left them in perpetual comas. Because neither had documented their wishes about life-sustaining measures, the courts would not allow their families to disconnect life-support equipment. Cases like these led to California's 1976 Natural Death Act, which made "Resuscitate" or "Do Not Resuscitate" (DNR) orders a part of many patients' health care planning, often in the form of a "living will," or a "durable power of attorney for health care" granted to a trusted family member or friend. Although the public has been slow to embrace these documents, a 1991 federal law requires hospitals to

offer new patients the opportunity to complete them (though this effort is often perfunctory). The Robert Wood Johnson Foundation funded a five-year, $28-million project to increase the use of advance directives with more than 9,000 seriously ill patients, but it too was a flop. Almost half of the DNR orders were written just prior to death, and most physicians remained ignorant about their patients' preferences. SUPPORT Principal Investigators. "A Controlled Trial to Improve Care for Seriously Ill Hospitalized Patients: The Study to Understand Prognoses and Preferences for Outcomes and Risks of Treatments (SUPPORT)," *JAMA* 274 (1995), pp. 1591–98.

161   feel like night and day: Meisal, A., Snyder, L. Quill, T. "Seven legal barriers to end-of-life care," *JAMA* 284 (2000), pp. 2495–2501, and Luce, J.M., Alpers, A. "Legal aspects of withholding and withdrawing life support from critically ill patients in the United States and providing palliative care to them," *American Journal of Respiratory and Critical Care Medicine* 162 (2000), pp. 2029–32.

162   two months later: This case is more fully described and discussed in an article in our Quality Grand Rounds series: Lynn, J., Goldstein, N.E. "Advance care planning for fatal chronic illness: Avoiding commonplace errors and unwarranted suffering," *Ann Intern Med* 138 (2003), pp. 812–18.

162   chance at six-month survival: Lynn, J., Harrel, F., Cohn, F. et al. "Prognosis of seriously ill hospitalized patients on the days before death: Implications for patient care and public policy," *New Horizons* 5 (1997), pp. 56–61; Claessens, M.T., Lynn, J., Zhong, Z., et al. "Dying with lung cancer or chronic obstructive pulmonary disease: Insights from SUPPORT," *Journal of the American Geriatrics Society* 48 (2000), pp. S146–153.

163   advance directives with them: Danis, M, Southerland, L.I., Garrett, J.M., et al. "A prospective study of advance directives for life-sustaining care," *NEJM* 324 (1991), pp. 882–88.

165   enough to have been fatal: Forester, A.J., Murff, H.J., Peterson, J.F., et al. "The incidence and severity of adverse events affecting patients after discharge from the hospital," *Ann Intern Med* 138 (2003), pp. 161-67.

165   nobody wants to pay for the service: Dudas, V., Bookwalter, T., Kerr, K.M., Pantilat, S.Z. "The impact of follow-up telephone calls to patients after hospitalization," *Am J Med* 111 (2001), pp. 26S–30S.

167-8 safety of hospitalized patients: Bob actually coined the term *hospitalist* in Wachter, R.M., Goldman, L. "The emerging role of "hospitalists" in the American health care system," *NEJM* 335 (1996), pp. 514–17.

168   too often simply indispensable: The ICU literature is summarized in Pronovost, P.J., Angus, D.C., Dorman, T., et al. "Physician staffing patterns and clinical outcomes in critically ill patients: A systematic review," *JAMA* 288 (2002), pp. 2151–62; the hospitalist literature is summarized in Wachter, R.M., Goldman, L. "The hospitalist movement 5 years later," *JAMA* 287 (2002), pp. 487–94.

174   "Health care is composed of...": Commitee on Quality Health Care in America, Institute of Medicine. *Crossing the Quality Chasm*, p. 78.

175   erroneously received prior to transfer: Our doctors scrambled to figure out if the patient had suffered a neurological catastrophe en route from the smaller facility or if his condition was the result of some mix-up in medication. Everyone breathed a huge sigh of relief when, after a frantic call to the community hospital, we learned of the paralytic medication.

175   by a factor of three: Peterson, L.A., Brennan, T.A., O'Neil, A.C., et al. "Does housestaff discontinuity of care increase the risk for preventable adverse events?" *Ann Intern Med* 121 (1994), pp. 866–72; Peterson, L.A., Orav, E.J., Teich, J.M., et al. "Using a computerized sign-out program to improve continuity of inpatient care and prevent adverse events," *Joint Commission Journal of Quality Improvement* 24 (1998), pp. 77–87. The importance of "bridging gaps" is nicely described in Cook, R.I., Render, M., Woods, D.D. "Gaps in continuity of care and progress on patient safety," *BMJ* 320 (2000), pp. 791–94.

177   giants of health care: For the Kaiser Permanente story, see Lawrence, D. *From Chaos to Care: The Promise of Team-Based Medicine* (New York: Perseus Publishing, 2002).

CHAPTER 11: SEE ONE, DO ONE, TEACH ONE

187   might have done some good: Bob later learned there was little they could have done to save Mr. Adams, even if he had reported his concerns immediately—the therapies for a massive pulmonary embolism (blood thinners, like heparin) available in the early '80s just didn't work that fast. Still, if heparin had been started immediately and the patient had been taken at once to the ICU, aggressive treatment might have increased his chances from nil to maybe 10 percent—long odds, but still better than the alternative.

187-8 "In medicine, we have long faced...": Gawande, A. *Complications: A Surgeon's Notes on an Imperfect Science* (New York: Metropolitan Books, 2002), p. 24.

189   "On the one hand...": Bosk, C.L. *Forgive and Remember: Managing Medical Failure* (Chicago: University of Chicago Press, 1979), p. 3.

192   "The way you learn as an intern...": ibid., p. 53.

192   "I know a lot of patients complain...": ibid., p. 11.

196   became a hallowed tradition: For more on the history of residency training, see Ken Ludmerer's superb *Time to Heal: American Medical Education from the Turn of the Century to the Era of Managed Care* (New York: Oxford University Press, 1999).

196-7 "How did earlier generations of physicians...": Strub, W.M. "Current resident work hours: Too many or not enough," *JAMA* 287 (2002), p. 1802.

197-8 "...have come with a cost...": Drazen, J.M., Epstein, A.M. "Rethinking medical training—the critical work ahead," *NEJM* 347 (2002), pp. 1271–72.

198   legally drunk in every state: Dawson, D., Reid, K. "Fatigue, alcohol and performance impairment," *Nature* 388 (1997), p. 235.

198   the norm for medical residents: Linde, L., Bergstorm, M. "The effect of one night without sleep on problem-solving and immediate recall," *Psychological Research* 54 (1992), pp. 127–36; and Polzella, D.J. "Effects of sleep deprivation on short-term recognition memory," *Journal of Experimental Psychology and Human Learning and Memory* 104 (1975), pp. 194–200.

199   and strange-looking numbers: Two excellent reviews of the research are Gaba, D.M., Howard, S.K. "Fatigue among clinicians and the safety of patients," *NEJM* 347 (2002), pp. 1249–55; and Veasey, S., Rosen, R., Barzansky, B., et al. "Sleep loss and fatigue in residency training. A reappraisal," *JAMA* 288 (2002), pp. 1116–24. Also see Jacques, C.H., Lynch, J.C., Samkoff, J.S. "The effects of sleep loss on cognitive performance of resident physicians," *Journal of Family Practice* 30 (1990), pp. 223–29.

200   in both tired and rested conditions: Engel, W., Seime, R., Powell, V., D'Alessandri, R. "Clinical performance of interns after being on call," *Southern Medical Journal* 80 (1987), pp. 761–63 (regarding ER residents); Christensen, E.E., Deitz, G.W., Murry, R.C., Moore, J.G. "The effect of fatigue on resident performance," *Radiology* 125 (1977), pp. 103–05 (regarding the radiologists).

200   most residents were driving alone: Steele, M.T., Ma, O.J., Watson, W.A., et al. "The occupational risk of motor vehicle collisions for emergency medicine residents," *Academic Emergency Medicine* 6 (1999), pp. 1050–53.

200   "If the law judges us unsafe to drive…": Jeffers, R., Jeys, L. "Tired surgical trainees: Unfit to drive but fit to operate?" *BMJ* 324 (2002), p. 173.

201   Experts disagree as to why this happened: Asch, D.A., Parker, R.M. "The Libby Zion case: One step forward or two steps backwards?" *NEJM* 318 (1988), pp. 771–75.

202   resulting in the boy's death: Pankranz, H. "Witness: Doctor dozed: Technician testifies in boy's ear-surgery death," *Denver Post* 15 Sept 1995, p. A1.

202   "The public could interpret…": Philibert, I., Friedmann, P., Williams, W.T., for the members of the ACGME Work Group on Resident Duty Hours. *JAMA* 288 (2002), pp. 1112–14.

204   after ten hours for a mandatory break: The potential harm from fatigued truckers and other drivers was highlighted in Dement, W.C. "The perils of drowsy driving," *NEJM* 337 (1997), pp. 783–84.

206   violating the work-hours limits: *State Health Department Cites 54 Teaching Hospitals for Resident Working-Hour Violations.* Albany: New York State Department of Health, 26 June 2002.

206   "Teaching hospitals can recruit and train…": Weinstein, D.F. "Duty hours for resident physicians—tough choices for teaching hospitals," *NEJM* 347 (2002), pp. 1275–78.

206   "Junior attendings are fearing for their lives": Quote is of Jeffrey Upperman, MD, junior faculty member at Children's Hospital of Pittsburgh, in Croasdale, M. "ACGME gives final nod to 80-hour workweek," *American Medical News* 10 Mar 2003.

206-7 For Yale, see Croasdale, "ACGME gives final nod…" and "Yale surgery accreditation," *NYT* 9 May 2002, p. B6. For Hopkins, see Kohn, D. "Hopkins residency program loses accreditation over labor rules. Some say board made example of med school," *Baltimore Sun* 27 Aug 2003.

207   "Nobody likes a whistleblower": Lamberg, L. "Long hours, little sleep. Bad medicine for physicians in training?" *JAMA* 287 (2002), pp. 303–06. Quote is of Michael Suk, orthopedics surgery resident at Montefiore Medical Center.

CHAPTER 12: HUBRIS AND TEAMWORK

209   The Lighthouse Parable: This possibly apocryphal story was most famously used in Stephen R. Covey's *The 7 Habits of Highly Effective People* (New York: Simon & Schuster, 1989).

210   only a third of the time: Diem, S.J., Lantos, J.D., Tulsky, J.A. "Cardiopulmonary resuscitation on television: Miracles and misinformation," *NEJM* 334 (1996), pp. 1578–82.

210   wildly inflated TV survival rate: Ebell, M.H., Becker, L.A., Barry, H.C., Hagen, M. "Survival after in-hospital cardiopulmonary resuscitation: A meta-analysis," *JGIM* 13 (1998), pp. 805–16; and Fisher, G.S., Tulsky, J.A., Rose, M.R. et al. "Patient knowledge and physician predictions of treatment preferences after discussion of advance directives," *JGIM* 13 (1998), pp. 447–54.

217   contact with particularly offensive doctors: Rosenstein, A.H. "Nurse-physician relationships: Impact on nurse satisfaction and retention," *American Journal of Nursing* 102 (2002), pp. 26–34.

217   care for the aging Baby Boom generation: "The hospital nursing workforce shortage: Immediate and future," *TrendWatch*. Vol. 3., No. 2. (Washington D.C.; American Hospital Association, June 2001), pp. 1–8; *The Healthcare Workforce Shortage and its Implications for America's Hospitals*. Long Beach, Calif: First Consulting Group, Fall 2001; Spratley, E., Johnson, A. Sochalski, J., et al. "The registered nurse population: findings from the National Sample Survey of Registered Nurses: Mar 2000," Washington, D.C.: Health Resources and Service Administration, Feb 2002; Hecker, D.E. "Occupational employment projections to 2010," *Monthly Labor Review* Nov 2001, pp. 57–84.

217   "What is exceptional in nursing…": Abel-Smith, B. *A History of the Nursing Profession* (New York: Springer, 1960).

217   "Most healthcare workers entered...": AHA Commission on Workforce for Hospitals and Health Systems. *In Our Hands: How Hospital Leaders Can Build a Thriving Workforce* (Chicago: American Hospital Association, Apr 2002).

218   leave their jobs in coming year: Spratley, "The registered nurse population..."; also Aiken, L.H., Clarke, S.P., Sloane, D.M., et al. "Nurses' reports on hospital care in five countries," *Health Affairs (Millwood)* 20 (2001), pp. 43–53.

218   dissatisfaction increased 23 percent and 15 percent, respectively: Steinbrook, R. "Nursing in the crossfire," *NEJM* 346 (2002), pp. 1757–66; Aiken, L.H., Clarke, S.P., Sloane, D.M., et al. "Hospital nurse staffing and patient mortality, nurse burnout, and job dissatisfaction," *JAMA* 288 (2002), pp. 1987–93; Needleman, J., Buerhaus, P., Mattke, S., et al. "Nurse-staffing levels and the quality of care in hospitals," *NEJM* 346 (2002), pp. 1715–22.

220   "People don't understand...": Buresh, B., Gordon, S. *From Silence to Voice: What Nurses Know and Must Communicate to the Public* (Canadian Nurses Association, 2000). Quoted in Corbett, S. "The Last Shift," *NYT Magazine* 16 Mar 2003, pp. 58 61.

220   "Nurses prevent bad things...": Ibid.

222   survived a hard-fought operation: "Associated Press: Doctors fined for scuffling in operating room," *San Jose Mercury News* 28 Nov 1993, p. 7A.

223   everyone else goes down as well: Sexton, J.B., Thomas, E.J., Helmreich, R.L. "Error, stress, and teamwork in medicine and aviation: cross sectional surveys," *BMJ* 320 (2000), pp. 745–49.

224   pointing out mistakes made by the captain: Beaty, D. *The Naked Pilot: The Human Factor in Aircraft Accidents* (London: Airlife Publications, 1996), p. 38.

224-6 Captain van Zantent's background is described in "Pair of 747s Collide in Worst Air Disaster of All Time." www.super70s.com/Super70s/Science/Transportation/Aviation/AirDisasters/77-03-27(Tenerife).asp (last accessed March 2, 2005).

225   "On hearing this, the KLM flight...": *Secretary of Aviation (Spain) Report on Tenerife Crash.* Oct 1978. Aircraft Accident Digest (ICAO Circular 153-AN/56), pp. 22–68.

227   just now being tried in medicine: Helmreich, R.L., Wilhlem, J.A., Gregorich, S.E., Chidester, T.R. "Preliminary results from evaluation of cockpit resource management training: Performing ratings of flight crews," *Aviation, Space, and Environmental Medicine* 61 (1990), pp. 576–79. In a seven-year study of near-misses relayed to the Aviation Safety Reporting System, 70 percent of aviation errors were linked to poor information transfer and questionable personal interactions in the cockpit. See Billings, C.E., Reynard, W.D. "Human factors in aircraft incidents: Results of a 7-year study," *Aviation, Space, and Environmental Medicine* 55 (1984), pp. 960–65. Observations also showed, not surprisingly, that crews who

had not previously worked together suffered higher accident rates than those who had. Even though a vast study of more than 17,000 ICU patients showed that strong teamwork, good coordination, and positive conflict resolution are strongly associated with better critical care outcomes, medicine has been slow to embrace this obvious cure to at least one cause of our error epidemic. See Shortell, S.M., Zimerman, J.E., Rousseau, D.M., et al. "The performance of intensive care units: Does good management make a difference?" *Medical Care* 32 (1994), pp. 508–25.

227-8 "How do we prevent...": Interview with John Nance, March 3, 2000. At www. bookreporter.com/authors/au-nance-john.asp (Last accessed March 2, 2005).

228   lives of thirteen young firefighters: The Mann Gulch incident was first described in *Young Men and Fire* by Norman MacLean (Chicago: University of Chicago Press, 1992). The analysis of the incident was published by Karl Weick in a paper, "The Collapse of Sensemaking in Organizations: The Mann Gulch Disaster," *Administrative Science Quarterly* 38 (1993), pp. 628–53; and his book, *Sensemaking in Organizations* (Thousand Oaks, Calif.: Sage Publications, 1995). The incident was famously described, and analogized to patient safety, by Don Berwick in his essay, *Escape Fire: Lessons for the Future of Healthcare*, published by the Commonwealth Fund, 2002.

230   times are below one hour: Cannon, C.P., Gibson, C.M., Lambrew, C.T., et al. "Relationship of symptom-onset-to-balloon time and door-to-balloon time with mortality in patients undergoing angioplasty for acute myocardial infarction," *JAMA* 283 (2000), pp. 2941–47.

230   "We do loads of practice...": The Pitstop Story. Featuring Jacques Villeneuve and Alistair Gibson. www.jacques.villeneuve.com/express/2001/article69.htm (last accessed March 2, 2005).

231   mutual respect—among caregivers: Gittell, J.H., Fairfield, K.M., Bierbaum, B., et al. "Impact of relational coordination on the quality of care, post-operative pain and functioning, and the length of stay: A nine-hospital study of surgical patients," *Medical Care* 38 (2000), pp. 807–19.

CHAPTER 13: THE OTHER END OF THE STETHOSCOPE

237   unwittingly promote—medical errors: This case was analyzed in our medical errors journal, *AHRQ WebM&M*, by Drs. Bernard Lo and James Tulsky in July 2003. See "Code Status Confusion" at http://webmm.ahrq.gov/spotlightcases.aspx?ic=25 (last accessed March 2, 2005).

238   from a patient's perspective: Braddock, C.H., Edwards, K.A., Hasenburg, N.M., et al. "Informed decision making in outpatient practice: Time to get back to basics," *JAMA* 282 (1999), pp. 2313–20.

238   patient's own recitation of his clinical complaint: Langewitz, W., Denz, M., Keller, A., et al. "Spontaneous talking time at start of consultation in outpatient clinic: Cohort study,"

BMJ 325 (2002), pp. 682–83.

239-40 only 10 percent of the cases: Tulsky, J.A., Chesney, M.A., Lo, B. "How do medical residents discuss resuscitation with patients?" *JGIM* 10 (1995), pp. 436–42.

240 in North Carolina and Pittsburgh: Fischer, G.S., Tulsky, J.A., Rose, M.R., et al. "Patient knowledge and physician predictions of treatment preferences after discussion of advance directives," *JGIM* 13 (1998), pp. 447–54; and Tulsky, J.A., Fischer, G.S., Rose, M.R., Arnold, R.M. "Opening the black box: How do physicians communicate about advance directives?" *Ann Intern Med* 129 (1998), pp. 441–49.

241 "A poorly worded conversation...": Tulsky, J.A., Chesney, M.A., Lo, B. "See one, do one, teach one? House staff experience discussing do-not-resuscitate orders," *Arch Intern Med* 156 (1996), pp. 1285–89.

242 outcomes in diseases like diabetes: For prevalence of low health literacy, see Gazmararian, J.A., Baker, D.W., Williams, M.V., et al. "Health literacy among Medicare enrollees in a managed care organization," *JAMA* 281 (1999), pp. 545–51; and Williams, M.V., Parker, R.M., Baker, D.W., et al. "Inadequate functional health literacy among patients at two public hospitals," *JAMA* 274 (1995), pp. 1677–82. For poor health outcomes in diabetes: Schillinger, D., Grumbach, K., Piette, J., et al. "Association of health literacy with diabetes outcomes," *JAMA* 288 (2002), pp. 475–82.

244 had put them two weeks earlier: We thank our colleague, Dr. Dean Schillinger, for sharing this case with us.

245 used instead of professional interpreters: Flores, G., Laws, M.B., Mayo, S.J., et al. "Errors in medical interpretation and their potential clinical consequences in pediatric encounters," *Pediatrics* 111 (2003), pp. 6–14.

245-6 urging patients to "Speak Up!": Joint Commission on Accreditation of Healthcare Organizations.

246 "In the traditional medical model...": Landro, L. "Steps that you can take to safeguard your care," *WSJ* 13 Mar 2003.

246 cross the room to the sink: Lipsett, P.A., Swoboda, S.M. "Handwashing compliance depends on professional status," *Surgical Infections (Larchmont)* 2 (2001), pp. 241–45.

247 no towels required: Parienti, J.J., Thibon, P., Heller, R., et al. "Hand-rubbing with an aqueous alcoholic solution vs traditional surgical hand-scrubbing and 30-day surgical site infection rates: A randomized equivalence study," *JAMA* 288 (2002), pp. 72227; and Bissett, L. "Can alcohol hand rubs increase compliance with hand hygiene?" *British Journal of Nursing* 11 (2002), pp. 1072, 1074–77.

248 just what the doctor ordered: Kaufman, J. "Caveat Emptor," *New York* 2 Dec 2002, pp. 28, 30.

251   "When Dr. Jaggers was done...": http://members.cox.net/myrossprocedure/ RPExp/exp06.html (posted January 1, 1999, last accessed March 2, 2005).

253   Alfred Hitchcock, not Frank Capra: The description of the Duke case is drawn from a number of sources. Among the most helpful were: Draper, M. "A hopeful heart," *The News and Observer* 10 Jan 2003, p. 1; Shamp, J. "Duke transplant error requires NASA-like probe, agency says," *The Herald Sun* 19 Feb 2003, p. A1; Landro, L. "Transplant mistake pushes hospitals to prevent errors," *WSJ* 20 Feb 2003, p. 1; Barclay, L. "ABO incompatibility in heart-lung transplant: An expert interview with Robert A. Metzger, MD," available at http://www.medscape.com/viewarticle/449763. 21 Feb 2003 (last accessed March 2, 2005); Altman, L.K. "Even the elite hospitals aren't immune to errors," *NYT* 23 Feb 2003, p. 16; Archibold, R.C. "Girl in transplant mix-up dies after two weeks," *NYT* 23 Feb 2003, p. 16; Gettleman, J., Altman, L.K. "Grave diagnosis after 2nd transplant," *NYT* 23 Feb 2003, p. A11; Altman, L.K. "Doctors discuss transplant mistake," *NYT* 23 Feb 2003, p. A11; Vedantam. S. "Surgical expertise, undone by error," *WP* 24 Feb 2003, p. A1; Adler, J. "'A tragic error,'" *Newsweek* 3 Mar 2003, pp. 20–25; Kher, U., Cuardos, P. "A miracle denied," *Time* Magazine 3 Mar 2003, p. 61; *60 Minutes*. CBS-TV 16 Mar 2003; Comarow, A. "Jesica's story: One mistake didn't kill her—the organ donor system was fatally flawed," *U.S. News & World Report* 28 July 2003, pp. 51–72. Additional sources include several media statements released by Duke, and other information on the Duke University Medical Center and UNOS websites.

255   who *was* a perfect fit: According to Comarow in *U.S. News & World Report*, "it isn't terribly unusual for a suitable candidate not to appear on the match-run list," but the reasons for this in general—or in Jesica's specific case—remain obscure.

262-3 "First, patients are unintentially harmed...": Vincent, C. "Understanding and responding to adverse events," *NEJM* 348 (2003), pp. 1051–56.

263   honesty is always the best policy: Karman, S.S., Hamm, G. "Risk management: extreme honesty may be the best policy," *Ann Intern Med* 131 (1999), pp. 963–67.

263   "Everything you read...": Gallagher, T.H., Waterman, A.D., Ebers, A.G., et al. "Patients' and physicians' attitudes regarding the disclosure of medical errors," *JAMA* 289 (2003), pp. 1001–07.

264   had told them about it: Wu, A.W., Folkman, S., McPhee, S.J., Lo, B. "Do house officers learn from their mistakes?" *JAMA* 265 (1991), pp. 2089–94; and Blendon, R.J., DesRoches, C.M., Brodie, M., et al. "Views of practicing physicians and the public on medical errors," *NEJM* 347 (2002), pp. 1933–40.

264   "[I'd want the doctor...]": Gallagher, "Patients' and physicians' attitudes...," p. 1004.

264   "You would love to be just straightforward...": ibid., p. 1005.

265   "Her doctors continue to monitor her progress…": Adler, J., "'A tragic error,'" p. 24.

265   "In our efforts to identify organs…": ibid.

266   "This is an example…": Comarow, "Jesica's story"

266   fatigued and inadequately supervised: Robins, N. *The Girl Who Died Twice: Every Patient's Nightmare: The Libby Zion Case and the Hidden Dangers of Hospitals* (New York: Delacorte, 1995).

267   Mount Sinai Hospital: Shapiro, D.W. "NY liver donor dies," *Professional Liability Newsletter* 32 (2002), p. 1.

267   Linda McDougal: "Breasts removed by mistake; paperwork slip-up blamed," 21 Jan 2003. Available at www.cnn.com/2003/HEALTH/01/20/cnna.mastectomy.mistake/ index.html (last accessed March 2, 2005).

268   favor the former over the latter: The quality comparisons are in Rosenthal, G.E., Harper, D.L., Quinn, L.M. Cooper, G.S. "Severity-adjusted mortality and length of stay in teaching and nonteaching hospitals: Results of a regional study," *JAMA* 278 (1997), pp. 485–90; Ayanian, J.Z., Weissman, J.S. "Teaching hospitals and quality of care: A review of the literature," *Milbank Quarterly* 80 (2002), pp. 569–93; Polanczyk, C.A., Lane, A., Coburn, M., et al. "Hospital outcomes in major teaching, minor teaching, and nonteaching hosptials in New York state," *Am J Med* 112 (2002), pp. 255–61.

Teaching hospitals tend to document errors and complications better than do nonteaching hospitals, which can create the appearance of being more error-prone. Teaching hospitals also have higher "rescue rates" (i.e., preventing or decreasing the harm after an adverse event). This means that, among patients who do suffer complications of medical care, the outcomes are better at teaching hospitals, which further bolsters the case that higher rates of adverse events at teaching hospitals (when present) reflect more compulsive documentation, not poorer quality. See Silber, J.H., Williams, S.V., Krakauer, H., Schwartz, J.S. "Hospital and patient characteristics associated with death after surgery: A study of adverse occurrence and failure to rescue," *Medical Care* 30 (1992), pp. 615–29; Silber, J.H., Rosenbaum, P.R., Schwartz, J.S., et al. "Evaluation of the complication rate as a measure of quality of care in coronary artery bypass graft surgery," *JAMA* 274 (1995), pp. 317–23; Aiken, L.H., Clark, S.P., Sloan, D.M., et al. "Hospital nurse staffing and patient mortality, nurse burnout, and job dissatisfaction," *JAMA* 288 (2002), pp. 1987–93.

268   *the* major source of errors: Altman, L.K. "Even the elite hospitals aren't immune to errors," *NYT* 23 Feb 2003, p. 16.

270   "It was the mirror held up…": Millenson, M.L. "Pushing the profession," pp. 57–63.

CHAPTER 15: WHETHER REPORTS?

275   the diagnostic wheels turn: These are classic descriptions of porphyria (the urine turning color) and carcinoid syndrome (the wheezing and rash).

276   "Precisely because of its technological wonders...": Hilfiker, D. "Mistakes," in *On Doctoring*. Reynolds, R. and Stone, J., eds. (New York: Simon & Schuster, 1991), pp. 376–87.

277   errors they committed themselves: Pierluissi, E., Fischer, M.A., Campbell, A.R., Landefeld, C.S. "Are medical errors discussed in Morbidity and Mortality Conferences?" *JAMA* 290 (2003), in press.

277   "I felt a sense of shame...": Gawande, *Complications*, p. 61.

278   "After the case of Mr. Will...": Bosk, *Forgive and Remember*, pp. 140–41.

279   "You are supposed to give...": Gallagher, "Patients' and physicians' attitudes," p. 1005.

279   "putting on the hair shirt...": Bosk, *Forgive and Remember*, p. 144.

280   "You know that there's no one looking...": Bosk, *Forgive and Remember*, p. 145.

281   achieve the required degree of trust: Hutchinson, A. "Patient safety: research and practice lessons from the United States: Report of a study visit September to November 2002," White paper presented at the second annual AHRQ patient safety conference, Arlington, VA. 2–4 Mar 2003.

283   track record for dealing with them: Reported at the Annual Meeting of the American College of Preventive Medicine, Feb 2003.

284   so far none has passed): "House passes bill to track medical errors voluntarily," *WSJ* 12 Mar 2003.

285   stakes are higher—are investigated: Hutchinson, "Patient safety...," p. 14.

286   resolve or eliminate the problem: "Aircraft Accident Report: Trans World Airlines Boeing 727-231, Berryville, Virginia, Dec 1, 1974" (Washington D.C.: National Transportation Safety Board; 1975), Report NTSB-AAR-75-16.

286   in the aviation system: FAA. *Aviation safety action programs* (Washington, D.C.: FAA, 1999), Advisory Circular 120-66A; Reason, *Managing the risks*, pp. 196–205; Billings, C.E., Reynard, W.D. "Human factors in aircraft incidents: Results of a 7-year study," *Aviation, Space, and Environmental Medicine* 55 (1994), pp. 960–65; Billings, C.E. "Some hopes and concerns regarding medical event-reporting systems. Lessons from NASA Aviation Safety Reporting System," *Archives of Pathology and Laboratory Medicine* 122 (1998), pp. 214–15; Barach, P., Small, S.D. "Reporting and preventing medical mishaps: Lessons from

nonmedical near-miss reporting systems," *BMJ* 320 (2000), pp. 759–63; and Thomas E.J., Helmreich, R.L. "Will airline safety models work in medicine?" In Rosenthal, *Medical Error*, pp. 217–34. Quotes are from FAA Advisory Circular; Aviation Safety Reporting Program. FAA AC No. 00-46; May 1975.

287   decreased tenfold over the past twenty years: "Accidents and Accident Rates by NTSB Classification, 1983 through 2002, for U.S. Air Carriers Operating under 14 CFR 121," Table 2.

288   reports back to participating institutions: Provonost, P. "Intensive Care Safety Reporting System," report at the second annual AHRQ patient safety conference, Arlington, Va., 2–4 Mar 2003; and Dr. Peter Pronovost, personal communication, 3 Oct 2003.

289   "This is one of the few businesses…": Gallagher, "Patients' and physicians' attitudes," p. 1005.

289   "Virtually every practitioner…": Wu, A.W. "Medical error: The second victim: The doctor who makes the mistake needs help too," *BMJ* 320 (2000), pp. 726–27.

290   network of hospitals, clinics, and nursing homes: Landro, L. "New push after transplant tragedy: Hospitals search for ways to prevent errors, help doctors learn from others," *WSJ* 20 Feb 2003, p. 1.

CHAPTER 16: MALPRACTICE

295   transferring the patient downstairs: The best analogy would be if you had a heart attack a few minutes from the hospital. If you were very—but not desperately—ill, it might make sense for your spouse to drive you to the ER rather than wait there for the ambulance.

296   "…that's why I'm leaving medicine.": This case was first presented in our series, Quality Grand Rounds: Brennan, T.A., Mello, M.M. "Patient safety and medical malpractice: a case study," *Ann Intern Med* 139 (2003), pp. 267–73.

297   weaves them into a single system: This section on malpractice is drawn from a number of sources, but we particularly relied upon Alan Merry and Alexander McCall Smith's superb book, *Errors, Medicine and the Law* (Cambridge: Cambridge University Press, 2001).

298   check at his local bank: ibid., p. 24; Anon. "Surgeon who left an operation to run an errand is suspended," *NYT* 9 Aug 2002, p. A13.

298   morphine during house calls: Stewart, J.B. *Blind Eye: How the Medical Establishment Let a Doctor Get Away with Murder* (New York: Simon & Schuster, 1999); O'Neill, B. "Doctor as murderer," *BMJ* 320 (2000), pp. 329–30.

299   "All too often…": Merry, *Errors, Medicine, and the Law*, p. 173.

299   "The tendency in such circumstances…" : Ibid., pp. 103–04.

299   "Apportioning blame has no material role...": Reason, *Managing the Risks*, p. 208; Johnston, N. "Do blame and punishment have a role in organizational risk management?" *Flight Deck*. Spring 1995, pp. 33–36.

300   and were more careful: West, D.W., Levine, S., Magram, G., et al. "Pediatric medication order error rates related to the mode of order transmission," *Archives of Pediatric and Adolescent Medicine* 148 (1994), pp. 1322-26.

303   "is not an extraordinary or unusual creature...": *Arland v. Taylor* [1955] OR 131 at 152; cited in Merry, *Errors, Medicine, and the Law,* p. 181.

303   "It is essential that the law...": ibid., p. 132.

304   and the system better: Blumenthal, D. "Making medical errors into 'medical treasures.'" *JAMA* 272 (1994), pp. 1867-68.

305   without jeopardizing quality care: Kessler, D., McClellan, M. "Do doctors practice defensive medicine?" *Quarterly Journal of Economics* 111 (1996), pp. 353–90.

305   no evidence that they commit fewer errors: Mello, M.M., Brennan, T.A. "Deterrence of medical errors: Theory and evidence for malpractice reform," *University of Texas Law Review* 80 (2002), pp. 1595–1638; Dewees, D., Trebilcock, M. "The efficacy of the tort system and its alternatives: A review of empirical evidence," *Osgoode Hall Law Journal* 30 (1992), pp. 57–138; Blendon, R.J., Schoen, C., DesRoches, C., et al. "Common concerns amid diverse systems: Health care experiences in five countries," *Health Affairs (Millwood)* 22 (2003), pp. 106–21.

305   negligent care file claims: Localio, "Relation between malpractice claims...," pp. 245–51; and Studdert, "Negligent care and malpractice...," pp. 250–60.

306   or even the patient's family: Brennan, "Patient safety and medical malpractice"; and Brennan, T.A. Quality Grand Rounds conference, UCSF Medical Center, 4 Dec 2002.

306   New York Harbor: *United States v. Carroll Towing.* 159 F 2d 169 (147).

306   61 percent of the time: "Current award trends in personal injury, 2002 edition. Jury Verdict Research," *American Medical News* 14 Apr 2003, p. 9.

307   risks of being sued: Hickson, G.B., Federspiel, C.F., Pichert, J.W., et al. "Patient complaints and malpractice risk," *JAMA* 287 (2002), pp. 2951–57.

307   a sense of humor: Levinson, W., Roter, D.L., Mullooly, J.P., et al. "Physician-patient communication," *JAMA* 277 (1997), pp. 553-59.

307   leaves much to be desired: Brennan, T.A. Quality Grand Rounds conference, UCSF Medical Center, 4 Dec 2002.

308   doctor has done nothing wrong: Localio, "Relation between malpractice claims," pp. 245–51; and Studdert, "Negligent care and malpractice," pp. 250–60.

309   "both lopsided and mismatched": in Studdert, "Incidence types of adverse events."

310   speeders fly by unscathed: Weiler, P.C., Hiatt, H.H., Newhouse, J.P., et al. *A Measure of Malpractice: Medical Injury, Malpractice Litigation, and Patient Compensation* (Cambridge: Harvard University Press, 1993), p. 75.

310   doubled since 1997: DeFrances, C.J., Smith, S.K., Langan, P.A., et al. *Civil Jury Cases and Verdicts in Large Counties.* Bureau of Justice Statistics Special Report. (Washington, D.C.; U.S. Department of Justice, Office of Justice Programs; 1995), NCJ-154346, pp. 1–14; "Trends in Personal Injury Awards," *Jury Verdict Research,* 2002.

310   to find a new doctor: *LAT* 4 Mar 2002.

310   nursing homes spend billions more: Treaster, J.B. "Malpractice insurance: no clear or easy answers," *NYT* 5 Mar 2003, pp. C1, C3; Armstrong, J. "Malpractice rates leading doctors to drop coverage," *Physicians Financial News* 15 May 2002.

310   Las Vegas's major trauma center: *WP* 4 July 2002.

310   "Physicians are generally very independent...": Albert, T. "N.J. physicians stop work in biggest liability protest yet," *American Medical News* 17 Feb 2003, pp. 46:1–2.

311   "our own proselytizing...": Quote from Troy Brennan at the December 4, 2002 Quality Grand Rounds conference at UCSF.

311   one-third the national average: "NAIC Profitability by Line by State, 2001," presented before the House Judiciary Committee by PIAA, June 2002.

312   her breast biopsy specimen: Stolberg, S.G. "Lobbyists on both sides duel in the medical malpractice debate," *NYT* 12 Mar 2003, p. A19.

312   of keeping doctors in business: No federal malpractice cap was enacted during this 2003 legislative passion play, but the state of Florida passed its own cap of $500,000. See James, J. "Legislature approves malpractice overhaul," *Miami Herald* 14 Aug 2003, p. 1A. A July 2003 study by researchers at the Agency for Healthcare Research and Quality demonstrated a relationship between the presence of pain-and-suffering malpractice caps and the supply of physicians in a given state. Hellinger, F.J., Encinosa, W.E. "The impact of state laws limiting malpractice awards on the geographic distribution of physicians," 3 July 2003.

313   a 1990 study by Troy Brennan... : Brennan, T.A., Localio, A.R., Leape, L.L., et al. "Identification of adverse events during hospitalization," *Ann Intern Med* 112 (1990), pp. 221-26.

313   "to my knowledge, it was never discussed..." : Brennan, "Patient safety and medical malpractice."

313   "From the public's point of view...": Mohr, J.C. "American malpractice litigation in historical perspective," *JAMA* 283 (2000), pp. 1731–37; Millenson, "Pushing the profession," pp. 57–63.

Interestingly, in societies that lack a respected legal system to redress these concerns, families may be more likely to extract their own "justice." In the late 1990s, a Beijing neurosurgeon was attacked by a man whose father had died after an operation to remove a brain tumor. The attacker struck the doctor with a mirror, severing nerves and tendons and probably preventing him from ever practicing his delicate art again. Four months later, a fifty-five-year-old farmer, dissatisfied with the results of eye surgery, returned to the Third Municipal Hospital in Chongquing and set off a bomb, killing himself, his physician, and three bystanders. And these were only two of 525 medical assault cases reported in the People's Republic during the previous few years. These cases were examined by our former UCSF colleague, Dr. Jerry Lazarus, who spent three years teaching medicine in Beijing. His conclusions are illuminating: "It has everything to do with the culture of punishment in contemporary Chinese medicine. 'Kill one to save a hundred,' said an associate professor at one of China's leading medical schools. 'We use punishment to ensure quality.' As a result, hospitals and doctors don't admit mistakes. A high-ranking medical leader at another institution whispered, 'We have no medical errors because if you make a mistake your career is over.' (Lazarus, G. "Sick and tired of their own system Chinese lash out at doctors long before SARS," *WP* 4 May 2003, p. B04).

314   "Health care professionals and patients...": Gulland, A. "Doctors must be free of the 'confetti of interference,'" *BMJ* 325 (2002), p. 1190.

CHAPTER 17: ACCOUNTABILITY

318   can be missed by the scanner: This case took place in the early 1990s; modern CAT scanners are less apt to miss cerebellar pathology, though MRI is still better at imaging this region.

320   accept the patient in transfer: In fact, this kind of remote monitoring by specialized experts is becoming more common, and seems to work. A system pioneered at Johns Hopkins beams video images and all pertinent patient data (vital signs, blood tests, medication doses, X-rays) to a specialist in intensive care medicine sitting at a console like a NASA controller. There is good evidence that ICUs that can't afford to have their own critical care specialists on site (and there is a huge shortage of trained intensivists in the U.S.) but use this remote monitoring system have far better results than those who go without the specialists' input (Angus, D.C., Kelley, M.A., Schmitz, R.J., et al. "Caring for the critically ill patient. Current and projected workforce requirements for care of the critically ill and patients with pulmonary disease: can we meet the requirements of an aging population?" *JAMA* 284 (2000), pp. 2762–70 (for the intensivist shortage); and Rosenfeld, B.A., Dorman T., Breslow, M.J., et al. "Intensive care unit telemedicine: Alternate paradigm for providing continuous intensivist care," *Critical Care Medicine* 28 (2000), pp. 3925–31 (for remote ICU monitoring)).

321   "There is no accountability": Discussion with the authors, March 3, 2003.

322   "This is the way...": Reason, *Managing the Risks*, p. 211.

324   "When a skilled, decent...": Gawande, *Complications*, p. 95.

324-5 "Amid the uproar...": Wolfe, S.M. "Bad doctors get a free ride," *NYT* 4 Mar 2003, p. A27.

325   longer than their younger counterparts: Kershaw, S. "In insurance cost, woes for doctors and women," *NYT* 29 May 2003, p. A16.

325   "Seeing them get away with it...": Reason, *Managing the Risks,* p. 212.

326   "The professional's last line of defense...": Bosk, *Forgive and Remember,* p. 171.

CHAPTER 18: ATTACKING A NEW DISEASE

329   take on the gay population: Centers for Disease Control. "Pneumocystis Pneumonia— Los Angeles." *MMWR* 5 June 1981, pp. 250-52.

330-1 actually one in 300: Gerberding, J. "Incidence and prevalence of human immunodeficiency virus, hepatitis B virus, hepatitis C virus, and cytomegalovirus among health care personnel at risk for blood exposure; final report from a longitudinal study," *Journal of Infectious Diseases* 172 (1995), pp. 1410–17.

331   Written up in the *New England Journal of Medicine:* Gerberding, J.L., Hopewell, P.C., Kaminsky, L.S., Sande, M.A. "Transmission of hepatitis B without transmission of AIDS by accidental needlestick," *NEJM* 312 (1985), pp. 5657.

331-2 "The dominant feature...was silence...": Mann, J. M., "AIDS: A Worldwide Pandemic", in *Current Topics in AIDS*, Vol. 2, Gottlieb, M.S., Jeffries, D.J., Mildvan, D., et al., eds. (New York: John Wiley & Sons, 1989).

332   80 percent drop in mortality: www.cdc.gov/hiv/stats/hasr1302/table21.htm (last accessed March 2, 2005).

334   had begun to dominate it: Wachter, R.M. *The Fragile Coalition: Science, Activists, and AIDS* (New York: St. Martin's Press, 1991).

334-5 a giant condom in 1991: At this writing, the best-known patient safety advocacy group is probably Persons United Limiting Substandards and Errors in health care (PULSE), a group funded by a Long Island mother whose child died after a tonsillectomy. ACT UP was the AIDS group that pulled off the condom stunt; the condom was printed with the message: "A condom to stop unsafe politics. Helms is deadlier than a virus."

CHAPTER 19: WHAT CAN POLICYMAKERS DO?

338   committees all over the country: Shojania, K.G., Duncan, B.W., McDonald, K.M., Wachter, R.M., eds. *Making Health Care Safer: A Critical Analysis of Patient Safety Practices.* Evidence Report/Technology Assessment No. 43 from the Agency for Healthcare Research

and Quality: AHRQ Publication No. 01-E058 (2001). The IOM report was supported by grants from the Commonwealth Fund and the National Resource Council; the latter is the funding arm of the National Academy of Sciences and receives significant federal support.

339   such accidents have already happened: Gosbee, J., Gosbee, L.L. "Flying object hits MRI," *AHRQ WebM&M*, http://webmm.ahrq.gov/cases.aspx?ic=4, (last accessed March 2, 2005); Chaljub, J., Kramer, L.A., Johnson, R.F. III, et al. "Projectile cylinder accidents resulting from the presence of ferro-magnetic nitrous oxide or oxygen tanks in the MR suite," *American Journal of Roentgenology* 177 (2001), pp. 27–30.

339   "Medicine used to be simple...": Chantler, C. "The role and education of doctors in the delivery of health care," *Lancet* 353 (1999), pp. 1178–81.

344   overall claims records showed improvement: Brennan, "Patient safety and medical malpractice"

344   "I've been proselytizing..." : Quote from Troy Brennan at the December 4, 2002 Quality Grand Rounds conference at UCSF.

345-6 compensation scheme too expensive and cumbersome: Merry, *Errors, Medicine and the Law*, p. 223–29.

346   "an army of administrators and case managers...": ibid., p. 225–26.

346   effective and highly popular: Rosenthal, M.M. *Dealing with Medical Malpractice: The British and Swedish Experience* (London: Tavistock, 1987).

346   benefits of a nonadversarial process: Studdert, D.M., Brennan, T.A., Thomas, E.J. "What have we learned since the Harvard Medical Practice Study," in Rosenthal, *Medical Error*, pp. 3–33; Studdert, D.M., Brennan, T.A. "No-fault compensation for medical injuries. The prospect for error prevention," *JAMA* 286 (2001), pp. 217–23.

346   "Societies, just like the operators of hazardous systems...": Reason, *Managing the Risks*, p. 188.

CHAPTER 20: A CULTURE OF SAFETY

348   can do some great things: This model is described by CDC director Julie Gerberding in one of our *Quality Grand Rounds* articles: Gerberding, J.L. "Hospital-onset infections: a patient safety issue," *Ann Intern Med* 137 (2002), pp. 665–70.

349   patient identification and medication errors: Metzger, J., Forten, J. *Computerized Physician Order Entry in Community Hospitals: Lessons from the Field*. Prepared by the California HealthCare Foundation and First Consulting Group (2003).

349   political leaders give the go-ahead: Bates, D.W., Gawande, A.A. "Improving safety with information technology," *NEJM* 348 (2003), pp. 2526–34.

350   preventable errors in California hospitals *each week*: This cost of retrofitting estimate comes from a comprehensive report by RAND, commissioned by the California HealthCare Foundation: Mead C, Kulick J, Hillestad R. *Estimating the Compliance Costs for California SB1953* (2001). Forty-seven of the earthquake deaths in hospitals occurred with the collapse of the VA hospital in Sylmar during the 1971 San Fernando Valley earthquake. The estimate of 100 medical error deaths in California hospitals per week comes from the lower bounds of the Harvard Medical Practice Study/IOM estimate of 44,000 deaths/year in the U.S. California has one-ninth of the population of the United States, and thus would be expected to have 4,900 deaths per year, or 94 deaths per week. The legislation, of course, is intended to ensure that hospitals would remain standing to treat the injured during a major quake, but there have been virtually no reported deaths in the past century attributed to damaged hospitals that were unable to care for quake victims. See Schultz, C.H., Koenig, K.L., Lewis, R.J.. "Implications of hospital evacuation after the Northridge, California earthquake," *NEJM* 348 (2003), pp. 1349–55.

350   perhaps the most vital step: Singer, S.J., Gaba, D.M., Geppert, J.J., et al. "The culture of safety: results of an organization-wide survey in 15 California hospitals," *Quality and Safety in Health Care* 12 (2003), pp. 112–18.

351   mortality rate of one in four: Wolfe T. *The Right Stuff* (New York: Farrar, Straus, Giroux, 1979), p. 22; "Drinking..." is on p. 37. Dr. Atul Gawande first highlighted this comparison between the Mercury astronauts and modern physicians in a speech to the Association for Surgical Education on May 6, 2000: *Focus on Surgical Education* 17 (2000), p. 12–19. *The Right Stuff* has been criticized as being overly melodramatic: In fact, Yeager was a disciplined flier and not a showboater—the X-plane fliers were often rushed into testing unproven technologies and exceeding impossible limits by the Cold War imperatives of the day. Many journalists were surprised to learn years later that Yeager, when driving to work, never exceeded the speed limit and said he regularly "pissed off" motorists stuck behind him on narrow desert highways.

351   "An experienced zombie would do fine...": Wolfe, *The Right Stuff*, p. 181.

352   what they call "cookbook medicine": Reinertsen, J.L. "Zen and the art of physician autonomy maintenance," *Ann Intern Med* 138 (2003), pp. 992–95.

It is important to add that an unfettered embrace of a robotic system in which physicians lose the capacity to improvise or personalize their care would be disastrous. Even in commercial aviation—which has wholeheartedly embraced a more systematic, regimented approach— the successful pilot knows when to break the mold. On July 19, 1989, United Flight 232, a McDonnell Douglas DC-10, suddenly lost all three of its hydraulic systems. The designers of the plane considered this situation so unlikely (less than one-in-a-billion chance) that they had not designed any emergency procedures for it. As Captain Alfred Haynes later recalled: "That left us at 37,000 feet with no ailerons to control roll, no rudders to coordinate a turn, no elevators to control pitch, no leading edge devices to help us slow down, no trailing edge flaps to be used in landing, no spoilers on the wings to slow us down in flight or help braking on the ground, no nosewheel steering, and no brakes. That did not leave us a great deal to work with." Haynes and his copilots improvised a solution, alternating the throttles first on the right-, then left-sided engines to skid the aircraft through the air in descending 'S' turns, like a skier traversing a steep slope. Their improvisation saved the lives of nearly 200 people. (Haynes, A.C. "United 232: Coping with the loss of all flight controls," *Flight Deck* 3 (1992), pp. 5–21. The Flight 232 story is described in Reason, *Managing the Risks*, p. 79). Future health care providers must have the training and the blessing to try innovative approaches when the standard operating procedures won't do. But that cannot be their daily diet.

CHAPTER 21: A SYSTEM OF SAFETY

355   James Reason tells a moving story: Reason, *Managing the Risks*, pp. 15–16; the *Legasov Tapes*, transcript prepared by the U.S. Department of Energy (1988). The original material appeared in *Pravda* shortly after Legasov's death.

356   these by themselves are not insurmountable: Shojania, *Making Health Care Safer*; Shojania, K.G., Duncan, B.W., McDonald, K.M., Wachter, R.M. "Safe but sound: Patient safety meets evidence-based medicine," *JAMA* 288 (2002), pp. 508–513. The evidence on CPOE is becoming increasingly persuasive; at this point, our main concern is that it comes from a handful of pioneering institutions (namely Boston's Brigham and Women's Hospital and Indiana's Regenstrief Medical Center) where highly motivated leaders and researchers have made a huge institutional investment in making it work. Whether an off-the-shelf CPOE system will improve safety at the average community hospital, a rural hospital, or a cash-strapped county hospital remains to be seen.

357   potentially effective therapy, AZT, was published: Yarchoan, R., Klecker, R.W., Weinhold, K.J., et al. "Administration of 3'-azido-3'deoxythymidine, an inhibitor of HTLV-III/LAV replication, to patients with AIDS or AIDS-related complex," *Lancet* 1 (1986), pp. 575–80. AZT was approved for use by the FDA in March 1987.

358   improved quality and patient safety: Jha, A.K., Perlin, J.B., Kizer, K.W., Dudley, R.A. "Effect of the transformation of the Veterans Affairs Health Care System on the quality of care," *NEJM* 348 (2003), pp. 2218–27; and Bagian, J.P., Lee, C., Gosbee, J., et al. "Developing and deploying a patient safety program in a large health care delivery system: You can't fix what you don't know about," *Joint Commission Journal of Quality Improvement* 27 (2001), pp. 522–32.

358   to one in 200,000: Adams, A.P. "Standards and postgraduate training" and Armstrong, R.F. "Monitoring in Anesthesia," in Walker, J.S. ed. *Quality and Safety in Anesthesia* (London: BMJ Publishing, 1994), pp. 31, 173.

359   activists upon which to build their programs: Wachter, R.M. "AIDS, activism, and the politics of health," *NEJM* 326 (1992), pp. 128–33.

360   "Now killing fewer patients?": Boodman, S.G. "No end to errors: Three years after a landmark report found pervasive medical mistakes in American hospitals, little has been done to reduce death and injury," *WP* 3 Dec 2002, p. F1.

361   "Cognizant organizations understand...": Reason, *Managing the Risks*, pp. 114, 37.

CHAPTER 22: WHAT CAN PATIENTS DO?

363   and be subjected to more risks: Barker, K.N., Flynn, E.A., Pepper, G.A., et al. "Medication errors observed in 36 health care facilities," *Arch Intern Med* 162 (2002), pp. 1897–1903. In this study of several thousand medication administrations at a variety of facilities, 19 percent of the administered doses had some sort of error associated with them, but only 7 percent of errors (equivalent to about 1 percent of the total) were potentially harmful. See also Bates, D.W., Cullen, D.J., Laird, N., et al. "Incidence of adverse drug events and potential adverse drug events: Implications for prevention: ADE Prevention Study Group," *JAMA* 274 (1995), pp. 29–34. This study showed that the risk of dying from a medication was about 1 in 2,000, and most of these deaths were from drug side effects rather than errors.

367   we're a few years away from that: Eysenbach, G. "Consumer health informatics," *BMJ* 320 (2000), pp. 1713–16; Larkin, H. "Permanent record: allowing patients to post their own medical records on the Internet is becoming big business," *American Medical News* 8 Nov 1999, pp. 21–22; Schoenfelt, S. "New possibilities for patient information storage in a technological age," *Journal of the American Health Information Management Association* 69 (1998), pp. 50–54; and Chin, T. "Think tank touts portable EMRs for patients," *American Medical News* 11 Nov 2002.

AFTERWORD

373   worried that DNR wristbands would stigmatize patients: The concern about stigma relates to the observation that, although a DNR order is only meant to signify that a patient wishes to decline CPR, patients fear (sometimes for good reason) that clinicians will abandon them and withhold therapies or tests that the patients *would* like to receive.

373   "Before you wear your cool yellow LiveStrong wristband...": Hayes, S. "Wristbands called patient safety risk," *St. Petersburg Times* 10 Dec 2004, p. 1A.

374   even safer five years from now: From a survey using the computerized audience response system at the 8th annual "Management of the Hospitalized Patient" conference, San Francisco, October 2004.

374   only 17 percent thought it was better: Kaiser Family Foundation / Agency for Healthcare Research and Quality / Harvard School of Public Health *National Survey on Consumers' Experiences with Patient Safety and Quality Information*, November 2004.

374   they are unlikely to be repeated: The studies are Brennan, T.A., Leape, L.L., Laird, N.M., et al. "Incidence of adverse events and negligence in hospitalized patients: Results of the Harvard Medical Practice Study I," *NEJM* 324 (1991), pp. 370–76; and Thomas, E.J., Studdert, D.M. Burstin, H.R., et al. "Incidence types of adverse events and negligent care in Utah and Colorado," *Medical Care* 38 (2000), pp. 261–71. They are described more fully in Chapter 3.

375   and workforce and training issues: Bob presented much of this material, including the grades, in more academic prose in: Wachter, R.M., "The end of the beginning: patient safety five years after 'To Err is Human'," *Health Affairs (Millwood)* 2004 Nov 30, available at http://

content.healthaffairs.org/cgi/reprint/hlthaff.w4.534v1 (last accessed January 16, 2005).

375   to see how care is actually delivered: This method, called the "Tracer Methodology," is described in "Tracer methodology: how it can help you improve quality," *Healthcare Benchmarks and Quality Improvement* 11 (2004), pp. 61-63.

376   "I had two main ones...": Quote is from commercial airline pilot Yo Hoffner, who, with a number of colleagues, has begun to do leadership and teamwork training in health care as part of a company called MachOne Leadership.

376   all the reports that *were* submitted: Pérez-Peña, R. "Law to rein in hospital errors is widely abused, audit finds," *NYT* 29 Sept 2004, p. A1.

377   no persuasive evidence that supports this association: Cullen, D.J., et al., "The incident reporting system does not detect adverse events: a problem for quality improvement," *Joint Commission Journal of Quality Improvement* 21 (1995), pp. 541-48.

377   "I'm distressed at the amount of attention...": Quote is from Institute for Healthcare Improvement teleconference, November 17th 2004. Available at www.ihi.org.

378   leading to a near-disastrous drug error: The Cedars-Sinai and Beth Israel cases are described in Chapter 4. A good general article on computer-induced errors is Ash, J.S., Berg, M., and Coiera, E. "Some unintended consequences of information technology in health care: the nature of patient care information system-related errors," *Journal of the American Informatics Association* 11 (2004), pp. 104-12. The heart attack case is Tang, P.C. "Electronic err", AHRQ WebM&M, available at http://webmm.ahrq.gov/cases.aspx?ic=79 and the moving patient case is Lindenauer, P. "Moved too soon," *AHRQ WebM&M*, available at http://webmm.ahrq.gov/cases.aspx?ic=77 (both cases published in October 2004 and last accessed January 16, 2005).

378   well built and implemented: the VA experience is described in Greenfield, S. and Kaplan, S.H., "Creating a culture of quality: the remarkable transformation of the Department of Veterans Affairs health care system," *Ann Intern Med* 141 (2004), pp. 316-18.

379   stronger and more consistent federal support: Brailer's quote is from Lohr, S. "Health care technology is a promise unfinanced," *NYT* 3 Dec 2004, p. C5.

381   will fall from slim to none: The Florida initiative is described in Albert, T. "State reform ballot wins set stage for further battles," *AMA News* 22/29 Nov 2004, p. 1.

381   or nurses are under-trained: Aiken, L.H., et al., "Hospital nurse staffing and patient mortality, nurse burnout, and job dissatisfaction," *JAMA* 288 (2002), pp. 1987–93; Needleman, J., et al., "Nurse-staffing levels and the quality of care in hospitals," *NEJM* 346 (2002), pp. 1715–22; Rogers, A.E., et al., "The working hours of hospital staff nurses and patient safety," *Health Affairs (Millwood)* 23 (2004), pp. 202-12; and Aiken, L.H., et al., "Educational levels of hospital nurses and surgical patient mortality," *JAMA* 290 (2003), pp. 1617-23.

382   free up dollars to meet the ratios: Hackenschmidt, A., "Living with nurse staffing ratios: early experiences," *Journal of Emergency Nursing* 30 (2004), pp. 377-79.

382   or 30 hours per shift): Weinstein, D.F. "Duty hours for resident physicians—tough choices for teaching hospitals," *NEJM* 347 (2002), pp. 1275–78.

382   and a state of-the-art IT system: Landrigan, C.P., et al., "Effect of reducing interns' work hours on serious medical errors in intensive care units," *NEJM* 351 (2004), pp. 1838-48. This was the study in which residents wore electrodes on their heads; its results were pending when we first described the study in Chapter 11. The survey that found that residents are more likely to have car crashes or close calls on the way home after overnight shifts is Barger, L.K., Cade, B.E., Ayas, N.T., et al., "Extended work shifts and the risk of motor vehicle crashes among interns," *NEJM* 352 (2005), pp. 125-34.

382   boards are requiring periodic recertification: For example, see Wasserman, S.I., Kimball, H.R., and Duffy, F.D., "Recertification in Internal Medicine: a program of continuous professional development. Task Force on Recertification," *Ann Intern Med* 133 (2000), pp. 202-8.

383   can improve both performance and safety: Morey, J.C., et al., "Error reduction and performance improvement in the emergency department through formal teamwork training: evaluation results of the MedTeams project," *Health Services Research* 37 (2002), pp. 1553-81. For simulator training, see Lee, S.K., et al., "Trauma assessment training with a patient simulator: a prospective, randomized study," *Journal of Trauma* 55 (2003) pp. 651-57.

APPENDIX IV

399   patient safety practices with the best supporting evidence: Shojania, K.G., Duncan, B.W., McDonald, K.M., Wachter, R.M., eds. *Making Health Care Safer: A Critical Analysis of Patient Safety Practices.* Evidence Report/Technology Assessment No. 43 from the Agency for Healthcare Research and Quality: AHRQ Publication No. 01-E058; 2001. Available at http://www.ahrq.gov/clinic/ptsafety/

399   In general, more is better: A more detailed review of these relationships is Halm, E.A., Lee, C., Chassin, M.R. "Is volume related to outcome in health care? A systematic review and methodologic critique of the literature," *Ann Intern Med* 137 (2002), pp. 511–20. The authors point out that many of the studies citing specific volume thresholds are methodologically weak. Nevertheless, the overall premise that "practice makes perfect" remains largely unchallenged.

400   whether their patient had a urinary catheter: Saint, S., Wiese, J., Amory, J.K., et al. "Are physicians aware of which of their patients have indwelling urinary catheters?" *Am J Med* 109 (2000), pp. 476–80.

401   they worry about blame or are convinced it won't do any good: Reason, *Managing the Risks*, pp. 196–205.

402   associated with better ICU outcomes: This intensivist literature is summarized in Pronovost, P.J., Angus, D.C., Dorman, T., et al. "Physician staffing patterns and clinical outcomes in critically ill patients: A systematic review," *JAMA* 288 (2002), pp. 2151–62. The telemedicine study is Rosenfeld, B.A., Dorman, T., Breslow, M.J., et al. "Intensive care unit telemedicine: Alternate paradigm for providing continuous intensivist care," *Critical Care Medicine* 28 (2000), pp. 3925–31. The hospitalist studies are Auerbach, A.D., Wachter, R.M., Katz, P., et al. "Implementation of a voluntary hospitalist service at a community teaching hospital: Improved clinical efficiency and patient outcomes," *Ann Intern Med* 137 (2002), pp. 859–65; Meltzer, D., Manning, W.G., Morrison, J., et al. "Effects of physician experience on costs and outcomes on an academic general medicine service: Results of a trial of hospitalists," *Ann Intern Med* 137 (2002), pp. 866–74. The hospitalist literature is summarized in Wachter, R.M., Goldman, L. "The hospitalist movement 5 years later," *JAMA* 287 (2002), pp. 487–94.

402   Ratios of more than 6:1 or 7:1...: The patient-to-nurse relationships were shown by Aiken, L.H., Clarke, S.P., Sloane, D.M., et al. "Hospital nurse staffing and patient mortality, nurse burnout, and job dissatisfaction," *JAMA* 288 (2002), pp. 1987–93. The RN ratios were shown in Needleman, J., Buerhaus, P., Mattke, S., et al. "Nurse-staffing levels and the quality of care in hospitals," *NEJM* 346 (2002), pp. 1715–22. Finally, the bachelor's degree study was Aiken, L.H., Clark, S.P., Cheung, R.B., et al. "Educational levels of hospital nurses and surgical patient mortality," *JAMA* 290 (2003), pp. 1617-23.

402   There is good evidence that the involvement of clinical pharmacists...: The literature on clinical pharmacists is summarized in Kaushal, R., Bates, D.W. "The clinical pharmacist's role in preventing adverse drug events," in Shojania, *Making Health Care Safer*. A more recent study found a 78 percent fall in medication-related adverse events when pharmacists rounded with hospital ward teams: Kucukarslan, S.N., Peters, N., Mlynarek, M., Nafziger, D.A. "Pharmacists on rounding teams reduce preventable adverse drug events in hospital general medicine units," *Arch Intern Med* 163 (2003), pp. 2014-18.

403   benefit of this kind of training: The literature on simulators is summarized in Jha, A.K., Duncan, B.W., Bates, D.W. "Simulator-based training and patient safety," and Pizzi, L., Goldfarb, N., and Nash, D.B. "Crew Resource Management and its applications in medicine." Both chapters in Shojania, *Making Health Care Safer*. One study did show impressive improvements in safety and teamwork after ER staff underwent teamwork training: Morey, J.C., Simon, R., Jay, G.D., et al. "Error reduction and performance improvement in the emergency department through formal teamwork training: evaluation results of the MedTeams project." *Health Services Research* 37 (2002), pp. 1553-81.

INDEX

Abbreviations, dangerous, 380-382

Accountability, 315-326

    case, 315-321

    credentials committees and, 322-323, 325

    malpractice payout statistics and, 324-325

    state licensing boards and, 324-325

Accreditation Council for Graduate Medical
    Education (ACGME), 202, 205, 206, 382

Acker, Michael, 266

ACT UP, 334

Adverse drug events (ADEs), 72

Advocacy groups, 333-334

Agency for Healthcare Research and Quality
    (AHRQ), 287-288, 338-339, 384

AHRQ Web M&M, 23, 287-288

AIDS epidemic, 329-335, 337, 338, 357-59

Aiken, Linda, 218

Airline industry. *See* Aviation

Alzheimer's disease, 359

Amish, 381

American Academy of Orthopedic Surgeons, 132

American Hospital Association, 217

Amputation errors, 121-124

And the Band Played On (Shilts), 333

Annals of Internal Medicine, 23, 41

Anonymous reports, 281

Apologies, 264-265

Arbit, Ehud, 125-131

Armstrong, Lance, 334, 373

Arndt, David, 298

Artificial intelligence (AI), 115-118

Artis, Johnnie, 126

Association of Operative Registered Nurses, 137

Astronauts, 351

Attending physicians. *See* Trainee errors

Automatic behavior, 88-92

    See also Slips

Automobile industry, 92-93

Availability effect, 106

Aviation:

    error reporting system, 286-287

    failure mode and effects analysis (FMEA),
        348-349

    recertification in, 150

    regulation of, 31-32

    Russian airliner case, 116-117

    safety improvements in, 350-352

    teamwork in, 222-228, 230

    Tenerife crash, 224-226

Aviation Safety Reporting System (ASRS),
    286-287

Ayyappan, Rajeswari, 125-130, 267, 268

Bar-coding systems, 94-97, 356, 358

Barnard, Christiaan, 109

Bay Area Reporter, 329, 331

Bayes, Thomas, 112, 119

Bayesian reasoning, 112-113

Bayes' theorem, 112

Bazell, Robert, 56

Becher, Elise, 41, 46

Bell, Joseph, 109

Benamy, Jane,* 315-317

Bennett, Kent,* 101-103, 120

Berra, Yogi, 99

Berwick, Ann, 97

Berwick, Don, 58, 97, 334, 377

Beth Israel Deaconess Hospital, 78-79, 378

Bilateral symmetry, 124-125

Bioterrorism, 405

Blakeney, Barbara, 220

Blame, culture of, 301-304

Bleich, Howard, 115

Born on the Fourth of July (Kovic), 358

Bosk, Charles, 157-158, 189, 192, 277-278, 326

Boston Globe, 78, 378

Boutique hospitals, 146

Brailer, David, 379

Brennan, Troy, 307-309, 311-313

Brigham and Women's Hospital, 73, 74, 440

British Medical Journal, 69

British Royal Air Force, 147

Bush, George W., 373, 378

    State of the Union, 378

California hospitals, 349-350, 382, 410

California Nurses Association, 382

Camus, Albert, 347

Minoxidil, 71

Miscommunications. *See* Communications errors

Misdiagnoses. *See* Diagnostic errors

Mission Rehearsal Exercise, 152

Mistakes, intolerance of, 157

Mistakes vs. slips, 88-90

Morbidity and Mortality Conferences (M&Ms), 141-142, 273, 276-281, 290

Morris, Joan,* 29-41, 45, 241

Morrison, Jane,* 30-32, 38

Morris wrong patient case, 29-41

    list of seventeen individual errors in, 378-379

    systems approach to errors and, 45-47

Morton Thiokol, 48

Mount Sinai Hospital, 267

Mueller, Robert, 47

Nader, Ralph, 237

Nance, John, 227-228

NASA, 47-50, 53, 78, 290, 351

NASCAR pit crews, 230

National Health Information Technology Coordinator, 379

National Institutes of Health, 339

National Practitioner Data Bank (NPDB), 309, 324

Near-miss errors, 274

Neurosurgeons, malpractice and, 310, 311

New England Journal of Medicine, 139, 275, 331

New England Organ Bank (NEOB), 255

New technique skill acquisition, 148-156

New Yorker, 156-158

New York Hospital, 101, 266

New York State Department of Health, 205

New York State Patient Occurrence Report and Tracking System (NYPORTS), 285

New York Times, The, 131, 136, 201, 270, 376

New Zealand, 345-346

Nicklaus, Jack, 156-157, 231

No-fault system, 342-346

Noncommunication, culture of, 46

Nuland, Sherwin, 109-110

Nurses:

    charge, 36-37

    dissatisfaction among, 217-218

    head, 36

    medication slips and. *See* Medication slips

patient flow chaos and, 31-33

-physician relationship, 216-220

retained sponges and. *See* Retained sponges

role of, 220

shortage of, 217-220, 381

-to-patient ratios, 218, 382

Objects, retained. *See* Retained sponges

Obstetricians, malpractice and, 310, 311

O'Leary, Dennis, 246

Openness, transition from secrecy to, 337-338

Open reports, 282

"Operate Through Your Initials" (American Academy of Orthopedic Surgeons), 132

Oregon Health Sciences University, 265

Osler, Sir William, 109, 113, 156

Our Bodies, Ourselves, 237

Overconfidence, 108, 223-224, 350

Paracelsus, 83

Paternalism, 237

Patient action, 26

Patient activists, 333-334

Patient autonomy movement, 237-238

Patient demographics, 103

Patient flow chaos, 31-33

Patient IDs, checking, 45

Patients:

    informed consent and. *See* Informed consent

    safety initiatives. *See* Patient safety initiatives

    similar sounding names, 33

Patient Safety Director, 348

Patient safety initiatives, 363-368

    handoff errors and, 365-366

    informed consumers, 367-368

    list of, 383-388

    medical records, 366-367

    medication errors, 363-364

Pauling, Linus, 109

Personality of physician, malpractice suits and, 306-307

Pfizer, 71

Pharmacia & Upjohn, 71

Phonetic alphabet, 176

"Physical Genius: What do Wayne Gretsky, Yo-Yo Ma, and a Brain Surgeon Named Charlie Wilson Have in Common?" (Gladwell), 156-158

ACKNOWLEDGMENTS

Quite the opposite of James Reason's Swiss cheese model of error, we have been blessed by a series of lucky breaks, discerning critics, insightful predecessors, and unstinting supporters.

About four years ago, we decided to create a series of case-based articles on medical error, *Quality Grand Rounds*. This idea—which involved airing our field's dirty laundry in a major medical journal—was considered professional heresy, but we and our coeditors (Dr. Sanjay Saint and Amy Markowitz) searched anyway for a patron to support the work and a journal to host it. Dr. Mark Smith and his California HealthCare Foundation became our Medici, sticking with us through thick and thin. Drs. Harold Sox and Cynthia Mulrow, editors of the *Annals of Internal Medicine*, had the nerve to publish the series. Later, the U.S. Agency for Healthcare Research and Quality—Nancy Foster, Marge Keyes, and Drs. Gregg Meyer, Dan Stryer and Carolyn Clancy—gave us the chance to expand the concept into a full-fledged journal, *AHRQ WebM&M*. We thank all of these people and their superb organizations for their support.

To produce the articles for both series, we engaged many of the world's patient safety experts. Working with them has been an education and a joy. We hope we've done justice to their work—and to the work of the many other authors and thinkers who have inspired and influenced us: particularly Drs. Lucian Leape, Don Berwick, David Bates, Joanne Lynn, Atul Gawande, Rod Hayward, Tim Hofer, Alan Merry, Julie Gerberding, Troy Brennan, Arnie Milstein, and Mark Chassin; Professors Charles Bosk, Paul Cleary, Karl Weick, Alexander McCall Smith, and James Reason; and the late John Eisenberg, Amos Tversky, and Jonathan Mann, each of whom died too young.

In the summer of 2002, Denise Grady of *The New York Times* wrote a wonderful piece about our first *Quality Grand Rounds* article ("The Wrong Patient"), and Webster Stone, who had just launched a dynamic and eclectic publishing house called Rugged Land, saw in it the makings of a book. Web's passion and tough love have been pivotal to creating these pages, and the rest of the Rugged Land crew—particularly Jeanine Pepler, Chris Min, Zoe Feigenbaum, and Nate Allard—have been a delight to work with, as has our agent, Amy Rennert. Jay Wurts helped coach us out of our professorial introspection and into a style that, we hope, hit the sweet spot between the dramatic and the instructive. Sitting in Jay's living room—as he challenged us to "dolly in" on the people, and then "wide-angle" out on the issues ("how exactly did things get to be this way!")—was like having our own graduate writing seminar, without the trip to Iowa. We are indebted to him, to Jeremy Blachman and Amy Markowitz, who edited the book, to Adam Bousiakis and the staff at Café XO (where most of the book was written), and to several individuals who critiqued earlier drafts of specific chapters: Drs. Michael Lesh and Don Redelmeier, Capt. Bill Rutherford, Dean Kathy Dracup, Mary Whitney, and Stephen Fried.

We have been blessed by a wealth of professional support at home. Our colleagues at the University of California, San Francisco, particularly our chair, Dr. Lee Goldman, our manager, Kathleen Kerr, and UCSF Medical Center's leadership—Mark Laret, Dr. Ted Schrock, and Brigid Ide—have been unstinting advocates for our work; less committed leaders would have seen only risk and controversy and pulled the plug. The Society of Hospital Medicine, representing the nation's hospitalists, has worked tirelessly to improve the safety of hospitalized patients, and has been a marvelous professional home to us. And our UCSF hospitalist colleagues and chief residents have been with us every step of the way—always ready to bounce around an idea and to forgive our absences, both physical and cognitive, while we worked on the book. The fact that even these superb, empathic physicians can commit occasional errors is proof positive that we will not curb our epidemic of medical mistakes by trying to mint better physicians—there simply are none.

Our families—Amy, Douglas, and Benjy for Bob, and Lauren and Ali for Kaveh— have nurtured us and held down our home fronts, even as we exchanged e-mails at two in the morning. Their love is our fuel.

Finally, our greatest debt is to the many patients and caregivers who have shared their stories with us. In doing so, they hoped only that they might help keep a stranger out of harm's way. This book is our small attempt to do justice to their remarkable charity.

Also by **ROBERT M. WACHTER**

Hospital Medicine
The Fragile Coalition: Scientists, Activists, and AIDS

Also by **KAVEH G. SHOJANIA** and **ROBERT M. WACHTER**

Making Health Care Safer: A Critical Analysis of Patient Safety Practices